Veterinary Science and Medicine

nova
science publishers
www.novapublishers.com

Veterinary Science and Medicine

Combating Canine Cancers with Phytochemicals
Katrin Sak, PhD
2021. ISBN: 978-1-53619-716-7 (Softcover)
2021. ISBN: 978-1-53619-809-6 (eBook)

Veterinary Herbal Pharmacopoeia
Sun-Chong Wang
2020. ISBN: 978-1-53617-947-7 (Hardcover)
2020. ISBN: 978-1-53617-948-4 (eBook)

Entrepreneurship and Social Responsibility in Veterinary Medicine: Concepts and Applications
Katia Denise Saraiva Bresciani
and José Antonio Soares
2017. ISBN: 978-1-53610-939-9 (OBook)

Mammary Glands: Anatomy, Development and Diseases
Edmund B. Rucker (Editor)
2014. ISBN: 978-1-62948-853-0 (Hardcover)
2014. ISBN: 978-1-62948-856-1 (eBook)

Salmonella Pathogenesis and Progression in the Development of Human and Veterinary Non-Typhoidal Salmonella Vaccines against Human Salmonellosis
Rahul M. Nandre and John Hwa Lee
2014. ISBN: 978-1-63321-882-6 (Softcover)
2014. ISBN: 978-1-63321-941-0 (eBook)

More information about this series can be found at
https://novapublishers.com/product-category/series/veterinary-science-and-medicine/

Selwyn Arlington Headley
Editor

Infectious and Parasitic Diseases of Animals in Developing Countries

nova
science publishers
www.novapublishers.com

DOI: 10.52305/KRDF2922.

NOTICE TO THE READER

Library of Congress Cataloging-in-Publication Data

Names: Headley, Selwyn Arlington, editor.
Title: Infectious and parasitic diseases of animals in developing countries / Selwyn Arlington Headley (editor), Professor, Laboratory of Animal Pathology, Department of Veterinary Preventive Medicine, Universidade Estadual de Londrina, Brazil.
Description: New York : Nova Science Publishers, [2023] | Series: Veterinary science and medicine | Includes bibliographical references and index. |
Identifiers: LCCN 2023000569 (print) | LCCN 2023000570 (ebook) | ISBN 9798886975048 (hardcover) | ISBN 9798886975772 (adobe pdf)
Subjects: LCSH: Communicable diseases in animals--Developing countries. | Veterinary parasitology--Developing countries. | Communicable diseases in animals--South America. | Veterinary parasitology--South America.
Classification: LCC SF781 .I485 2023 (print) | LCC SF781 (ebook) | DDC 636.089/690091724--dc23/eng/20230215
LC record available at https://lccn.loc.gov/2023000569
LC ebook record available at https://lccn.loc.gov/2023000570

Published by Nova Science Publishers, Inc. † New York

Contents

Preface

Infectious and Parasitic Disease of Animals in Developing Countries is a unique book as it presents a list of important animal diseases that occur in developing nations and is written predominantly by experienced scientists from several developing countries. This is the origin and the main objectives that were considered in the preparation of this book as it provides high-quality literature of international standards for veterinary students, practicing veterinarians, and veterinary diagnosticians in developing and under-developed countries written by scientists/professors from these regions.

This is of fundamental importance, since most books on infectious and parasitic diseases of domestic animals, used worldwide in universities and other institutions, are written predominantly by American and/or European-based authors/scientist and frequently reflects the American and/or European views of specific diseases, which does not always coincide with the manifestations of these diseases in developing countries. Consequently, this book offers an alternative view of important diseases of animals based on the experience of scientists from developing countries.

It is our intention that *Infectious and Parasitic Disease of Animals in Developing Countries* serves as a complementary text for these specific diseases so that veterinary students and veterinarians from developing countries may easily identify these disease processes in domestic and/or wild animals.

Selwyn Arlington Headley, DVM, MSc, PhD
Editor

Chapter 1

Neurological Diseases of Ruminants in Brazil: Preliminary Differential Diagnosis

Júlio Augusto Naylor Lisbôa[1,*]
and Gustavo Rodrigues Queiroz[2]
[1] Department of Veternary Clinics, CCA,
State University of Londrina, Londrina, Paraná, Brazil
[2] Pitágoras University, UNOPAR, Arapongas, Paraná, Brazil

Introduction

The ruminant practitioner is usually faced with difficulties in managing cases of neurological diseases for the following reasons:

1) There are several disorders;
2) They are easily confused with each other because the clinical manifestations are similar and there are no pathognomonic signs;
3) In exceptional cases it is possible to establish the clinical or therapeutic diagnosis;
4) Imaging exams are limited, expensive, and restricted to large institutions;
5) Most diseases result in death without response to treatment attempts;
6) The confirmation of the diagnosis is established after death and depends on the application of specific laboratory tests on tissue samples of central nervous system (CNS).

* Corresponding Author's Email: janlisboa@uel.br.

In: Infectious and Parasitic Diseases of Animals in Developing Countries
Editor: Selwyn Arlington Headley
ISBN: 979-8-88697-504-8

In most cases, gross lesions are absent, the necropsy is inconclusive, requiring a histopathological examination.

The relevance of these diseases is incontestable. They are frequent, especially in cattle, and many of the most important neurological diseases can occur in the form of outbreaks, causing death to many animals within a short period of time. This causes significant economic losses and the need for a quick differential diagnosis so that effective measures of control and prevention and, less frequently, therapeutics can be adopted.

It is correct to say that the complete and successful investigation in these cases depends on the collaborative work of professionals specialized in different areas, especially the clinician and the pathologist. The clinician, without the assistance of the pathologist, has limited possibility of concluding the diagnosis. The pathologist, in turn, despite playing a decisive role in defining the diagnosis, faces the challenge of the time required for processing and examining the collected tissue samples. Working together is advantageous because information from well-interpreted clinical evidence can direct the attention of the histopathological examination to the areas of greatest interest, that is, those most likely to be affected in the CNS. Faster and more efficient results can be expected from this type of professional interaction, which is both positive and desirable.

The clinician can contribute with relevant information if he is able to perform the clinical examination applied to the nervous system and to interpret the manifestations and characterize the neurological syndrome(s) present, associating these with the possible location(s) of the lesion(s) in the CNS. He must be aware of the most frequent diseases that occur in the region in which he is working and must have sufficient knowledge about their epidemiological aspects and most likely clinical characteristics, such as onset, course, neurological syndromes, and outcome (time to death). The large animal clinician must be able to recognize toxic plants with direct effects on the CNS, with hepatotoxic potential and with myotoxic potential that occur in the region where he is located. He must be able to prepare a preliminary rational list of suspicions and, based on this, collect, and refer biological samples (cerebrospinal fluid – CSF, blood, and serum) for specific laboratory assays. The results of these tests may reinforce or eliminate suspicions and, eventually, confirm diagnoses even before death.

This text aims to present information related to the applied practice of these diagnostic procedures performed before death. The most frequent neurological diseases of ruminants in Brazil will be highlighted and information will be provided on whether it is possible or not to differentiate these based on clinical criteria. Finally, the results of laboratory tests that reinforce suspicions or confirm the diagnosis will be reviewed. This information is valuable for the clinician who works in the field, enabling him to formulate a more reduced and rational list of differential diagnoses. In addition, they can guide coherent therapeutic decisions and the guidance of sensible preliminary preventive measures.

Although they are decisively important for defining the diagnosis in most cases, methods of confirmation after death using CNS tissue, such as the pattern of histopathological lesion, special staining methods, identification of the presence of antigens (immunohistochemistry and direct immune-fluorescence), molecular identification (polymerase chain reaction) and the pathogen involved (microbiological and cellular cultures), are beyond the scope of this review. Readers will, however, be able to obtain this specific information from the original studies.

Neurological Diseases of Ruminants in Brazil

Information from surveys on the occurrence of neurological diseases in ruminants is more numerous in cattle and is scarce in small ruminants. The authors of this review are unaware of case series studies on these diseases in buffaloes. The surveys in cattle were concentrated in the last decade and covered the states of Rio Grande do Sul (Barros 2009; Konradt et al. 2017; Sanches et al. 2000; Santos et al. 2018), Paraíba, Pernambuco, and Rio Grande do Norte, grouped as the semi-arid region of the Northeast (Galiza et al. 2010), Mato Grosso do Sul (Pupin et al. 2019; Ribas et al. 2013), Minas Gerais (Oliveira et al. 2016), Goiás (Terra et al. 2018), and Paraná (Queiroz et al. 2018). Alternatively, surveys in sheep were done only in the semi-arid region of the Northeast (Guedes et al. 2007), and in the states of Rio Grande do Sul (Cecco et al. 2021; Konradt et al. 2017; Rissi et al. 2010a; 2010c) and Mato Grosso do Sul (Almeida et al. 2013). A very small number of observations have been reported in goats (Guedes et al. 2007; Konradt et al. 2017; Rosa et al. 2013).

The greater interest in cattle is due to the greater occurrence of these diseases and this certainly facilitates the gathering of a significant number of observations. It is natural that they occur more frequently in cattle since the herd is much larger than that of other ruminant species. In addition, it can be speculated that the cattle farmer may be more interested in requesting the veterinary service to clarify the diagnosis than the sheep farmer or goat farmer.

In any case, epidemiological surveillance for neurological diseases in cattle needs to be intensified due to bovine spongiform encephalopathy (BSE), a disease that causes the imposition of barriers to meat exports. It is as important to prove that BSE does not occur in Brazil as it is to demonstrate which neurological diseases are prevalent. The epidemiological surveillance chain for herbivore rabies is well structured and carried out by the official health defense services of each state. However, the differential diagnosis for other diseases represents a much greater challenge, as it depends on the application of varied and specific laboratory methods for each disease. In this sense, all these case studies in cattle are very relevant because they provide up-to-date epidemiological information.

Considering the results of case studies that investigated *neurological diseases in cattle* regardless of age and without excluding any specific disease, it is possible to gather observations in 1,532 animals raised in the states of Rio Grande do Sul (Barros 2009), Paraíba, Pernambuco, and Rio Grande do Norte (Galiza et al. 2010), Mato Grosso do Sul (Ribas et al. 2013), Goiás (Terra et al. 2018), and Paraná (Queiroz et al. 2018), and to freely establish the frequency distribution. It is clear that the result presented below is not representative of the entire country and does not cover the Southeast and North regions. Furthermore, it should be considered that there are important regional, state and local particularities that determine specific differences in the prevalence of certain diseases. However, this is the available information and can be understood as a general concept.

Inflammatory diseases of the CNS of cattle, represented mainly by encephalitis and rarely by myelitis, are predominant and represent 50% of all cases (Figure 1). Among them, those caused by viral agents are very frequent (44.5%) and those caused by bacteria have a low prevalence (5.5%). Rabies is the most prevalent disease (28%) and this was confirmed in all studies, appearing as the most frequent (Barros 2009; Galiza et al. 2010; Terra et al. 2018) or second in frequency (Queiroz et al. 2018; Ribas et al. 2013). Encephalitis caused by bovine alphaherpesvirus 5 (BoAHV5), and eventually by BoAHV1, is the second most important disease in this group, representing 10% of all cases. This was consistently demonstrated in surveys from the states of Rio Grande do Sul (Barros 2009), Mato Grosso do Sul (Ribas et al. 2013), Goiás (Terra et al. 2018), and Paraná (Queiroz et al. 2018), but not in the semi-arid region of the Northeast (Galiza et al. 2010). The cases of non-specific non-suppurative meningoencephalitis, in which the causative agent has not been defined, appear in third place of importance among inflammatory diseases (4% of all cases). It is consistent to suppose that bovine herpesvirus

(BoAHV5 and/or BoAHV1) was involved in most of these cases, but, for different reasons, it was not confirmed by specific laboratory methods. Finally, malignant catarrhal fever (MCF) represents 2.4% of all cases, appearing in all surveys, especially those in the state of Rio Grande do Sul (Barros 2009) and the semi-arid region of the Northeast (Galiza et al. 2010) (Figure 2).

Among the encephalitis or myelitis of bacterial origin, there is an emphasis on brain, spinal cord, or spinal canal abscesses with spinal cord compression (2.8% of all cases) and cases of suppurative meningoencephalitis not organized in the form of abscesses (1.4% of all cases). Histophilosis, also called thromboembolic or thrombotic meningoencephalitis, represents 0.8% of cases and had a higher prevalence in the study done in the state of Paraná (Queiroz et al., 2018). Finally, listeriosis represents only 0.6% of cases, having been observed in almost all states, and always with a low prevalence (Barros 2009; Galiza et al. 2010; Oliveira et al. 2016; Queiroz et al. 2018; Terra et al. 2018) (Figure 2).

This fact is relevant because listeriosis is identified as the main cause of encephalitis in cattle in temperate countries and cold climates in the northern hemisphere (Morin 2004). For this reason, it receives justified prominence in traditional textbooks from these countries. Based on the evidence from Brazilian surveys, we can say that listeriosis is certainly a disease of minor importance in cattle from Brazil. Even in a study of specific cases of bacterial CNS diseases, carried out in the state of Rio Grande do Sul, listeriosis represented 14% of bacterial encephalitis and 1.8% of all cases of inflammatory CNS diseases in cattle (Konradt et al. 2017). Very similar results were observed in the case series study of neurological diseases in calves up to one year of age, carried out in the state of Rio Grande do Sul. Excluding tetanus from bacterial diseases, listeriosis represented 13% of bacterial encephalitis and 1.8% of all cases (Santos et al. 2018).

Toxic diseases rank second in importance (36% of cases) (Figure 1). We must clarify that tetanus and botulism were arbitrarily computed within this group of diseases, since neurological dysfunctions are caused by bacterial toxins. Among these diseases, botulism (16.7% of all cases), which had a very high prevalence in the study of the state of Mato Grosso do Sul (Ribas et al. 2013), and hepatic encephalopathy secondary to poisoning by hepatotoxic plants (11.5% of all cases), notably *Senecio brasiliensis*, whose occurrence was very high in the study of the state of Rio Grande do Sul (Barros 2009), can be highlighted (Figure 3).

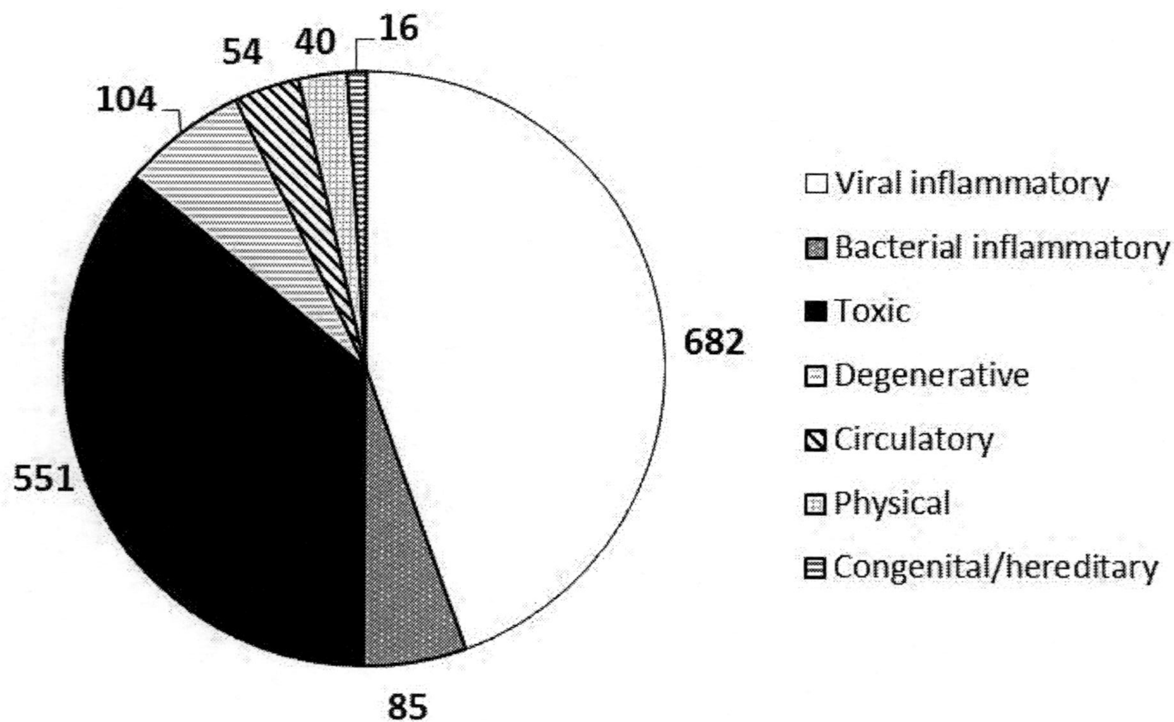

Figure 1. Causes of neurological diseases in cattle in Brazil. Grouping of case studies done in the states of Rio Grande do Sul (Barros 2009), Paraíba, Pernambuco, and Rio Grande do Norte (Galiza et al. 2010), Mato Grosso do Sul (Ribas et al. 2013), Goiás (Terra et al. al. 2018), and Paraná (Queiroz et al. 2018).

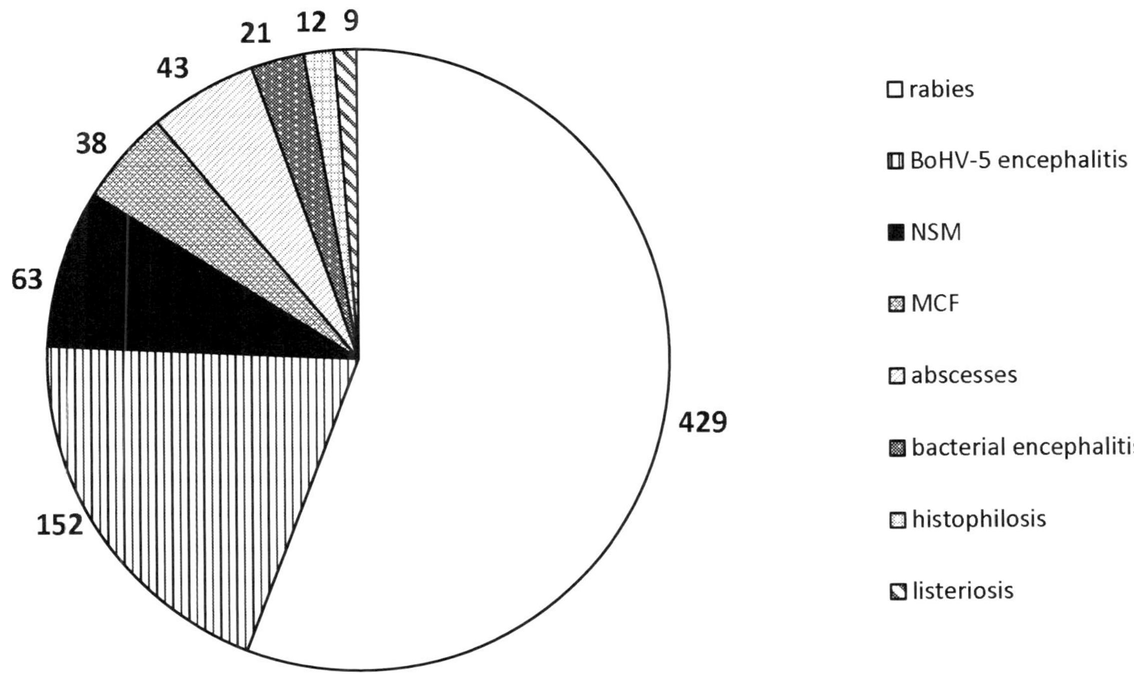

Figure 2. Inflammatory CNS diseases of cattle in Brazil. Grouping of case studies done in the states of Rio Grande do Sul (Barros 2009), Paraíba, Pernambuco,and Rio Grande do Norte (Galiza et al. 2010), Mato Grosso do Sul (Ribas et al. 2013), Goiás (Terra et al. 2018), and Paraná (Queiroz et al. 2018). *NSM: nonsuppurative meningoencephalitis; MCF: malignant catarrhal fever.*

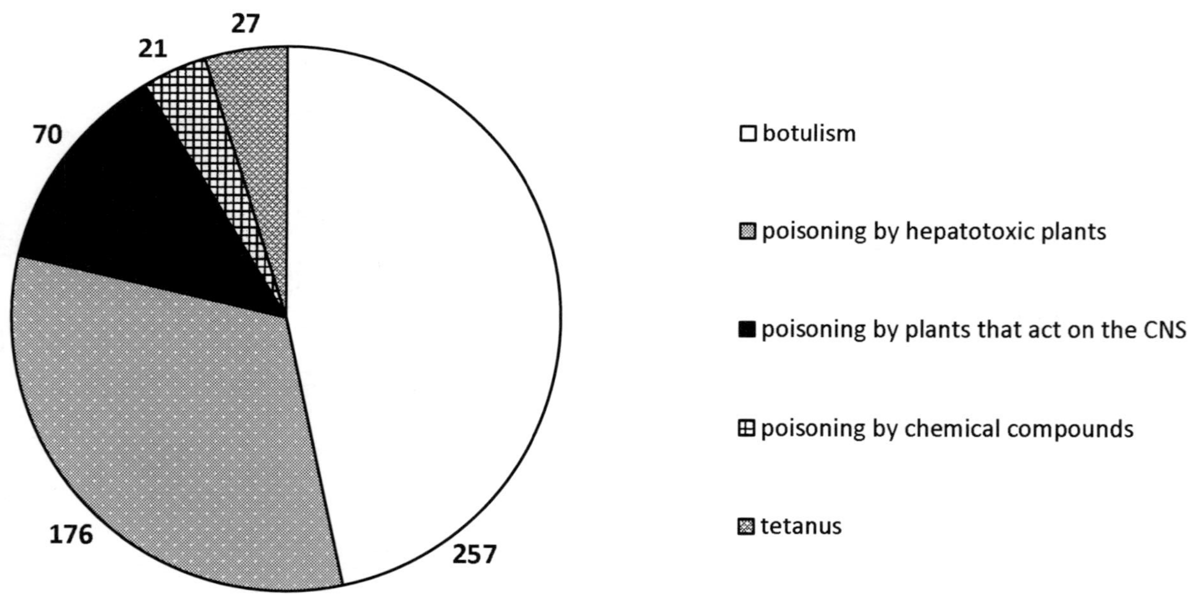

Figure 3. Toxic diseases that determine neurological dysfunctions in cattle in Brazil. Grouping of case studies done in the states of Rio Grande do Sul (Barros 2009), Paraíba, Pernambuco, and Rio Grande do Norte (Galiza et al. 2010), Mato Grosso do Sul (Ribas et al. 2013), Goiás (Terra et al. 2018), and Paraná (Queiroz et al. 2018).

Poisoning by plants with direct action on the CNS represent 4.5% of all cases and were observed mainly in the studies from the states of Rio Grande do Sul (Barros 2009) and Paraná (Queiroz et al. 2018). Plant poisonings are relevant causes of neurological disease in cattle and collectively represent almost half of the occurrences of toxic causes (44.6%) and 16% of all cases. Intoxication by chemical compounds, considering the possibilities of intoxication by urea (ammonia) (Terra et al. 2018), nitrite, sodium chloride (NaCl), carbamate or organophosphate (Queiroz et al. 2018), has a reduced occurrence (1.3% of all cases). In specific situations, however, they can assume outstanding importance within a herd when they occur in the form of an outbreak, causing the rapid death of a large number of animals. Differently from what is observed in equids, tetanus generally occurs with reduced frequency in cattle (1.7% of all cases).

By definition, polioencephalomalacia is a pathological process that results in necrosis of the gray matter of the brain, which occurs in different diseases, such as altered thiamine metabolism, excess sulfur intake, NaCl intoxication associated with water deprivation, lead poisoning. and BoHV-5 meningo-encephalitis (Sant'Ana et al. 2009a). In the present review, the term polioencephalomalacia (PEM) will be used to represent a disease caused by altered thiamine metabolism or excessive sulfur intake. The other diseases that determine this type of alteration in the brain can be confirmed by specific methods, guaranteeing the differential diagnosis.

PEM is a relevant degenerative neurological disease in cattle and represents 6.8% of all cases (Figure 1). It was diagnosed in all state surveys, with emphasis on the states of Mato Grosso do Sul (Ribas et al. 2013) and Goiás (Terra et al. 2018), where the frequency of occurrence was 13% and 17%, respectively. In other studies, the disease occurred at lower rates, ranging from 1.8% to 3.8% of cases (Barros 2009; Galiza et al. 2010; Queiroz et al. 2018; Santos et al. 2018). In the survey carried out in the state of Minas Gerais, in which rabies cases were not included, PEM represented 11% of all investigated cases (Oliveira et al. 2016).

Cerebral babesiosis is caused by infection by *Babesia bovis* and occurs with a frequency of 3.5% in Brazilian grouped surveys. It is presented in this review as a circulatory cause of neurological disease in cattle (Figure 1). It was observed in all the studies done in all states, except for Goiás (Terra et al. 2018), with low rates, ranging between 0.9 and 2.1%. In the state of Rio Grande do Sul, the situation is different, reaching frequencies of 6.5% of cases in cattle of all ages (Barros 2009) and 16% of cases in calves up to 12 months of age (Santos et al. 2018). In the study from state of Minas Gerais, in which rabies was excluded, the disease occurred in 12.3% of cases (Oliveira et al. 2016). It is a more relevant disease in regions with a colder climate, characterized as zones of enzootic instability for bovine hemoparasitosis (anaplasmosis and babesiosis), where the population of the tick vector *Rhipicephalus microplus* fluctuates a lot throughout the months of the year. On the other hand, the movement of cattle from areas of instability (cold climate) to areas of enzootic stability (warm climate) is an important risk factor.

Finally, head and spine injuries determining secondary neurological dysfunctions can occur with a frequency equivalent to 2.6% of all cases (Figure 1).

Table 1. Main neurological diseases in cattle presented in descending order of occurrence

Order	%	Disease
1	28.0	Rabies
2	16.7	Botulismo
3	11.5	Hepatic encephalopathy (hepatotoxic plant poisoning)
4	9.9	BoAHV5 meningoencephalitis
5	6.8	Polioencephalomalacia
6	4.5	Poisoning by plants with direct action on the CNS
7	4.0	Non-suppurative meningoencephalitis (causing agent not determined)
8	3.5	Cerebral babesiosis
9	2.8	CNS (brain or spinal cord) or spinal canal abscesses
10	2.6	Trauma to the skull or spine
11	2.4	Malignant catarrhal fever
12	1.7	Tetanus
13	1.4	Bacterial meningoencephalitis (not organized into an abscess)
14	1.3	Poisoning by various chemical compounds
15	1.0	Congenital and/or hereditary CNS disorders
16	0.8	Histophilosis
17	0.6	Listeriosis

Grouping of case studies done in the states of Rio Grande do Sul (Barros 2009), Paraíba, Pernambuco, and Rio Grande do Norte (Galiza et al. 2010), Mato Grosso do Sul (Ribas et al. 2013), Goiás (Terra et al. al. 2018), and Paraná (Queiroz et al. 2018).

The main neurological diseases of cattle are shown in Table 1 in descending order of occurrence. It cannot be forgotten that there are relevant conditions that influence the regional prevalence and incidence of these diseases. Considering the data published by the Brazilian Ministry of

Agriculture, Livestock and Supply[1], on the cases of rabies diagnosed in domestic herbivorous species in each state and each year, it is correct to say that this is, in fact, the main neurological disease of cattle in Brazil, occurring in all states of the country. The wide distribution of this disease is due to the extensive geographic distribution of the transmitter hematophagous bat *Desmodus rotundus*, present and well adapted to the different ecosystems existing in Brazil (Dognani et al. 2016; Langohr et al. 2003; Lima et al. 2005; Reis et al. 2003).

On the other hand, it should be considered that the occurrences of botulism and hepatic encephalopathy, mainly due to *Senecio brasiliensis* intoxication, must be overestimated in this grouped series. These two diseases occurred with very high frequencies in the surveys of the states of Mato Grosso do Sul (Ribas et al. 2013) and Rio Grande do Sul (Barros 2009), respectively, but this does not represent the current situation in other states or regions. Botulism, for example, represented 30% of cases with a diagnosis concluded in Mato Grosso do Sul (Ribas et al. 2013), but its frequency was always lower in the surveys of the other states: 6.3% in the semi-arid region of Northeast (Galiza et al. 2010), 5.9% in Goiás (Terra et al. 2018), 3.4% in Paraná (Queiroz et al. 2018), and 0.9% in Rio Grande do Sul (Barros 2009). In a more recent survey from the state of Mato Grosso do Sul, botulism occurred with a frequency more compatible with other studies in the country, representing 6.2% of cases, while rabies was confirmed as the most prevalent disease (20.8% of cases) and BoHV-5 encephalitis (6.2% of cases) tied with botulism for second place (Pupin et al. 2019). Hepatic encephalopathy, in turn, was observed exclusively in surveys in Rio Grande do Sul, representing 24% of cases (Barros 2009), and Paraná, representing 5.9% of cases (Queiroz et al. 2018). Poisoning by *Senecio brasiliensis*, the main responsible for these cases of hepatic encephalopathy, can only be expected in the southern states and in São Paulo, due to the geographic distribution of this invasive plant (Tokarnia et al. 2012).

In the specific case of toxic plants, neurological dysfunctions can be caused by plants that cause acute or chronic liver injury (hepatic encephalopathy), and by plants that have toxic principles that directly affect the CNS. The latter can be grouped into:

- Plants that cause diseases due to storage in neurons;
- Plants that cause tremorgenic syndrome;

[1] https://www.gov.br/agricultura/pt-br/assuntos/sanidade-animal-e-vegetal/saude-animal/programas-de-saude-animal/raiva-dos-herbivoros-e-eeb/DADOSRAIVAATE2015.pdf/view.

- Plants that cause lesions located in the CNS;
- Plants with other neurological actions; and
- Plants that harbor mycotoxin-producing fungi acting on the CNS (Tokarnia et al. 2012).

In Brazil, there are 31 species of toxic plants that affect the CNS currently recognized, and most of these cause disease in ruminants. The latest review on the subject is available for consultation (Riet-Correa et al. 2017). The geographic distributions of these plants vary considerably, which explains such different prevalence in different states or regions of the country. In this review, this subject will not be explored in depth, despite its undeniable relevance among the neurological diseases of ruminants. Interested readers can find detailed and up-to-date information on plants, areas in which they occur, toxic principles, clinical signs and evolution, lesions, and diagnosis in the texts by Tokarnia et al. (2012), Riet-Correa et al. (2017), and Morais et al. (2019).

Regarding to plant poisoning, myotoxic plants such as *Senna occidentalis* and *Senna obtusifolia* are also worth mentioning. They do not cause neurological disorders but cause skeletal muscle necrosis and functional disability, which determines permanent recumbency. For this reason, they must be included in the list of differential diagnoses of neurological diseases in cattle. In addition, cattle intoxicated with *Senna obtusifolia* may have hepatic encephalopathy, since the plant also has hepatotoxic effect (Queiroz et al. 2012).

From the point of view of epidemiological and economic importance, we must highlight the diseases that can occur in the form of outbreaks, causing the death of many cattle. Rabies is even more important because it is a zoonosis. Bovine diseases that can occur as outbreaks include rabies, botulism, hepatic encephalopathy, BoAHV-5 meningoencephalitis, PEM, poisoning by plants with direct action on the CNS, cerebral babesiosis, MCF, and histophilosis. Isolated cases of these diseases can also be seen. On the contrary, the diseases that exclusively or more frequently appear as isolated cases are trauma, tetanus, bacterial meningoencephalitis, and listeriosis. In cases of diseases of the first group, guidelines for control and prevention measures are indispensable. This is not true for cases of trauma and bacterial meningoencephalitis (whether organized as abscesses or not), as they commonly affect a single bovine in the herd.

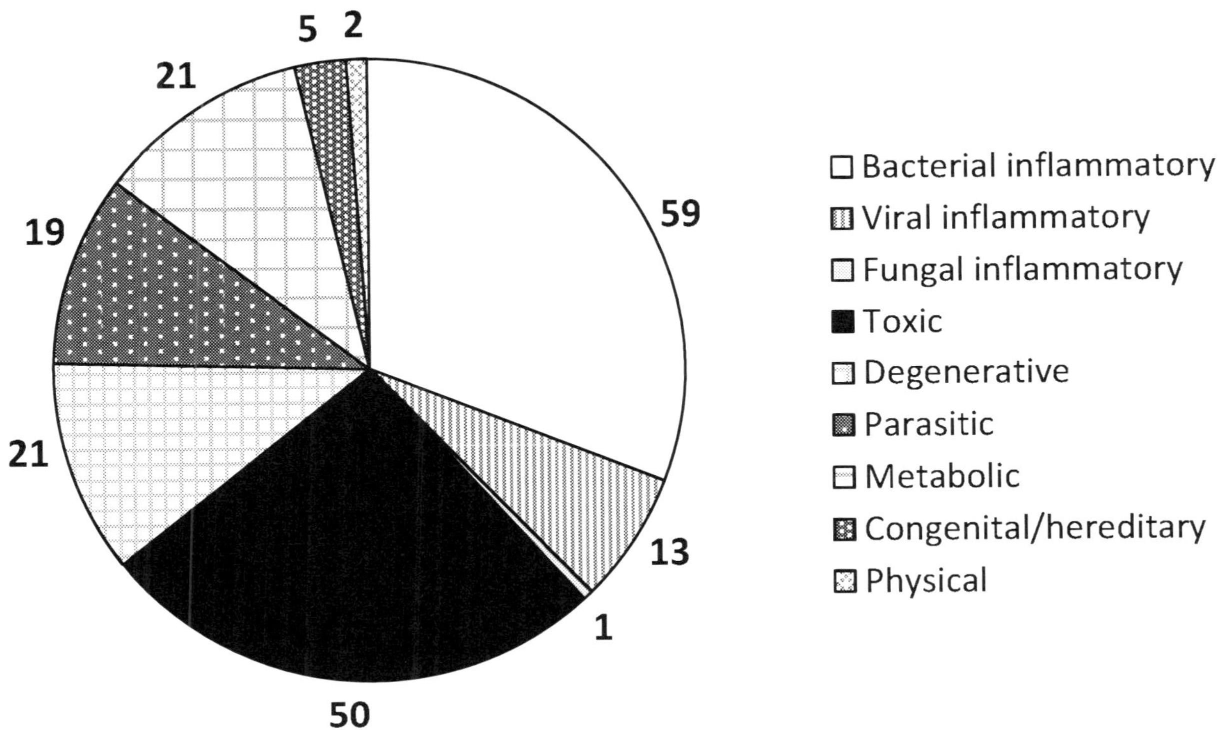

Figure 4. Causes of neurological diseases in sheep. Grouping of case studies done in the states of Paraíba (Guedes et al. 2007), Rio Grande do Sul (Cecco et al. 2021; Rissi et al. 2010a; 2010c), and Mato Grosso do Sul (Almeida et al. 2013), totaling 191 cases.

Among the *neurological diseases of sheep* registered in Brazil, inflammatory diseases caused by bacterial infection stand out and, unlike cattle, viral encephalitis has little epidemiological importance (Figure 4).

In the case series study on meningoencephalitis and myelitis, done in the state of Rio Grande do Sul with the three ruminant species, diseases caused by bacteria affected only 13% (28/219) of cattle with CNS inflammation. On the other hand, they occur in 90% (19/21) of sheep and 100% (7/7) of goats, especially listeriosis. This disease affected only 1.8% (4/219) of cattle but was very common in sheep (38%; 8/21) and goats (71%; 5/7) (Konradt et al. 2017). This proves that listeriosis is of little importance in cattle in Brazil, but has an outstanding epidemiological relevance in small ruminants. Abscesses located in the CNS are the first important cause in this group of diseases in sheep and rabies is the only viral encephalitis diagnosed (Table 2).

Table 2. Main neurological diseases in sheep presented in descending order of occurrence

Order	%	Disease
1	12.5	Abscesses in CNS (brain or spinal cord) or in spinal canal
2	10.4	Tetanus
3	9.9	Listeriosis
4	9.4	Coenurosis
4	9.4	Poisoning by plants with direct action on the CNS or hepatotoxic
5	8.9	Pregnancy toxemia
6	8.3	Bacterial meningoencephalitis or myelitis (not organized into an abscess)
7	5.7	Rabies
8	5.2	Polioencephalomalacia
9	3.6	Poisoning by closantel
9	3.6	Scrapie

Grouping of case studies done in the states of Paraíba (Guedes et al. 2007), Rio Grande do Sul (Cecco et al. 2021; Rissi et al. 2010a; 2010c), and Mato Grosso do Sul (Almeida et al. 2013), totaling 191 cases.

Toxic causes are primarily represented by tetanus (10.4% of cases) and by poisonings due to plants with direct action on the CNS or hepatotoxic plants, causing hepatic encephalopathy (9.4% of cases). The only parasitic cause is coenurosis, the larval form of *Taenia multiceps*, called *Coenurus cerebralis*, whose cyst develops inside the brain, expanding, occupying space, and compressing the adjacent structures. This disease has a very high frequency (9.4% of cases), but it is overestimated due to the high prevalence in the study carried out in Rio Grande do Sul (Rissi et al. 2010a). The dog is the definitive host of the parasite and the direct contact with the sheep in the pasture areas is the primary risk factor. The disease only occurs in places where dogs are used as sheep herders. Therefore, it has epidemiological relevance in the southern region of the country, notably the state of Rio Grande do Sul. It probably does not occur in other regions. Finally, PEM also occurs in sheep with a frequency equivalent to 5.2% of cases.

In the series of neurological diseases in sheep admitted to the large animal internal medicine service of the Veterinary Hospital of the Universidade Estadual de Londrina, in the last 26 years, tetanus (44.4%) and post-caudectomy ascending bacterial myelitis (16.7%) are highlighted. Many of these cases of tetanus also occurred after caudectomy, particularly when using the tourniquet procedure with an elastic rubber ring. Tail amputation has fallen into disuse in the state of Paraná, ascending myelitis has been reduced to almost zero and tetanus has become more sporadic. Other diseases diagnosed were bacterial meningoencephalitis (8.3%), pregnancy toxemia (8.3%), urea (ammonia) intoxication (8.3%), hepatic encephalopathy due to poisoning by hepatotoxic plants (5.5%), listeriosis, PEM, and CNS abscesses (2.8% each).

The only case series studies on *neurological diseases in goats* that the authors of the present review are aware of were carried out in the semi-arid region of the Northeast, mainly in the state of Paraíba (Guedes et al. 2007), and in the state of Rio Grande do Sul (Rosa et al. 2013). Two other studies carried out in Rio Grande do Sul also provided information but included a very small number of animals (Konradt et al. 2017; Rissi et al. 2010b). Therefore, observations of these diseases diagnosed in Brazil can be considered scarce for this species.

In the study from Rio Grande do Sul, listeriosis was the most important disease, reaching 36% of cases (Rosa et al. 2013). In the northeastern semiarid region, the following disorders were reported: tetanus (23.4% of cases), rabies, CNS abscesses, listeriosis, poisoning by plants with direct action on the CNS, and trauma to the skull or spine (8.8% of cases each), enzootic ataxia, pregnancy toxemia, and meningitis (5.9% of cases). PEM was also observed (2.9% of cases).

In the large animal internal medicine service of the Veterinary Hospital of the Universidade Estadual de Londrina, Paraná, neurological diseases in goats occurred in a reduced number and tetanus (26.7%), bacterial meningo-encephalitis (20%), poisoning by plants with direct action on the CNS (20%), CAEV encephalitis in kids (13.3%), PEM (13.3%), and neonatal hypo-glycemia (6.7%) were diagnosed.

It is necessary to alert the reader about some neurological diseases of ruminants that certainly had underestimated occurrences in the surveys reviewed. This is the case of metabolic diseases and congenital diseases. The metabolic diseases that determine neurological dysfunction and occur in Brazil are hypocalcemia puerperal paresis (HPP) in cows, pregnancy toxemia, and hypocalcemia in ewes and goats at the end of gestation, the nervous form of ketosis in cows in early lactation, and hypoglycemia/hypothermia in newborn lambs and kids. The practitioner whose routine is focused on dairy cattle may frequently encounter HPP and ketosis, assume the clinical suspicion with the diagnosis confirmed due to the response to treatment. For this reason, the cases do not appear in the sample surveys reviewed. In addition, beef cattle represented the largest contingent of occurrences in the five main series studies grouped in this review (Barros 2009; Galiza et al. 2010; Queiroz et al. 2018; Ribas et al. 2013; Terra et al. 2018). It is understandable, therefore, that diseases that specifically affect dairy cows would be underestimated.

It is also coherent to admit that the cases of pregnancy toxemia or hypocalcemia in pregnant ewes and goats could have been included as metabolic disease and were excluded from the series of neurological diseases in the surveys. In many of these animals, depression is profound and obviously characterizes cerebral cortex dysfunction.

Regarding neonates, and particularly perinates, who have neurological disorders, it is understandable that the farmer considers them non-viable animals and decides to shorten their lives without requesting the veterinary service to clarify the diagnosis.

Neurological Syndromes Observed in the Main Diseases: Applied Preliminary Differential Diagnosis

Tetanus is the only neurological disease in which an accurate clinical diagnosis is possible, since it has characteristic manifestations: generalized muscle rigidity (limbs, neck, and head) and hyperesthesia. Excitement may occur, but there are no other signs of cerebral syndrome, except for the possibility of seizure in very severe and advanced cases (Figure 5). Exposure of the third eyelid, common in horses, is not always present in ruminants.

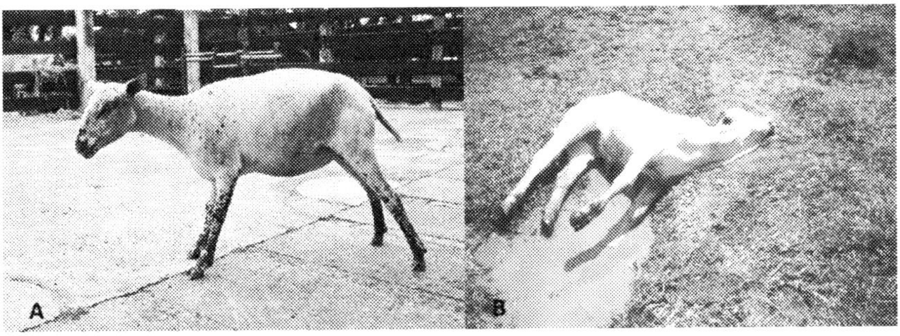

Figure 5. Sheep with tetanus at an early stage, presenting muscle stiffness in the limbs and neck, erect ears, erect tail, base-wide stance (forelimbs projected forward and hindlimbs projected backwards), difficult walking with rigid gait (little or no flexion of the limb joints) and mild degree of hyperesthesia; individual case in the herd (A). Steer affected by polioencephalomalacia with permanent recumbency, spasticity of the limbs, opisthotonus, depression (decreased mentation) alternating with episodes of mild hyperesthesia, tongue flaccidity, and bilateral amaurosis; individual case in the herd (B). The steer had been castrated 10 days ago. However, it cannot be confused with tetanus due to the presence of signs of brain syndromes, notably amaurosis.

Few diseases other than tetanus can be diagnosed based only on clinical criteria. Head trauma is accompanied by signs of acute brain syndromes due to the occurrence of diffuse cerebral edema and must be distinguished from other diseases in which these manifestations are present. However, it can be assumed as a definite diagnosis if the occurrence is reported by the person who attended and/or if there are apparent injuries to the skull.

The same applies to spinal injuries that cause spinal cord syndromes characterized by limb incoordination (ataxia and/or paresis) due to spinal cord compression. The report of the occurrence, the acute course, and the evidence of bone alterations (deviations, misalignments and/or abnormal mobility and crackling of the vertebrae) are elements that guarantee the diagnosis. Cases of poisoning by organophosphates, carbamates and urea (ammonia) are characterized by sudden onset of excitation, generalized muscle tremors, sialorrhea, incoordination (ataxia), and seizure; and diarrhea, miosis, and bradycardia in the case of organophosphates. They can be assumed as a definite diagnosis if there is reliable information of recent ingestion (urea) or exposure (organophosphates and carbamate).

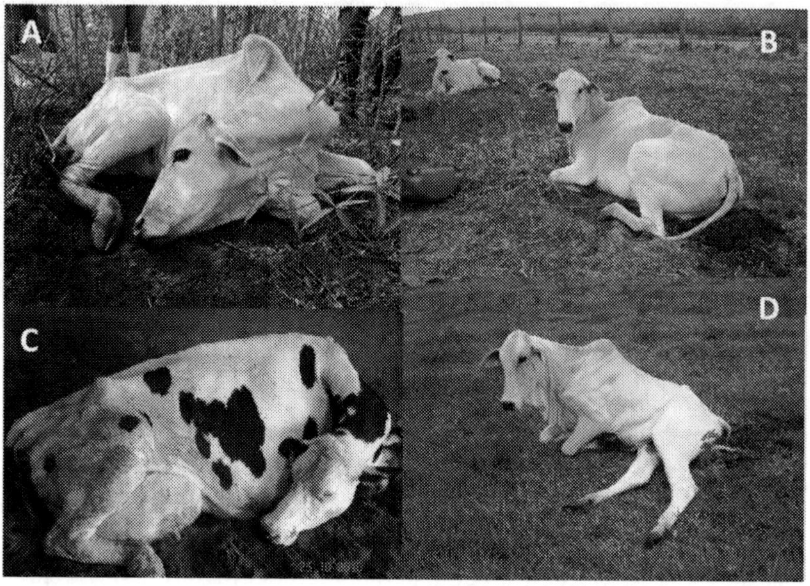

Figure 6. Cattle presenting muscle weakness (paresis) and permanent recumbency due to the inability to stand up, support weight and walk due to various causes. Heifer poisoned by *Acanthocladus brasiliensis* in an outbreak (A); Cows poisoned by *Senna obtusifolia* in an outbreak (B); Newly calved cow affected by hypocalcemic puerperal paresis; individual case (C); Heifer affected by botulism in the initial stage; individual case (D). Note that some cattle have altered consciousness (depression) and in these cases diseases that cause brain disorder should be suspected, especially with dysfunction of the cerebral cortex and/or midbrain (A and C). In cattle that show a normal response to environmental stimuli (B and D), hypotheses of spinal cord (myelopties), motor end plate, limb musculature (myopathies) and limb bones and joints dysfunctions should be considered. Remember that in some cases of rabies there may be paresis due to myelitis without signs of brain disorder at the beginning of the course, which will be obligatorily present and evident in the following days before death. Although botulinum toxin acts on the motor end plate and not on the CNS, cattle with botulism will show a decrease in the level of consciousness (depression) with the advance of the condition. Some of the cows poisoned by *Senna obtusifolia* showed depression due to hepatic encephalopathy resulting from hepatic necrosis.

Aside from these specific situations, what most commonly occurs is that these diseases are confused with each other and establishing a differential diagnosis is the mandatory challenge. In ruminants, encephalopathies are numerous and may occur in the form of outbreaks, whereas myelopathies are infrequent and usually affect isolated individuals. It is important to reinforce a concept: the first discrimination that the clinician must perform when starting the physical examination of an animal exhibiting neurological dysfunctions is whether it has brain (encephalopathy) or spinal (myelopathy) disorder. In the first case, there will be signs of cerebral, cerebellar, midbrain, or pontomedullary syndromes, combined (multifocal syndrome) or not with each other. In the second case, there will be exclusively limb incoordination (ataxia and/or paresis) of varying degrees, without changes in consciousness, behavior, and personality (Figure 6). In most of the diseases presented in Figures 1 and 2, there is injury and/or dysfunction of brain structures.

Based on the neurological syndromes and the course, the expected manifestations in each relevant disease will be presented below. It should be noted, however, that there will always be the possibility of variations and exceptions to the rule. Acute cerebral syndrome, accompanied or not by signs of other brain syndromes, is the pattern of the following diseases: BoAHV-5 meningoencephalitis (Elias et al. 2004; Lunardi et al. 2009; Rissi et al. 2009; Rissi et al. al. 2006; Salvador et al. 1998), PEM (Cunha et al. 2010; Mendes et al. 2007; Nakazato et al. 2000; Sant'Ana et al. 2009a), cerebral babesiosis (Antoniassi et al. 2009; Câmara et al. 2009; Rodrigues et al., 2005), MCF (Lemos et al. 2005; Macêdo et al. 2007; Marques et al. 1986; Mendonça et al. 2008; Rech et al. 2005), traumatic brain injury, lead poisoning, NaCl intoxication (Queiroz et al. 2018), histophilosis (Headley et al. 2015), and hepatic encephalopathy due to poisoning by plants that cause acute liver necrosis (Queiroz et al., 2013; Tokarnia et al. 2012). It can also occur in cases of diffuse bacterial meningoencephalitis. The signs of dysfunction are evident and marked from the beginning, since in many of these diseases there is diffuse cerebral edema (Figure 7).

The manifestation of signs of cerebellar, midbrain, and pontomedullary syndromes may be due to the presence of lesions located in these structures (cerebellum and brainstem), or to compression resulting from increased intracranial pressure. In the latter situation, the reduction of cerebral edema will result in attenuation or disappearance of the signs.

Signs of excitation (exaggerated neuronal activity) and/or deficiency (decreased neuronal activity) will be present in these diseases and may vary in severity over course. Signs of excitation, including the possibility of seizure, and the short course to death (12 to 36 hours) predominate in cases of cerebral babesiosis (Antoniassi et al. 2009; Câmara et al. 2009; Rodrigues et al. 2005) and hepatic encephalopathy due to poisoning by plants that cause acute liver necrosis (Queiroz et al. 2013; Tokarnia et al. 2012). Signs of depression are more common in BoAHV-5 meningoencephalitis (Elias et al. 2004; Lunardi et al. 2009; Rissi et al. 2006; Salvador et al. 1998), MCF (Lemos et al. 2005;

Macêdo et al. 2007; Marques et al. 1986; Mendonça et al. 2008; Rech et al. 2005), and histophilosis (Headley et al. 2015). In cases of PEM (Cunha et al. 2010; Mendes et al. 2007; Nakazato et al. 2000; Sant'Ana et al. 2009b), traumatic brain injury, lead poisoning, and NaCl intoxication, signs of excitation may predominate early in the course (Figures 5 and 7). In these diseases, death may occur between two and six days.

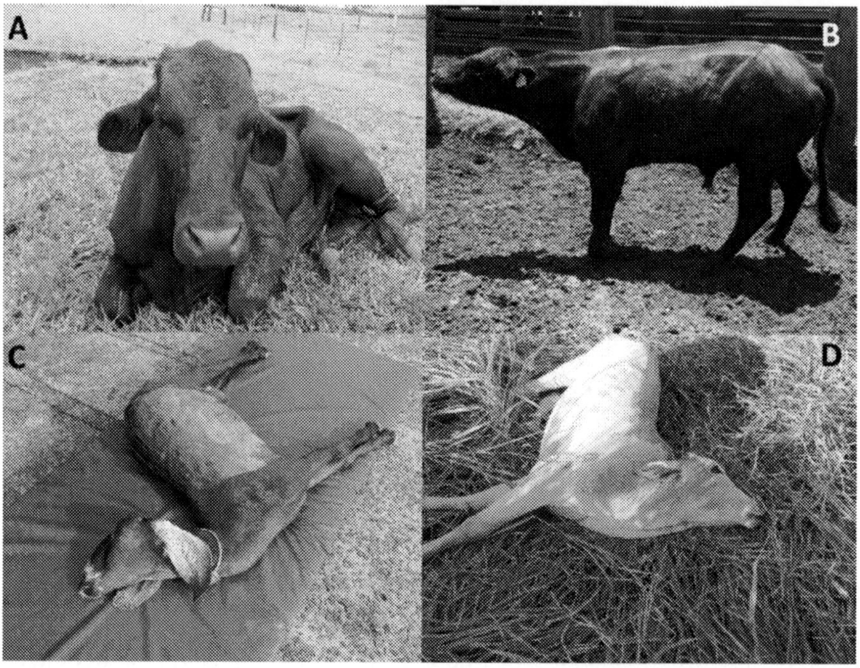

Figure 7. Neurological diseases with signs of acute brain syndromes. Calf with BoHV-5 meningoencephalitis showing depression, amaurosis, repeated involuntary movements of the head and right ear, and permanent sternal recumbency; course of 96 hours and occurrence in an outbreak (A); Calf with cerebral babesiosis showing excitement, generalized muscle tremors, stiff neck muscles with neck and head extension and proprioceptive deficit, progressing to seizure; course of 8 hours and individual case (B); Goat with bacterial meningoencephalitis showing depression, amaurosis, mydriasis, opisthotonus, rigidity of the limbs and permanent lateral recumbency; course of 24 hours and individual case (C); Steer with NaCl intoxication and water deprivation showing depression, amaurosis, dorsomedial strabismus, opisthotonus, mild degree of hyperesthesia with episodes of hyperextension and rigidity of the limbs, and permanent lateral recumbency; course of 36 hours and occurrence in an outbreak (D).

In the case of abscesses located in the brain, as in cenurosis, the signs of dysfunction may be less acute than those reported in previous diseases, mild at the beginning and worsening with time. This explains the longer course time.

The classic lesions of listeriosis are located at the brainstem, determining the predominant signs of pontomedullary and/or midbrain syndrome, notably asymmetric (unilateral) dysfunctions of the cranial nerves. Less frequently, there may be signs of acute cerebral syndrome (Morin 2004) due to the presence of multifocal lesions in the brain. Therefore, based on the most commonly displayed signs, listeriosis can be distinguished, with some ease, from the other aforementioned diseases.

The cases of hepatic encephalopathy due to poisoning by hepatotoxic plants that cause chronic liver damage (liver cirrhosis) are different from those above mentioned with acute liver damage that result in rapid death. The signs of cerebral syndrome may appear suddenly but are of less pronounced magnitude and the time to death is longer. Changes in behavior such as manias or bizarre and compulsive acts are frequently observed, but depression (decreased responses to environmental stimuli) is also common. Other signs are usually present and precede the onset of neurological dysfunctions, such as progressive weight loss, abdominal dilatation due to ascites, and chronic diarrhea (Tokarnia et al. 2012); jaundice is rarely found. Unlike acute hepatic necrosis, hepatic cirrhosis does not always result in hepatic encephalopathy. Therefore, in a herd outbreak, some animals will show signs of brain syndrome and others will not.

Animals poisoned by plants with direct action on the CNS that cause neuronal storage diseases generally show signs of cerebellar syndrome (Morais et al. 2019; Riet-Correa et al. 2017; Tokarnia et al. 2012). Localized or generalized muscle tremors with or without limb incoordination (ataxia) are manifestations related to the ingestion of plants that cause tremorgenic syndrome and plants that harbor fungi that produce certain toxins. In both cases, the cerebral cortex is usually not affected and changes in behavior and personality are not observed.

The presence of other clinical signs concomitant with neurological dysfunctions can also help the clinician to differentiate between diseases. Cattle with herpetic meningoencephalitis (BoAHV-5 or BoAHV-1 infections) may show signs of inflammation of the upper airways (bilateral nasal discharge, respiratory stridor, cough) and, rarely, pneumonia. However, in most cases, only signs of brain syndromes are present (Elias et al. 2004;

Lunardi et al. 2009; Rissi et al. 2006; Salvador et al. 1998), this can also be observed in histophilosis (Headley et al. 2015).

Finally, cattle with MCF may present a variety of digestive (stomatitis, mouth ulcerations, diarrhea), respiratory (bilateral nasal discharge, cough, dyspnea), ocular (keratitis with opacity and corneal ulcer, hypopyon, conjunctivitis, ocular secretion, decreased visual acuity), and cutaneous manifestations (crusted dermatitis of variable extent, dryness and peeling of the muffle and nostrils), dehydration, and weight loss (Lemos et al. 2005; Macêdo et al. 2007; Marques et al. 2007; Marques et al. al. 1986; Mendonça et al. 2008; Rech et al. 2005). In an outbreak of the disease, not all cattle will show signs of a neurological disorder. In the experience in the state of Paraná, the disease occurred as isolated cases in the herd and cattle showed exclusively neurological signs (Queiroz et al. 2018).

Rabies is a disease that, in most cases, causes death within five days. However, some animals may have a longer course of up to 10 days. Rabies is confused with any of the aforementioned neurological diseases (Langohr et al. 2003; Lima et al. 2005; Reis et al. 2003), as well as botulism, described below. Rabid animals may show signs of brain disorder from the beginning and in these, cases death is rapid. With this pattern of manifestations, rabies must be distinguished from all diseases that progress with acute brain syndromes (Figure 8). However, affected animals may initially present signs exclusive of spinal cord syndromes, with paraparesis that progresses to tetraparesis. In these cases, they may be able to stand up and walk with muscle weakness most evident at the hind limbs (paraparesis). As the disease progress to tetraparesis, affected animals adopt permanent sternal recumbency. Signs of brain syndromes will then appear, obligatorily, before death (Figure 8).

It is possible, therefore, that the rabid animal remains in sternal recumbency for a few days without showing any apparent signs of brain disorder. With this pattern of manifestations, rabies must be distinguished from spinal cord disorders in general, from muscle diseases with extensive lesions, as in cases of poisoning by *Senna occidentalis* and *S. obtusifolia* in cattle, and from botulism. This diversity of disease patterns in rabies is due to the type of route of the rabies virus within the CNS and its speed, causing myelitis and spinal cord dysfunctions before encephalitis whose outcome is death (Langohr et al. 2003; Lima et al. 2005).

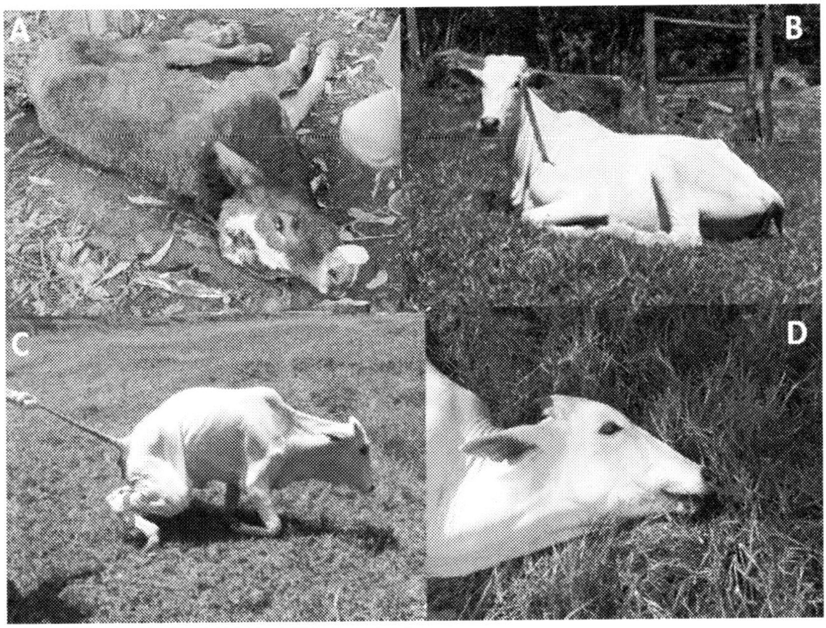

Figure 8. Rabid cattle. Signs of brain disorder may be present from the beginning of the condition (A), confusing them with other diseases that cause acute brain syndromes, or they may appear only at the end of the course (B, C and D), confusing them with botulism. The calf presented bilateral amaurosis, depression, nystagmus, tongue flaccidity, and tetraparesis with permanent lateral recumbency; course of 60 hours and outbreak in the herd (A). The tongue was not exposed originally, but remained after manual traction. The heifer was in permanent sternal recumbency for 48 hours and remained alert and without other signs of brain disorder since the beginning of its course; individual case (B). When stimulated, she made unsuccessful attempts to get up, showing more marked paresis in the hindlimbs (C). Two days later, she progressed to permanent lateral recumbency and depression (D).

When it is possible to follow disease progression, it is not difficult to distinguish rabies from myelopathies and myopathies since death does not occur quickly in these diseases. However, with respect to botulism, it can be difficult to differentiate the two diseases. Both diseases, rabies and botulism, are fatal and the course time to death is similar, up to 7 days. Very rare cases of botulism in cattle may have a chronic course with a non-fatal outcome. In botulism, generalized muscle weakness leads to permanent sternal recumbency. At the beginning, the animal is alert and does not show signs of brain disorder. As the disease progresses, the affected anima becomes depressed and evolves into lateral recumbency before death (Lisbôa et al. 1996) (Figure 9).

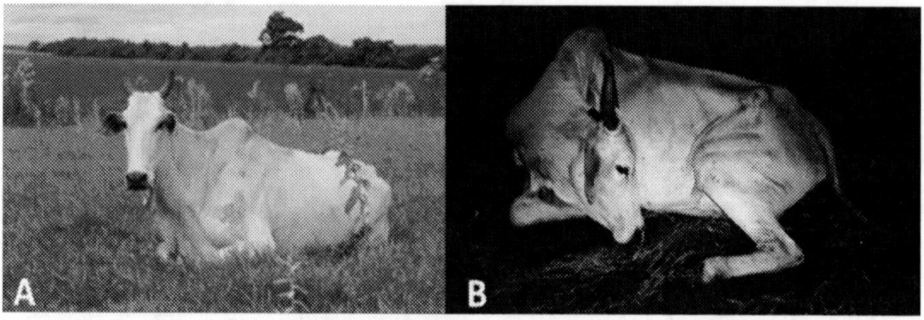

Figure 9. Cows with botulism. Generalized muscle weakness with permanent recumbency is the pattern since the onset of the condition. Decreased level of consciousness (depression) is not present at the beginning (A), but appears during the course (B). There are no other signs of brain disorder present, such as blindness, excitement, mania, and muscle tremors, and flaccidity of the tongue does not always occur. This is the expected pattern in the course of this disease and information about mental state and behavior at the beginning of the condition is essential for clinical reasoning. Cattle that have altered consciousness or other signs of brain disorder from the beginning are most likely not affected by botulism. It is important to emphasize that some cases of rabies may present this same pattern of manifestations and course.

The cause of mental depression in botulism is uncertain as the receptors for botulinum toxin are at the neuromuscular junction rather than the CNS. Aside from mental depression and tongue flaccidity, which may or may not be present, there are no other signs of brain disorder in botulism. This effectively differentiates botulism from other diseases of the brain and from rabies itself, when varied signs of brain syndromes are present (Figure 8A). This very important concept should be reinforced: botulism can be confused with cases of rabies (Figures 8B and C), myelopathy, and with cases of marked myopathy with extensive distribution (Figure 6B). Botulism, on the other hand, should never be confused with diseases that start with acute cerebral syndrome such as BoAHV-5 meningoencephalitis, PEM, cerebral babesiosis, MCF, traumatic brain injury, lead poisoning, NaCl intoxication, histophilosis, and hepatic encephalopathy (Figures 5B and 7).

Methods That Reinforce Suspicions or Confirm Diagnosis before Death

Some laboratory tests help in the differential diagnosis between neurological diseases before death. In the cerebrospinal fluid (CSF), the presence of pleocytosis (increased number of leukocytes; > 10 cells/mm^3) and the increased protein concentration (>40 mg/dL) confirm the existence of inflammatory processes in the brain or spinal cord (Câmara et al. 2020; Scott 2004). However, the absence of these changes does not, completely rule out a suspicion of encephalitis. Some cattle with rabies and histophilosis may have normal CSF (Curti et al. 2020; Queiroz et al. 2018). Alternatively, in BoAHV-5 encephalitis, pleocytosis with mononuclear cells (lymphocytes and macrophages) is always present and can be marked (> 50 cells/mm^3) (Lisbôa et al. 2009; Queiroz et al. 2018). In cases of bacterial encephalitis and myelitis, the elevation of protein content is usually very pronounced and pleocytosis with neutrophils is the marked alteration. In addition to the aforementioned cellular and biochemical changes, the elevation of the L-lactate concentration in the CSF (>3.6 mmol/L) is a reliable indicator of encephalitis in cattle (Curti et al. 2020).

The changes present in the CSF do not confirm the diagnosis, but they do confirm that there is inflammation and indicate the probable causative agent: viral or bacterial. This, in itself, already represents a huge step towards the preliminary differentiation between diseases. The presence of damaged red blood cells, in turn, indicates the existence of previous hemorrhage and reinforces the suspicion of traumatic injuries to the spine or skull. Finally, very high sodium concentrations (close to 200 mmol/L) in the CSF of cattle confirm the diagnosis of NaCl intoxication associated with water deprivation (Smith and George 2009).

The diagnosis of liver diseases that determine hepatic encephalopathy can be reinforced with the finding of increased serum activities of the gammaglutamyl transferase (GGT) and aspartate aminotransferase (AST), and increased concentration of bilirubin in the blood serum. In the case of muscle diseases, the increase in the activity of the creatine kinase (CK) in the blood serum confirms the presence of muscle injury and the values are very high (> 10,000 IU/L) in poisoning by *Senna obtusifolia* (Queiroz et al. 2012). Myoglobinuria (urine with blackish color) is also a common early manifestation of this disease. CK activity also increases in heavy cattle or buffaloes that remain recumbent for a long time, which can occur in a number of neurological diseases. This is due to muscle damage resulting from compression, decreased blood perfusion, and tissue hypoxia. In these cases, myoglubinuria is usually not present and the increase in serum CK activity is less pronounced.

Finally, a therapeutic diagnosis is possible in PEM, when an effective and rapid response to the administration of thiamine (vitamin B1) is observed

(Mendes et al. 2007). However, not all ruminants affected by PEM respond to treatment, and the absence of a response does not exclude this disease. As a rule of thumb for neurological diseases in general, the response to treatment is best when instituted as soon as possible after the appearance of signs of dysfunction (onset of the disease). Thiamine should be administered intramuscularly at a dose of 10 to 20 mg/kg, every 8 or 12 hours for the first two days and every 24 hours for the other two or three days, as needed (Mendes et al. 2007; Smith and Jorge 2009). Larger doses than these can be used on the first day and clinical improvement can be seen a few hours later. According to the authors' practical experience, cattle with BoHV-5 meningoencephalitis and ruminants with traumatic brain injury may also respond to thiamine treatment. However, the magnitude and speed of clinical improvement are smaller when compared to what occurs in PEM. In more advanced cases of PEM, response to thiamine treatment may or may not occur.

Conclusion

Given the above, it is possible to highlight that, even though neurological diseases are confused with each other, the clinician is able to perform the task of discriminating between them, with some success, based on clinical criteria and some specific laboratory findings. The recognition of the neurological syndromes present and the correct interpretation of the signs correlating them with the probable location of the lesions or dysfunctions in the structures of the CNS are the foundations for being able to elaborate a preliminary list of suspicions coherent, rational and as small as possible. The results of some laboratory tests, highlighting the importance of the changes present in the CSF, can decisively help in the differential diagnosis of neurological diseases in ruminants before death.

References

Almeida, T. L., K. B. Brum, R. A. A. Lemos, C. R. B. Leal, and F. A. Borges. 2013. "Doenças de ovinos diagnosticadas no Laboratório de Anatomia Patológica Animal da Universidade Federal de Mato Grosso do Sul (1996-2010) [*Sheep diseases diagnosed at Laboratory of Animal Pathology, Federal University of Mato Grosso do Sul, Brazil (1996-2010)*]." *Pesquisa Veterinária Brasileira* 33 (1): 21-29.

https://www.scielo.br/j/pvb/a/BYH4svLV7P3FVRwHSDnvPVt/?format=pdf&lang=pt.

Antoniassi, N. A. B., A. M. R. Corrêa, A. S. Santos, S. P. Pavarini, L. Sonne, P. M. Bandarra, and D. Driemeier. 2009. "Surto de babesiose cerebral em bovinos no estado do Rio Grande do Sul [*Cerebral babesiosis outbreak in bovines in the state of Rio Grande do Sul, Brazil*]." *Ciência Rural* 39 (3): 933-936. https://doi.org/10.1590/S0103-84782009000300049.

Barros, C. S. L. 2009. "Neuropatias bovinas emergentes [*Emerging bovine neuropathies*]." *Ciência Animal Brasileira* 10 (supl.1): 1-18. https://www.revistas.ufg.br/vet/article/view/7667/5440.

Câmara, A. C. L., J. A. Guimarães, A. C. Dantas, C. L. Mendonça, and J. A. B. Afonso. 2009. "Surtos de babesiose cerebral em bovinos leiteiros no nordeste brasileiro [*Cerebral babesiosis outbreaks in dairy cattle from Northeast Brazil*]." *Ciência Animal Brasileira* 10 (supl. 1): 619-624. https://www.revistas.ufg.br/vet/article/view/7873/5695.

Câmara, A. C. L., M. C. Gonzaga, T. M. Ziober, C. R. R. Queiroz, T. C. M. Fino, M. B. Castro, J. R. J. Borges, and B. Soto-Blanco. 2020. "Cerebrospinal fluid analysis in 58 ruminants showing neurological disorders." *Pesquisa Veterinária Brasileira* 40 (5): 346-354. https://doi.org/10.1590/1678-5150-PVB-6540.

Cecco, B. S., F. A. Molossi, L. C. Henker, M. P. Lorenzett, G. L. F. Correa, D. Driemeier, S. P. Pavarini, and L. Sonne. 2021. "Causes of death in sheep in Rio Grande do Sul, Brazil: analysis of 523 cases (2004-2019)." *Pesquisa Veterinária Brasileira* 41: e06886. https://doi.org/10.1590/1678-5150-PVB-6886.

Cunha, P. H. J., P. M. Bandarra, M. M. Dias, A. S. Borges, and D. Driemeier. 2010. "Surto de polioencefalomalacia por ingestão excessiva de enxofre na dieta em bezerros no Rio Grande do Sul [*Outbreak of polioencephalomalacia in cattle consuming high sulphur diet in Rio Grande do Sul, Brazil*]." *Pesquisa Veterinária Brasileira* 30 (8): 613-617. http://dx.doi.org/10.1590/S0100-736X2010000800001.

Curti, J. M., G. R. Queiroz, P. F. V. Pereira, M. C. Anjos, K. K. M. C. Flaiban, and J. A. N. Lisbôa. 2020. "L-lactate in cerebrospinal fluid can be used as a biomarker of encephalitis in cattle." *Canadian Journal of Veterinary Research* 84 (2): 146-152. https://www.ncbi.nlm.nih.gov/pmc/articles/PMC7088516/pdf/cjvr_02_146.pdf.

Dognani, R., E. J. Pierre, M. C. P. Silva, M. A. C. Patrício, S. C. Costa, J. R. Prado, and J. A. N. Lisbôa. 2016. "Epidemiologia descritiva da raiva dos herbívoros notificados no estado do Paraná entre 1977 e 2012 [*Epidemiology of rabies in large animals of Paraná, Brazil, from 1977 to 2012*]." *Pesquisa Veterinária Brasileira* 36 (12): 1145-1154. https://www.scielo.br/j/pvb/a/SBP3vqNWQVVnqbrwpgwGpKS/?format=pdf&lang=pt.

Elias, F., A. L. Schild, and F. Riet-Correa. 2004. "Meningoencefalite e encefalomalacia por Herpesvírus bovino-5: distribuição das lesões no sistema nervoso central de bovinos naturalmente infectados [*Bovine herpesvirus type-5 meningoencephalitis and malacia: histological lesions distribution in the central nervous system of naturally infected cattle*]." *Pesquisa Veterinária Brasileira* 24 (3): 123-131. https://doi.org/10.1590/S0100-736X2004000300003

Galiza G. J. N., M. L. C. R. Silva, A. F. M. Dantas, S. V. D. Simões, and F. Riet-Correa. 2010. "Doenças do sistema nervoso de bovinos no semiárido nordestino [*Diseases of the nervous system of cattle in the semiarid of Northeastern Brazil*]." *Pesquisa Veterinária Brasileira* 30 (3): 267-276. http://dx.doi.org/10.1590/S0100-736X2010000300014.

Guedes K. M. R., F. Riet-Correa, A. F. M. Dantas, S. V. D. Simões, E. G. M. Neto, V. M. T. Nobre, and R. M. T Medeiros. 2007. "Doenças do sistema nervoso central em caprinos e ovinos no semi-árido [*Diseases of the central nervous system in goats and sheep of the semiarid*]." *Pesquisa Veterinária Brasileira* 27 (1): 29-38. https://doi.org/10.1590/S0100-736X2007000100006.

Headley, S. A., A. P. F. R. L. Bracarense, V. H. S. Oliveira, G. R. Queiroz, W. Okano, A. F. Alfieri, K. K. M. C. Flaiban, J, A. N. Lisbôa, and A. A. Alfieri. 2015. "*Histophilus somni*-induced thrombotic meningoencephalitis in cattle from northern Paraná, Brazil." *Pesquisa Veterinária Brasileira* 35 (4): 329-336. http://dx.doi.org/10.1590/S0100-736X2015000400003.

Konradt, G., D. M. Bassuino, K. S. Prates, M. V. Bianchi, G. G. M. Snel, L. Sonne, D. Driemeier, and S. P. Pavarini. 2017. "Suppurative infectious diseases of the central nervous system in domestic ruminants." *Pesquisa Veterinária Brasileira* 37 (8): 820-828. https://doi.org/10.1590/S0100-736X2017000800007.

Langohr, I. M., L. F. Irigoyen, R. A. A. Lemos, and C. S. L. Barros. 2003. "Aspectos epidemiológicos, clínicos e distribuição das lesões histológicas no encéfalo de bovinos com raiva [*Epidemiology, clinical signs and distribution of lesions in the brain of rabid cattle*]." *Ciência Rural* 33 (1): 125-131. https://doi.org/10.1590/S0103-84782003000100020.

Lemos, R. A. A., R. R. Rech, E. B. Guimarães, A. Kadri, and I. S. Dutra. 2005. "Febre catarral maligna em bovinos no Mato Grosso do Sul e de São Paulo [*Malignant catarrhal fever in cattle from the states of Mato Grosso do Sul and São Paulo*]." *Ciência Rural* 35 (4): 932-934. http://dx.doi.org/10.1590/S0103-84782005000400030.

Lima, E. F., F. Riet-Correa, R. S. Castro, A. A. B. Gomes, and F. S. Lima. 2005. "Sinais clínicos, distribuição das lesões no sistema nervoso e epidemiologia da raiva em herbívoros na região nordeste do Brasil [*Clinical signs, distribution of the lesions in the central nervous system and epidemiology of rabies in northeastern Brazil*]." *Pesquisa Veterinária Brasileira* 25 (4): 250-264. http://dx.doi.org/10.1590/S0100-736X2005000400011.

Lisbôa J. A. N., A. J. Isernhagen, A. S. Borges, R. M. Amorim, M. R. S. Balarin, M. Lunardi, and A. A. Alfieri. 2009. "Hematological and cerebrospinal fluid changes in cattle naturally and experimentally infected with the bovine herpesvirus 5." *Brazilian Archives of Biology and Technology* 52: 69-76. https://doi.org/10.1590/S1516-89132009000700010.

Lisbôa, J. A. N., M. R. G. Kuchembuck, I. S. Dutra, R. C. Gonçalves, C. T. Almeida, and I. R. Barros Filho. 1996. "Epidemiologia e quadro clínico do botulismo epizoótico dos bovinos no estado de São Paulo [*Epidemiological and clinical aspects of the epi-zootic botulism of cattle in the state of São Paulo*]." *Pesquisa Veterinária Brasileira* 16 (2/3):

67-74. http://www.pvb.com.br/portal/download_artigo/Mjc5NXwyMDIyMDQwNzA5NTU1Nw.

Lunardi, M., M. P. Claus, J. A. N. Lisbôa, A. M. Amude, S. A. Headley, A. F. Alfieri, and A. A. Alfieri. 2009. "Neurological and epidemiological aspects of a BoHV-5 meningoencephalitis outbreak." *Brazilian Archives of Biology and Technology* 52 (spe): 77-85. http://dx.doi.org/10.1590/S1516-89132009000700011.

Macêdo, J. T. S. A., F. Riet-Correa, S. V. D. Simões, A. F. M. Dantas, and V. M. T. Nobre. 2007. "Febre catarral maligna em bovinos na Paraíba [*Malignant catarrhal fever in cattle in Paraíba, northeastern Brazil*]." *Pesquisa Veterinária Brasileira* 27 (7): 277-281. http://dx.doi.org/10.1590/S0100-736X2007000700004.

Marques, L. C., A. C. Alessi, G. H. Bechara, B. V. Tomaz, J. A. Marques, and L. Guerra. 1986. "Surto de febre catarral maligna em bovinos no estado de São Paulo [*Outbreak of malignant catarrhal fever in cattle in São Paulo*]." *Arquivo Brasileiro de Medicina Veterinária e Zootecnia* 38 (4): 719-729.

Mendes, L. C. N., A. S. Borges, J. R. Peiró, F. L. F. Feitosa, and C. R. Anhesini. 2007. "Estudo retrospectivo de 19 casos de polioencefalomalacia, em bovinos, responsivos ao tratamento com tiamina [*Retrospective study of 19 cases of polioencephalomalacia in cattle, responsive treatment with thiamine*]." *Arquivo Brasileiro de Medicina Veterinária e Zootecnia* 59 (1): 239-241. http://dx.doi.org/10.1590/S0102-09352007000100038.

Mendonça, F. S., R. G. S. Dória, F. B. Schein, S. H. Freitas, L. Nakazato, F. M. Boabaid, D. A. J. Paula, V. Dutra, and E. M. Colodel. 2008. "Febre catarral maligna em bovinos no estado de Mato Grosso [*Malignant catarrhal fever in cattle, Mato Grosso, Brazil*]." *Pesquisa Veterinária Brasileira* 28 (3): 155-160. http://dx.doi.org/10.1590/S0100-736X2008000300005.

Morais, R. M., N. S. Wicpolt, F. A. Molossi, D. Ogliari, A. M. Mori, V. Surkamp, and A. Gava. 2019. "Neurological diseases in cattle caused by plants and mycotoxins in Santa Catarina state, Brazil." *Pesquisa Veterinária Brasileira* 39 (4): 244-250. https://doi.org/10.1590/1678-5150-PVB-6024.

Morin, D. E. 2004. "Brainstem and cranial nerve abnormalities: listeriosis, otitis media/interna, and pituritary abscess syndrome." *Veterinary Clinics of North America, Food Animal Practice* 20 (2): 243-273. http://dx.doi.org/10.1016/j.cvfa.2004.02.007.

Nakazato, L., R. A. A. Lemos, and F. Riet-Correa. 2000. "Polioencefalomalacia em bovinos nos estados de Mato Grosso do Sul e São Paulo [*Polioencephalomalacia in cattle in the states of Mato Grosso do Sul and São Paulo*]." *Pesquisa Veterinária Brasileira* 20 (3): 119-125. http://dx.doi.org/10.1590/S0100-736X2000000300006.

Oliveira, T. S., V. Bull, R. Furtini, S. R. M. Drummnond, E. A. Costa, R. L. Santos, and T. A. Paixão. 2016. "Neurological diseases of cattle diagnosed by histopathology in Minas Gerais." *Brazilian Journal of Veterinary Pathology* 9 (2): 62-69. https://bjvp.org.br/wp-content/uploads/2016/07/v9-n2-4.pdf.

Pupin, R. C., P. V. Leal, J. P. L. Paula, C. C. Guizelini, T. B. M. Möck, R. A. A. Lemos, and D. C. Gomes. 2019. "Cattle diseases in Mato Grosso do Sul, Brazil: a 24-year survey (1995-2018)." *Pesquisa Veterinária Brasileira* 39 (9): 686-695. https://doi.org/10.1590/1678-5150-PVB-6384.

Queiroz G. R., P. F. V. Pereira, K. K. M. C. Flaiban, G. W. Di Santis, A. A. Alfieri, and J. A. N. Lisbôa. 2018. "Cerebrospinal fluid changes in cattle with rabies or with BoHV-5 meningoencephalitis and its correlation with the severity of CNS inflammatory process." *Research in Veterinary Science* 118 (6): 389–394. https://doi.org/10.1016/j.rvsc.2018.03.015.

Queiroz, G. R., R. A. M. Oliveira, K. K. M. C. Flaiban, G. W. Di Santis, A. P. F. R. L. Bracarense, S. A. Headley, A. A. Alfieri, and J. A. N. Lisbôa. 2018. "Diagnóstico diferencial das doenças neurológicas dos bovinos no estado do Paraná [*Differential diagnosis of neurologic diseases of cattle in the state of Paraná*]." *Pesquisa Veterinária Brasileira* 38 (7): 1264-1277. https://doi.org/10.1590/1678-5150-PVB-5429.

Queiroz, G. R., R. C. L. Ribeiro, F. T. N. M. A. Romão, K. K. M. C. Flaiban, A. P. F. R. L. Bracarense, and J. A. N. Lisbôa. 2012. "Intoxicação espontânea de bovinos por *Senna obtusifolia* no estado do Paraná [*Spontaneous Senna obtusifolia poisoning in cattle in the state of Paraná, Brazil*]." *Pesquisa Veterinária Brasileira* 32 (12): 1263-1271. http://dx.doi.org/10.1590/S0100-736X2012001200009.

Queiroz, G. R., R. C. L. Ribeiro, K. K. M. C. Flaiban, A. P. F. R. L. Bracarense, and J. A. N. Lisbôa. 2013. "Intoxicação espontânea por *Crotalaria incana* em bovinos no norte do estado do Paraná [*Spontaneous Crotalaria incana poisoning in cattle in the state of Paraná, Brazil*]." *Semina Ciências Agrárias* 34 (2): 823-832. https://www.uel.br/revistas/uel/index.php/semagrarias/article/view/12791/12588.

Rech, R. R., A. L. Schild, D. Driemeier, S. L. Garmatz, F. N. Oliveira, F. Riet-Correa, and C. S. L. Barros. 2005. "Febre catarral maligna em bovinos no Rio Grande do Sul: epidemiologia, sinais clínicos e patologia [*Malignant catarrhal fever in cattle in Rio Grande do Sul: epidemiology, clinical signs and pathology*]." *Pesquisa Veterinária Brasileira* 25 (2): 97-105. http://dx.doi.org/10.1590/S0100-736X2005000200006.

Reis M. C., J. N. Costa, A. P. C. Peixoto, L. J. C. Figueiredo, R. V. Menezes, M. M. Ferreira, and J. E. U. Sá. 2003. "Aspectos clínicos e epidemiológicos da raiva bovina apresentados na casuística da clínica de bovinos (Oliveira dos Campinhos, Santo Amaro, Bahia), Universidade Federal da Bahia, durante o período de janeiro de 1990 a dezembro de 1999 [*Clinical and epidemiologic aspects of bovine rabies diagnosed at the Bovine Clinics (Oliveira dos Campinhos, Santo Amaro, Bahia), Universidade Federal da Bahia, between January, 1990 and December, 1999 (case report)*]." *Revista Brasileira de Saúde e Produção Animal* 4 (1): 12-17.

Ribas, N. L. K. S., R. I. Carvalho, A. C. Santos, R. A. Valençoela, A. F. Gouveia, M. B. Castro, A. E. Mori, and R. A. A. Lemos. 2013. "Doenças do sistema nervoso de bovinos no Mato Grosso do Sul: 1082 casos [*Diseases of the nervous system of cattle in Mato Grosso do Sul, Brazil: 1082 cases*]." *Pesquisa Veterinária Brasileira* 33 (10): 1183-1194, 2013. http://dx.doi.org/10.1590/S0100-736X2013001000003.

Riet-Correa, F., R. M. T. Medeiros, J. A. Pfister, and F. S. Mendonça. 2017. "Toxic plants affecting the nervous system of ruminants and horses in Brazil." *Pesquisa Veterinária Brasileira* 37 (12): 1357-1368. https://doi.org/10.1590/S0100-736X2017001200001.

Rissi, D. R., F. N. Oliveira, R. R. Rech, F. Pierezan, R. A. A. Lemos, and C. S. L. Barros. 2006. "Epidemiologia, sinais clínicos e distribuição das lesões encefálicas em bovinos afetados por meningoencefalite por herpesvírus bovino-5 [*Epidemiology, clinical signs and distribution of the encephalic lesions in cattle affected by meningoencephalitis caused by bovine herpevirus-5*]." *Pesquisa Veterinária Brasileira* 26 (2): 123-132. http://dx.doi.org/10.1590/S0100-736X2006000200010.

Rissi, D. R., F. Pierezan, J. C. Oliveira Filho, R. A. Fighera, L. F. Irigoyen, G. D. Kommers, and C. S. L. Barros. 2010c. "Doenças de ovinos na região Central do Rio Grande do Sul: 361 casos [*Diseases of sheep from central Rio Grande do Sul State: 361 cases*]." *Pesquisa Veterinária Brasileira* 30 (1): 21-28. https://doi.org/10.1590/S0100-736X2010000100004.

Rissi, D. R., F. Pierezan, J. C. Oliveira-Filho, R. B. Lucena, P. M. S. Carmo, and C. S. L. Barros. 2010b. "Abordagem diagnóstica das principais doenças do sistema nervoso de ruminantes e equinos no Brasil [*Diagnostic approaches for the main neurological diseases of ruminants and horses in Brazil*]." *Pesquisa Veterinária Brasileira* 30 (11): 958-967. http://dx.doi.org/10.1590/S0100-736X2010001100010.

Rissi, D. R., R. A. Fighera, L. F. Irigoyen, G. D. Kommers, and C. S. L. Barros. 2010a. "Doenças neurológicas de ovinos na região Central do Rio Grande do Sul [*Neurological disease in sheep from central Rio Grande do Sul state, southern Brazil*]." *Pesquisa Veterinária Brasileira* 30 (3): 222-228. https://www.scielo.br/j/pvb/a/fWGgpH6C3GxS4zQGyHsgNxD/?format=pdf&lang=pt.

Rodrigues, A., R. R. Rech, R. R. Barros, R. A. Fighera, and C. S. L. Barros. 2005. "Babesiose cerebral em bovinos: 20 casos [*Cerebral babesiosis in cattle: 20 cases*]." *Ciência Rural* 35 (1): 121-125. https://www.scielo.br/j/cr/a/ChqKj9PLWTgLXWQB6WDtHSh/?format=pdf&lang=pt.

Rosa, F. B., R. A. Caprioli, T. M. Silva, G. J. N. Galiza, C. S. L. Barros, L. F. Irigoyen, R. A. Fighera, and G. D. Kommers. 2013. "Doenças de caprinos diagnosticadas na região Central no Rio Grande do Sul: 114 casos [*Diseases of goats diagnosed in the Central region of Rio Grande do Sul, Brazil: 114 cases*]." *Pesquisa Veterinária Brasileira* 33 (2): 199-204. https://www.scielo.br/j/pvb/a/6JktVdTcWLPLCx5n7CFYv3n/?format=pdf&lang=pt.

Salvador, S. C., R. A. A. Lemos, F. Riet-Correa, P. M. Roehe, and A. L. A. R. Osório. 1998. "Meningoencefalite em bovinos causada por herpesvírus bovino-5 no Mato Grosso do Sul e São Paulo [*Meningoencephalitis in cattle by bovine herpesvirus-5 in Mato Grosso do Sul and São Paulo*]." *Pesquisa Veterinária Brasileira* 18 (2): 75-82. https://doi.org/10.1590/S0100-736X1998000200007.

Sanches, A. W. D., I. M. Langohr, A. L. Stigger, and C. S. L. Barros. 2000. "Doenças do sistema nervoso central em bovinos no Sul do Brasil [*Diseases of the central nervous system in cattle of Southern Brazil*]." *Pesquisa Veterinária Brasileira* 20 (3): 113-118. http://dx.doi.org/10.1590/S0100-736X2000000300005.

Sant'Ana, F. J. F., D. R. Rissi, R. B. Lucena, R. A. A. Lemos, A. P. A. Nogueira, and C. S. L. Barros. 2009b. "Polioencefalomalácia em bovinos: epidemiologia, sinais clínicos e distribuição das lesões no encéfalo [*Bovine polioencephalomalacia: epidemiology, clinical signs and distribution of lesions in the brain*]." *Pesquisa Veterinária Brasileira* 29 (7): 487-497. http://dx.doi.org/10.1590/S0100-736X2009000700002.

Sant'Ana, F. J. F., R. A. A. Lemos, A. P. A. Nogueira, M. Togni, B. Tessele, and C. S. L. Barros. 2009a. "Polioencefalomalacia em ruminantes [*Polioencephalomalacia in ruminants*].” *Pesquisa Veterinária Brasileira* 29 (9): 681-694. https://www.scielo.br/j/pvb/a/NmmMJzMRHBXBYRj3PkZPtwj/?lang=pt&format=pdf.

Santos, B. L., P. Estima-Silva, A. C. B. Coelho, P. A. Oliveira, M. P. Soares, E. S. V. Sallis, F. R. P. Bruhn, and A. L. Schild. 2018. “Doenças do sistema nervoso central de bezerros no sul do Rio Grande do Sul: uma contribuição ao diagnóstico diferencial [*Central nervous system disease of calves in Southern Brazil: a contribution to the differential diagnosis*].” *Pesquisa Veterinária Brasileira* 38 (4): 685-691. https://doi.org/10.1590/1678-5150-PVB-5360.

Scott, P. R. 2004. “Diagnostic techniques and clinicopathologic findings in ruminant neurologic disease.” *Veterinary Clinics of North America, Food Animal Practice* 20 (2): 215-230. http://dx.doi.org/10.1016/j.cvfa.2004.02.004.

Smith, M. O., L.W. GEORGE. 2009. “Diseases of the nervous system.” In: Smith, B. P. *Large Animal Internal Medicine*. 4th ed. St. Louis: Mosby Elsevier. 972-1111.

Terra, J. P., G. R. Blume, R. E. Rabelo, J. T. Medeiros, C. G. N. Rocha, I. N. Chagas, M. S. Aguiar, and F. J. F. de Sant’Ana. 2018. “Neurological diseases of cattle in the state of Goiás, Brazil (2010-2017).” *Pesquisa Veterinária Brasileira* 38 (9): 1752-1760. https://doi.org/10.1590/1678-5150-PVB-5768.

Tokarnia, C. H., M. F. Brito, J. D. Barbosa, P. V. Peixoto, and J. Döbereiner. 2012. *Plantas Tóxicas do Brasil* [*Toxic Plants in Brazil*]. 2a. ed. Rio de Janeiro: Editora Helianthus. 566p.

Chapter 2

Histophilus somni-Associated Disease Syndromes in Ruminants from South America

Selwyn Arlington Headley*, DVM, MSc, PhD
Laboratory of Animal Pathology,
Department of Veterinary Preventive Medicine,
State University of Londrina, Paraná, Brazil

Introduction

Histophilus somni (HS) is a Gram-negative coccobacillus, that was formerly referred to as *Haemophilus somnus* (Corbeil 2007; Harris and Janzen 1989), and is, thus far, the only member of the genus *Histophilus* (Angen et al. 2003; Angen 2015). HS belongs to the *Pasteurellaceae* family, which includes other important bacteria of animal health and production, including *Pasteurella multocida*, *Mannheimia haemolytica*, *Actinobacillus pleuropneumoniae*, *A. lignieresii, and Glaesserella parasuis,* previously known as *Haemophilus parasuis* (Angen et al. 2003; Christensen et al. 2020). Although HS is within the *Pasteurellaceae* family, this organism does not have any close relationship with other species or genera of this family (Angen 2015). Additionally, phylogenetic studies based on the sequences of the 16S, RNA, and rpoB genes of bacteria, demonstrated that the organisms previously revered to as *Haemophilus somnus*, *Haemophilus agni* and *Histophilus ovis,* were indeed HS (Angen et al. 2003).

Since HS is a natural habitat of the respiratory and reproductive mucosa of healthy ruminants (Christensen et al. 2020), the mere presence or identification of this organism within these anatomic locations does not

* Corresponding Author's Email: selwyn.headley@uel.br.

In: Infectious and Parasitic Diseases of Animals in Developing Countries
Editor: Selwyn Arlington Headley
ISBN: 979-8-88697-504-8

necessarily imply disease. Nevertheless, HS is associated with a disease complex (collectively termed *histophilosis*) which can produce several clinical syndromes including thrombotic meningoencephalitis (TME), pleuritis, polysynovitis, arthritis, bronchopneumonia, septicemia, myocarditis, otitis media, infertility, abortion, and mastitis in affected ruminants (Corbeil 2007; Harris et al. 1989; Inzana and Corbeil 2004; Pérez et al. 2010). Furthermore, these syndromes are now referred to as the HS disease complex, HSDC (O'Toole and Sondgeroth 2016), with vasculitis being a typical manifestation of HS (Corbeil et al. 1986; Czuprynski et al. 2004; O'Toole et al. 2017).

The HSDC is well described in countries such as the USA (Ames 1987; Andrews et al. 1985; Dyer 2001; O'Toole et al. 2016; Ward et al. 1999), Canada (Corbeil et al. 1986; Gagea et al. 2006; Harris et al. 1989; Saunders and Janzen 1980; Van Donkersgoed et al. 1990), and Australia (Kessell et al. 2011; Lancaster et al. 1984). Furthermore, there are sporadic reports of HSDC in several countries including the UK (Wessels and Wessels 2005), Northern Ireland (Bryson et al. 1990; Cassidy et al. 1997), and Mexico (Diaz-Aparicio et al. 2009; Palomares et al. 2005; Perez-Romero et al. 2011). However, the current descriptions of HSDC within South America is sparse when compared with the vast investigations done in North America and other major cattle producing countries, suggesting that this pathogen is underdiagnoses or misdiagnosed in South America. Consequently, this chapter presents the clinical and pathological findings of HSDC with special emphasis on South America. Aspects related with the bacterial profile, host-parasite association, and pathogenicity of HS can be consulted elsewhere (Angen 2015; Corbeil 2007; Corbeil 2015; Czuprynski et al. 2004).

H. somni-Induced Bovine Respiratory Disease

The bovine respiratory disease (BRD) complex is multifactorial and multi-etiological disease entity that is associated with a wide range of infectious disease agents (Griffin et al. 2010; Taylor et al. 2010), together with managerial (Taylor et al. 2010) as well as environmental factors (Snowder et al. 2006; Taylor et al. 2010). Furthermore, BRD is the most important cause of livestock mortality in USA feedlots and contributes towards 16% of the number of non-predator losses to beef cattle (USDA 2011). In Brazil, the estimated morbidity due to BRD was \$6.31 million/annum, while BRD-associated mortality resulted in the loss of \$5.54 million/year (Baptista et al. 2017).

The participation of HS in the development of respiratory in Brazil was most likely initially diagnosed in 2013 in cattle with several clinical manifestations of HSDC (Headley et al. 2013). However, BRD *per se* due to HS was first reported in cattle (41.7%; 5/12) that had severe clinical manifestations of pulmonary discomfort and during which *H. somni* DNA was amplified from nasopharyngeal swabs (Headley et al. 2014). Since that initial description, we have demonstrated the association of *H. somni* with BRD in dairy (Oliveira et al. 2020) and feedlot cattle from several geographical regions of Brazil (Headley et al. 2017; Headley et al. 2018a; Magalhães et al. 2017). Furthermore, sheep from Southern Brazil with several disease syndromes, including respiratory discomfort, were also infected by *H. somni* (Headley et al. 2018b). Consequently, respiratory disease is the most frequent syndrome of HSDC currently diagnosed in ruminants from Brazil, and possibly Argentina (Moreira et al. 1987).

Cattle infected with pulmonary disease due to HS may demonstrate acute manifestation of pulmonary discomfort including dyspnea, extended head and neck, and audible noise when breathing (Baptista et al. 2017; Headley et al. 2018a), while some animals may die without clinical manifestations of pulmonary disease; similar clinical manifestations were described in pulmonary histophilosis in cattle from North America (O'Toole et al. 2016). Consequently, acute pulmonary histophilosis may result in death of affected cattle (Bryson et al. 1990; O'Toole et al. 2016), within 24 hours after the initial manifestations (Bryson et al. 1990).

Frequently, cattle with HS-associated BRD are concomitantly infected with viral and bacterial pathogens, such as bovine viral disease virus (BVDV), bovine respiratory syncytial virus (BRSV), bovine alphaherpesvirus 1 (BoAHV1), *P. multocida*, and *M. haemolytica* (Headley et al. 2014; Headley et al. 2017; Headley et al. 2018a; O'Toole et al. 2016). Recently, we have observed that a malignant catarrhal fever virus may be associated with BRD (Oliveira et al. 2021) and or pulmonary disease (Headley et al. 2020b) in cattle from Brazil. Although it is widely accepted that bacterial infections are generally secondary to a viral agent, the fact that HS can produce fatal pulmonary disease experimentally (O'Toole et al. 2016), suggests that the colonization of HS within the upper respiratory tract may inhibit viral infections (Corbeil 2015), considering that this pathogen is natural habitat of the respiratory system. Serological analyses suggest that cattle are infected and seroconvert within 14–21 days of entry into feedlots (O'Toole et al. 2016). However, there are no serological studies for HS in South America, consequently the number of cattle in contact or the frequency of infections with this bacterium in this continent remains unknown. The median onset for the development of fatal pneumonia is 12 days (Van Donkersgoed et al. 1990), and most feedlot cattle with HS-induced BRD from Brazil die within the first 30 days-on-feed (Baptista et al. 2017).

Cattle that succumb to HS-induced BRD may demonstrate the typical gross pathological pattern of fibrinous bronchopneumonia with pleuritis (Andrews et al. 1985; Headley et al. 2018a; Moreira et al. 1987). However, this gross pattern of pulmonary disease associated with infections induced by HS cannot be easily differentiated from the pulmonary diseases caused by *M. haemolytica* and *P. multocida* (Caswell and Williams 2016). Nevertheless, HS and *M. haemolytica* are frequently associated with fibrinous bronchopneumonia, while *P. multocida* is more frequently observed in suppurative bronchopneumonia of cattle (López and Martinson 2017). Furthermore, vasculitis may be the key to differentiate between these bacterial infections, in the absence of viral pathogens known to produce vasculitis, considering that vasculitis is the hallmark of infections due to HS (Czuprynski et al. 2004; Headley et al. 2013; O'Toole et al. 2017). However, a Canadian study that used metagenomic sequence analysis combined with the histological features of BRD demonstrated that there was a definite association between *M. haemolytica* and the development of fibrinous bronchopneumonia in feedlot cattle, while HS was more frequently associated with suppurative bronchopneumonia (Zhang et al. 2020). Since *M. haemolytica* and *P. multocida*-associated pulmonary infections in cattle are more widespread than those due to HS in Brazil, most cases of fibrinous and/or suppurative bronchopneumonia identified in cows are attributed to those of *M. haemolytica* and/or *P. multocida* and a diagnosis of pulmonary histophilosis is not further investigated. This may then explain the reduced number of cases of HS-related BRD diagnosed in Brazil and other South American countries.

The histopathologic pulmonary lesions observed in BRD due to HS, *M. haemolytica*, and/or *P. multocida* are somewhat superimposed or overlapping (Caswell et al. 2016), with lesions of HS varying between severe suppurative (Figure 1) to fibrinous bronchopneumonia (Andrews et al. 1985; Bryson et al. 1990; Castro et al. 2021). Therefore, an accurate interpretation of the histopathologic lesions induced by these organisms would require the concomitant utilization of additional diagnostic tools, such as immunehistochemistry (IHC), *in situ* hybridization (ISH), or molecular identification. Cases of HS-associated BRD that occurred in Brazil were essentially typical of purulent bronchopneumonia (Headley et al. 2013; Headley et al. 2017) and/or fibrinous bronchopneumonia (Headley et al. 2018a). However, since in some cases cattle from Brazil were concomitantly infected by *M. haemolytica* (Headley et al. 2018a), and IHC detection was not performed, the exact pattern of bronchopneumonia associated with HS in cattle from Brazil still has to be determined. Furthermore, cattle from Argentina with HS-associated pulmonary disease demonstrated suppurative bronchopneumonia, with pulmonary histophilosis confirmed by bacterial isolation (Moreira et al. 1987).

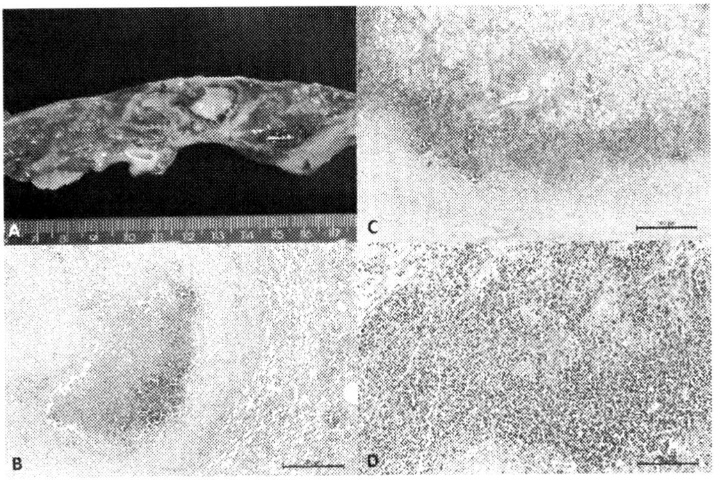

Figure 1. Suppurative bronchopneumonia induced by *Histophilus somni* in ruminants. Observe the accumulation of purulent exudate in the sectioned surface of the lung (A), and histopathologic demonstration of suppurative pneumonia (B-D).

It must be highlighted that molecular testing *per se* determines infection, while an *in situ* diagnosis confirms an active disease process (Fulton et al. 2012). Therefore, the production of a commercial antibody or protein for the utilization *in situ* diagnostic assays will drastically increase the cases of HSDC in South America.

It must be highlighted that the IHC diagnosis for HSDC is currently not extensively used worldwide, since commercial antibodies are not available, with *in situ* diagnosis being restricted to a few studies North America (Margineda et al. 2019; O'Toole et al. 2017; Tegtmeier et al. 1999). Consequently, the diagnosis of HSDC is widely based on the molecular identification of HS DNA associated with typical lesions in tissues, particularly vasculitis (Corbeil et al. 1986; Czuprynski et al. 2004; Headley et al. 2013). Although molecular testing is more sensitive than IHC and ISH for the identification of infectious disease pathogens (Castro et al. 2021; Fulton and Confer 2012), these two *in situ* diagnostic methods have the advantage over molecular testing to accurately demonstrate the intralesional accumulations of antigens and/or proteins of infectious disease agents within the histopathological patterns of pulmonary disease and are recommended when there is need to correlate histopathology with the intralesional identification of pathogens (Castro et al. 2021).

H. somni-Induced Thrombotic Meningoencephalitis

Thrombotic meningoencephalitis (TME) is a severe neurological disease of cattle caused by embolic bacterial dissemination of HS to the central nervous system (George 2015). TEM results in elevated fatality rates in affected herds and occurs predominantly in feedlot cattle relative to dairy or pastured cattle (Fecteau and George 2004). This manifestation of HS in cattle is well described in North America (Ames 1987; George 2015; O'Toole et al. 2016; Van Dreumel et al. 1970), Australia (Kessell et al. 2011), with few reports from Brazil (Headley et al. 2015a), Argentina (Descarga et al. 2002), and Uruguay (Romero et al. 2020). Additionally, there are descriptions of HS-induced TEM in sheep in associated with other HSDC in several countries including Australia (Philbey et al. 1991), Europe (Cassidy et al. 1997), Brazil (Headley et al. 2018b) and Uruguay (Romero et al. 2013). Since the clinical manifestations observed in sheep are quite similar to those observed in cattle, most descriptions will be done for cattle.

Clinically, cattle with TEM may develop fever, anorexia, depression, muscular weakness, reluctance to move, abnormal gait (George 2015; Panciera et al. 1968; Smith and Biberstein 1977), blindness, permanent recumbency (Ames 1987; Descarga et al. 2002; George 2015; Headley et al. 2015a), head tilt, nystagmus, strabismus, opisthotonos, and coma (George 2015; Headley et al. 2015a), motor incoordination, tetraparesis, and reduced tongue tonus (Headley et al. 2015a). Most TEM affected cattle die within 36 hours after the onset of clinical manifestations (Descarga et al. 2002; Fecteau et al. 2004; George 2015; Headley et al. 2015a; Panciera et al. 1968), some cattle may demonstrate neurological manifestations during several weeks (Headley et al. 2015a; MacDonald et al. 1973), while others are encountered dead without previous clinical manifestations (Ames 1987; Kennedy et al. 1960; MacDonald et al. 1973). The clinical evolution of TME observed in sheep varied between 1-11 days (Headley et al. 2018b; Romero et al. 2013), while some were found dead (Cassidy et al. 1997).

Nevertheless, the primary neurological manifestations of TME are depression, weakness, ataxia, paralysis, and coma (Ames 1987; George 2015; Kennedy et al. 1960). Probably, the most notable characteristic clinical manifestation of TEM in cattle is the sleepy appearance, where animals may be moving their heads up and down slowly with eyes closed or partially closed, which gave rise to the "sleeper syndrome" associated with this manifestation in cattle (George 2015). Additionally, the respiratory manifestation of HSDC may occur before the onset of the neurological disease (Ames 1987; Fecteau et al. 2004).

There seems to be distant differences between the pathological findings of TME in affected cattle from North American relative to the descriptions from South America. The typical gross lesions of TME as described in North America consists of several areas of hemorrhage and necrosis randomly distributed throughout the brain (Ames 1987; Kennedy et al. 1960; Panciera et al. 1968) with similar lesions possibly within the spinal cord (Ames 1987; George 2015; Panciera et al. 1968). Furthermore, the typical foci of necrosis are more frequently observed near the junction of the cortical grey and white matter of the cerebrum (Panciera et al. 1968). The characteristic histological lesions are severe multifocal necrosis with bacterial vasculitis within the brain and affected tissues (Ames 1987; Kennedy et al. 1960; Panciera et al. 1968). In addition to the typical brain lesion, cattle with TME frequently demonstrate systemic manifestation of disease with bronchopneumonia, renal infarcts, hemorrhagic enteritis, and lymphadenitis (George 2015; Headley et al. 2015a; MacDonald et al. 1973; Pérez et al. 2010).

However, in most confirmed cases of TME in cattle from South America, typical gross necrotic zones were not observed within the brain (Headley et al. 2015a; Margineda et al. 2019; Romero et al. 2020). However, there was severe congestion of meningeal vessels with multiple foci of brain hemorrhage (Headley et al. 2013), with extra neurological manifestations of systemic disease such as renal infarctions (Figure 2), bronchopneumonia, thrombosis frequently involving arteries of the *carotid rete miriabile,* and enteritis in cases from Brazil (Headley et al. 2013; Headley et al. 2015a), while fibrino-suppurative leptomeningitis, with ventriculitis and choroiditis were observed in Uruguay (Romero et al. 2020), and suppurative leptomeningitis in Argentina (Descarga et al. 2002; Margineda et al. 2019). These cases without typical brain necrosis have been referred to as atypical neurological manifestations of TEM (Ishikawa et al. 1984) and may be one of the factors for the reduced occurrence of TEM in Southern America, since most large animal veterinarians familiar with this disease would be expecting typical necrosis of the brain. Additionally, in most cases of TEM from South America thrombotic lesions were identified in other organs with confirmation of HS by molecular testing (Headley et al. 2015a) or by IHC (Margineda et al. 2019; Romero et al. 2020). In some of these cases from Brazil, and wide spread cerebral (Headley et al. 2015a),

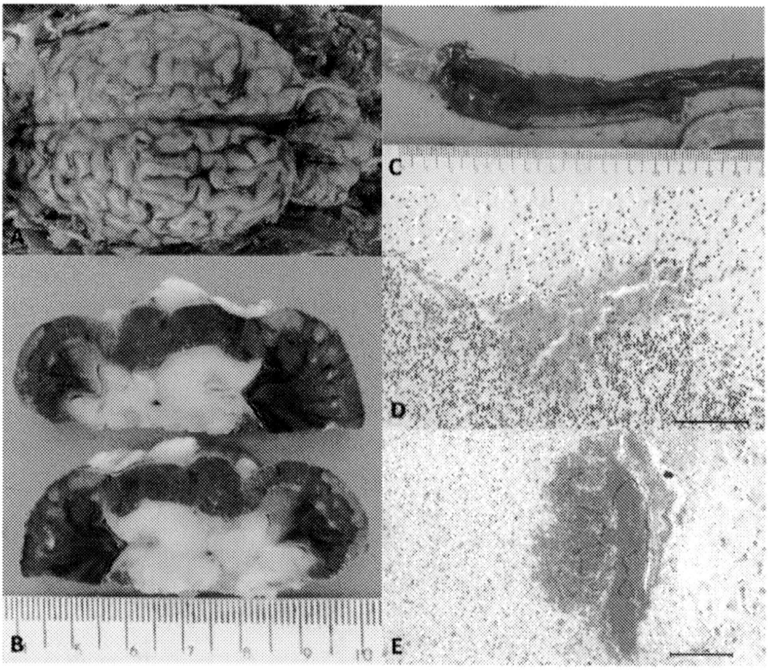

Figure 2. *Histophilus somni*-associated atypical thrombotic meningoencephalitis with extra-encephalitic lesions in a cow from Southern Brazil. There is marked congestion of cerebral vessels (A), renal infarcts (B), and hemorrhagic enteritis (C) grossly, with cerebellar (D) and cerebral (E) hemorrhages.

Consequently, diagnosticians from these regions must consider these alterations before a diagnosis of TEM is discarded, since it is rather unlikely that brain infarctions will be the key features in cattle from South America. Furthermore, it must be highlighted that the *carotid rete miriabile* is one of the anatomic regions of choice when evaluating neurological tissues for the possible participation of ovine gammaherpesvirus 2 (OvGHV2) induced sheep associated-malignant catarrhal fever (SA-MCF) in cattle (Headley et al. 2020a), where the typical lesion in SA-MCF is vasculitis with proliferative vascular lesions (Headley et al. 2021; Headley et al. 2020a), while thrombosis is the hallmark of TEM at the *carotid rete miriabile* (Headley et al. 2015a). Additionally, veterinary practitioners from Brazil investigating cattle with neurological disease manifestations must include bovine rabies, herpesvirus induced meningoencephalitis, SA-MCF, and HS as part of the differential diagnoses, since these are the most frequently occurring infectious neurological diseases of cattle in Brazil (Queiroz et al. 2018; Sanches et al. 2000; Terra et al. 2018). Moreover, from our experience in diagnostic pathology, cerebral necrosis in cattle from Brazil is more likely to be associated with herpesvirus induced meningoencephalitis (Figure 3) than other infectious disease pathogens of cattle.

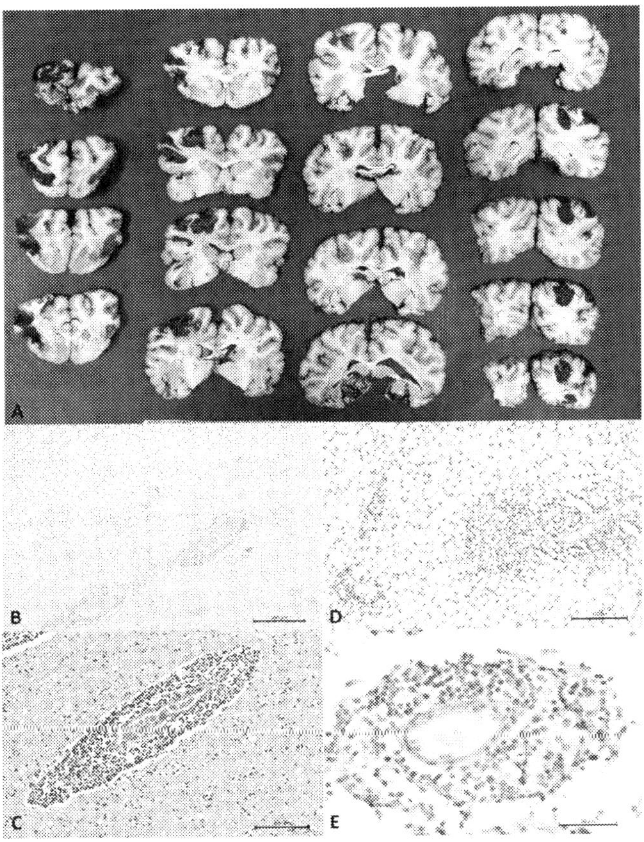

Figure 3. Bovine alphaherpesvirus 5 (BoAHV5)-induced necrotizing meningo-encephalitis in a cow from Southern Brail. Observe foci of necrosis throughout multiple serial sections of the brain (A), histopathologic demonstration of cerebral necrosis (B) with typical perivascular cuffings (C), and positive intralesional immunoreactivity to BoAHV5 antigens (D-E).

H. somni-Associated Myocardial Diseases

The occurrence of HS-related diseases in cattle from South America with emphasis on myocardial infections was revised (Margineda et al. 2019). Descriptions of HS-induced myocarditis were observed in cattle from Argentina (Margineda et al. 2019) and Brazil (Headley et al. 2013), and also in sheep from Brazil (Headley et al. 2018b). Myocardial infection is the most common manifestation of the sudden death syndrome in feedlot cattle within the HSDC (O'Toole et al. 2016) and is the principal cause of the death of feedlot calves (Haines et al. 2004). In cases from the USA, intralesional antigens of HS were detected IHC (O'Toole et al. 2017).

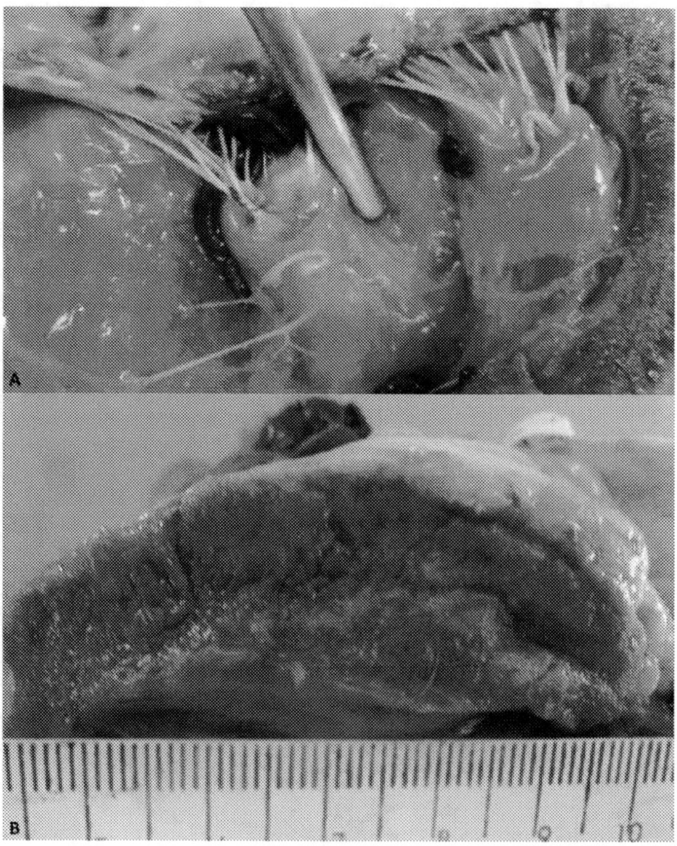

Figure 4. *Histophilus somni* induced myocarditis in a yearling calf. Observe white streaks at the pappilary muscle (A), and the pale area at the transverse section of the heart (B).

In acute cases, the affected cattle are found dead without any noticeable clinical manifestation (O'Toole et al. 2016). Alternatively, feedlot cattle chronically infected by HS may demonstrate clinical manifestations of heart failure with consequent ventral and submandibular edema (Guichon et al. 1988), depression, lethargy, and reduced growth (O'Toole et al. 2016); lesions may be restricted to the heart with or without pulmonary involvement (Haines et al. 2004). Gross lesions seem to be more frequent at the papillary muscles of the left ventricle (O'Toole et al. 2016; O'Toole et al. 2017; Pérez et al. 2010). In some of the cases observed in Brazil, there was sudden death, with pale streaks at the papillary muscle of the left ventricle grossly (Figure 4), which resulted in multifocal myocarditis with vasculitis by histopathology, during which HS DNA was amplified from multiple tissues (Headley et al. 2013), resulting in systemic manifestations of HSDC. In the cases from Argentina, three feedlot cattle died suddenly of acute multifocal myocarditis with lesions at the papillary muscles, after being 33 – 102 days on feed, had concomitant pulmonary disease, and contained intralesional antigens of HS by IHC (Margineda et al. 2019). Consequently, the myocardial manifestation of HS in cattle from South America is considerably similar to that observed in feedlot cattle from North America, Europe, and Australia.

H. somni and Reproductive Diseases

The identification of HS in the reproductive tracts must be considered in the absence and/or presence of associated clinical disease since this pathogen is a natural habitat of the reproductive tracts of ruminants (Kwiecien and Little 1991). Although infection of the reproductive tracts of male and female ruminants is an important manifestation of HSDC in ruminants (O'Toole et al. 2016), there are considerably few reports of HS-induced reproductive diseases from South America. Nevertheless, most of these reports were described in Brazil, in which HS was associated with abortions in cattle (Headley et al. 2015b; Scarcelli et al. 2004), endometritis in sheep (Rizzo et al. 2012), and identified within the semen of bulls (Dias et al. 2014). Furthermore, there is a report of HS-induced abortions in cattle from Argentina (Campero et al. 1993).

Most of the cases of spontaneous HS-associated abortions from Brazil were identified in fetuses between 120 – 270 days of gestation (Headley et al. 2015b; Scarcelli et al. 2004), from beef (Scarcelli et al. 2004) and dairy (Headley et al. 2015b) cattle herds located in several geographical regions of Brazil, and with varying clinical histories of reproductive problems (Headley et al. 2015b; Scarcelli et al. 2004). While the report of HS-induced abortion from Argentina occurred in a 120-day old fetus from a dairy herd with reproductive issues (Campero et al. 1993). Recently, we have identified that bovine fetuses previously known to be infected with HS (Headley et al. 2015b) were concomitantly infected with bovine gammaherpesvirus 2, and other reproductive disease pathogens of cattle (Headley et al. 2022).

The reproductive issues more frequently reported from cattle farms with animals infected by HS in South America included abortions (Campero et al. 1993; Headley et al. 2015b; Scarcelli et al. 2004), repeated estrus (Campero et al. 1993; Headley et al. 2015b), reduced conception rates, and stillbirths (Headley et al. 2015b). Fetuses infected with HS may demonstrate myocardial and renal hemorrhages, congestion of meningeal vessels, and hyperemia of intestinal mucosa grossly, with histopathological manifestations of necrotizing myocarditis with vasculitis, renal infarctions, hemorrhagic enteritis, and varying degrees of vasculitis, hemorrhage, and thrombosis of meningeal vessels (Headley et al. 2015b).

The identification of HS in the semen of bulls experimentally exposed (Dias et al. 2014) may pose a serious problem to the cattle industry in Brazil and South America, since most farms use some form of artificial insemination (AI). However, there is no mention if the bulls experimentally infected developed clinical manifestations of HS (Dias et al. 2014), but the finding of HS in semen must be considered as possible risk of infection in breeding centers where AI is routinely used. Nevertheless, HS was identified in the semen of rams with epididymitis (Palomares et al. 2005), and an elevated rate of HS was described in the semen of bulls from AI centers in Canada (Humphrey et al. 1982).

Conclusion

HSDC seems to be an emerging disease syndrome for ruminants in South America that may produce severe economic losses to the cattle industry. However, the few documented cases of this syndrome in South America may suggest that this disease is neglected, misdiagnosed, or underdiagnosed. Since the pulmonary manifestations of HSDC can be grossly confused with those induced by *Mannheimia haemolytica*, which is considered endemic and more prevalent than HS in South America, it is rather likely that most veterinary practitioners would confuse these pulmonary diseases resulting in misdiagnosis or underdiagnosis of HSDC. Furthermore, since most vaccines used in South America do not contain *H. somni*, mortality associated with this bacterial pathogen will continue to be a problem for the local cattle industry.

References

Ames, T. R. 1987. "Neurologic disease caused by *Haemophilus somnus*." *Veterinary Clinics of North America. Food Animal Practice* 3 (1): 61-73. https://doi.org/10.1016/s0749-0720(15)31179-8.

Andrews, J. J., T. D. Anderson, L. N. Slife, and G. W. Stevenson. 1985. "Microscopic lesions associated with the isolation of *Haemophilus somnus* from pneumonic bovine lungs." *Veterinary Pathology* 22 (2): 131-6. https://doi.org/10.1177/030098588502200206.

Angen, O., P. Ahrens, P. Kuhnert, H. Christensen, and R. Mutters. 2003. "Proposal of *Histophilus somni* gen. nov., sp. nov. for the three species incertae sedis '*Haemophilus somnus*,' '*Haemophilus agni*' and '*Histophilus ovis*'." *International Journal of Systematic and Evolutionary Microbiology* 53 (Pt 5): 1449-56. http://www.ncbi.nlm.nih.gov/pubmed/13130032.

Angen, Øystein. 2015. "Taxonomy of *Histophilus somni*." In *Histophilus somni. Current Topics in Microbiology and Immunology*, edited by T. Inzana. Switzerland: Springer.

Baptista, Anderson Lopes, Amanda Lima Rezende, Pedro de Almeida Fonseca, Geison Morel Nogueira, Selwyn Arlington Headley, Guilherme Lobato Menezes, Amauri Alcindo Alfieri, and João Paulo Elsen Saut. 2017. "Bovine respiratory disease complex associated mortality and morbidity rates in feedlot cattle from southeastern Brazil." *Journal of Infection in Developing Countries* 11: 791-799.

Bryson, D. G., H. J. Ball, M. McAliskey, W. McConnell, and S. J. McCullough. 1990. "Pathological, immunocytochemical and microbiological findings in calf pneumonias associated with Haemophilus somnus infection." *J Comp Pathol* 103 (4): 433-45. https://doi.org/10.1016/s0021-9975(08)80031-x.

Campero, C. M., A. R. Moreira, S. Daguerre, J. Bartolome, and E. Odriozola. 1993. "Aborto bovino asociado a *Haemophilus somnus*." *Veterinaria Argentina* 10: 404-409.

Cassidy, J. P., S. W. McDowell, G. A. Reilly, W. J. McConnell, F. Forster, and D. Lawler. 1997. "Thrombotic meningoencephalitis associated with *Histophilus ovis* infection in lambs in Europe." *Veterinary Record* 140 (8): 193-5. http://www.ncbi.nlm.nih.gov/pubmed/9061870.

Castro, Mariana Motta, T. E. S. Oliveira, and S. A. Headley. 2021. "Bovine respiratory disease in Brasil: a short review." *Semina: Ciências Agrárias* 42, no. 1 (3): 2081-2110. https://doi.org/(accepted).

Caswell, J. L., and K. J. Williams. 2016. "Respiratory system." In *Jubb, Kennedy, and Palmer's Pathology of Domestic Animals*, edited by M. G. Maxie, 465-591. Philadelphia: Saunders/Elsevier.

Christensen, Henrik, Janine Bossé, Øystein Angen, Niels Nørskov-Lauritsen, and Magne Bisgaard. 2020. "Immunological and molecular techniques used for determination of serotypes in *Pasteurellaceae*." In *Methods in Microbiology*, edited by Charles S. Pavia and Volker Gurtler, 117-149. Academic Press.

Corbeil, L. B. 2007. "*Histophilus somni* host-parasite relationships." *Animal Health Research Reviews* 8 (2): 151-60. https://doi.org/10.1017/S1466252307001417. http://www.ncbi.nlm.nih.gov/pubmed/18218158.

Corbeil, L. B. 2015. "Host immune response to *Histophilus somni*." In *Histophilus somni. Current Topics in Microbiology and Immunology*, edited by T. Inzana. Switzerland: Springer.

Corbeil, L. B., P. R. Widders, R. Gogolewski, J. Arthur, T. J. Inzana, and A. C. Ward. 1986. "*Haemophilus somnus*: bovine reproductive and respiratory disease." *Canadian Veterinary Journal* 27 (2): 90-3.

Czuprynski, C. J., F. Leite, M. Sylte, C. Kuckleburg, R. Schultz, T. Inzana, E. Behling-Kelly, and L. Corbeil. 2004. "Complexities of the pathogenesis of *Mannheimia haemolytica* and *Haemophilus somnus* infections: challenges and potential opportunities for prevention?" *Anim Health Res Rev* 5 (2): 277-82. https://doi.org/10.1079/ahr200483.

Descarga, C. O., H. G. Piscitelli, G. C. Zielinski, and A. L. Cipolla. 2002. "Thromboembolic meningoencephalitis due to *Haemophilus somnus* in feedlot cattle in Argentina." *Veterinary Record* 150 (26): 817. http://www.ncbi.nlm.nih.gov/pubmed/12120926.

Dias, Ferreira Francisca Elda, Cáris Maroni Nunes, Tânia Vasconcelos Cavalcante, Juliano Franco Souza, Silvia Minharro Barbosa, Andréa Azevedo Pires Castro, Felipe de Jesus Moraes Jr., Claúdia Marinovic Oliveira, and José Fernando Garcia. 2014. "Detecção de *Histophilus somni* (*Haemophilus somnus*) no sêmen bovino mediante reação em cadeia pela polimerase (PCR) [*Detection of Histophilus somni (Haemophilus somnus) in bovine semen using polymerase chain reaction (PCR)*]." *Revista Acadêmica: Ciências Agrárias e Ambientais* 12 (1): 11-16.

Diaz-Aparicio, E., V. R. Tenorio-Gutierrez, B. Arellano-Reynoso, I. Enriquez-Verdugo, and F. Aguilar-Romero. 2009. "Pathogenicity of different strains of *Histophilus somni* in the experimental induction of ovine epididymitis." *Canadian Journal of Veterinary Research* 73 (2): 157-60.

Dyer, N. W. 2001. "*Haemophilus somnus* bronchopneumonia in American bison (*Bison bison*)." *Journal of Veterinary Diagnostic Investigation* 13 (5): 419-21. http://www.ncbi.nlm.nih.gov/pubmed/11580065.

Fecteau, G., and L. W. George. 2004. "Bacterial meningitis and encephalitis in ruminants." *Veterinary Clinics of North America. Food Animal Practice* 20 (2): 363-77. https://doi.org/10.1016/j.cvfa.2004.03.002.

Fulton, Robert W., and Anthony W. Confer. 2012. "Laboratory test descriptions for bovine respiratory disease diagnosis and their strengths and weaknesses: Gold standards for diagnosis, do they exist?" *Canadian Veterinary Journal* 53 (7): 754-761. http://www.ncbi.nlm.nih.gov/pmc/articles/PMC3377458/.

Gagea, M. I., K. G. Bateman, T. van Dreumel, B. J. McEwen, S. Carman, M. Archambault, R. A. Shanahan, and J. L. Caswell. 2006. "Diseases and pathogens associated with mortality in Ontario beef feedlots." *Journal of Veterinary Diagnostic Investigation*, Jan, 18-28.

George, Leslie W. 2015. "Thromboembolic meningoencephalitis (*Histophilus somni* [formerly *Haemophilus somnus*] Infection; Sleeper Calves)." In *Large Animal Internal Medicine*, edited by Bradford P. Smith, 971-972. St. Louis, Missouri: Elsevier/Mosby.

Griffin, D., M. M. Chengappa, J. Kuszak, and D. S. McVey. 2010. "Bacterial pathogens of the bovine respiratory disease complex." *Veterinary Clinics of North America. Food Animal Practice* 26 (2): 381-94. https://doi.org/10.1016/j.cvfa.2010.04.004.

Guichon, P. T., J. Pritchard, and G. K. Jim. 1988. "*Haemophilus somnus* myocarditis in a feedlot steer." *Canadian Veterinary Journal* 29 (12): 1012-3.

Haines, D. M., K. M. Moline, R. A. Sargent, J. R. Campbell, D. J. Myers, and P. A. Doig. 2004. "Immunohistochemical study of *Hemophilus somnus*, *Mycoplasma bovis*, *Mannheimia hemolytica*, and bovine viral diarrhea virus in death losses due to myocarditis in feedlot cattle." *Canadian Veterinary Journal* 45 (3): 231-4.

Harris, F. W., and E. D. Janzen. 1989. "The *Haemophilus somnus* disease complex (Hemophilosis): A review." *Canadian Veterinary Journal* 30 (10): 816-22. http://www.ncbi.nlm.nih.gov/pubmed/17423440.

Headley, S.A., G. A. A. Lemos, A. M. Dall Agnol, A. A. C. Xavier, V. C. A. Depes, C. Y. Yasumitsu, T. E. S. Oliveira, L. E. Silva, T. C. Faccin, A. A. Alfieri, and J. A. N. Lisboa. 2021. "Ovine gammaherpesvirus 2 infections in cattle without typical manifestations of sheep-associated malignant catarrhal fever and concomitantly infected with bovine coronavirus." *Brazilian Journal of Microbiology*: 1-14. https://doi.org/10.1007/s42770-021-00653-6.

Headley, S.A., T. E. S. Oliveira, and C. W. Cunha. 2020a. "A review of the epidemiological, clinical, and pathological aspects of sheep-associated malignant catarrhal fever with emphasis on Brazil." *Brazilian Journal of Microbiology* 51: 1405–1432.

Headley, S.A., V. H. Oliveira, G. F. Figueira, D. E. Bronkhorst, A. F. Alfieri, W. Okano, and A. A. Alfieri. 2013. "*Histophilus somni*-induced infections in cattle from southern Brazil." *Tropical Animal Health and Production* 45 (7): 1579-1588. https://doi.org/10.1007/s11250-013-0402-7.

Headley, Selwyn A., Alfredo H. T. Pereira, Luciana C. Balbo, Giovana W. Di Santia, Ana P. F. R. L. Bracarense, Luiz F. C. Cunha Filho, Jackson Schade, Werner Okano, Priscilla F. V. Pereira, Fábio Morotti, Lucienne G. Preto-Giordano, Rogério A. Marcasso, Alice F. Alfieri, Júlio A. N. Lisbôa, and Amauri A. Alfieri. 2018b. "*Histophilus somni*-associated syndromes in sheep from Southern Brazil." *Brazilian Journal of Microbiology* 49 (3): 591-600. https://doi.org/https://doi.org/10.1016/j.bjm.2017.12.008. https://www.sciencedirect.com/science/article/pii/S1517838217305117.

Headley, Selwyn A., Alice F. Alfieri, Victor H. S. Oliveira, Edsel A. Beuttemmüller, and Amauri A. Alfieri. 2014. "*Histophilus somni* is a potential threat to beef cattle feedlots from Brazil." *Veterinary Record* 175 (10): 249. https://doi.org/10.1136/vr.102562.

Headley, Selwyn A., Ana Paula F. R. L. Bracarense, Victor H. S. Oliveira, Gustavo R. Queiroz, Werner Okano, Alice F. Alfieri, Karina K. M. C. Flaiban, Júlio A. N. Lisbôa, and Amauri A. Alfieri. 2015a. "*Histophilus somni*-induced thrombotic meningo-encephalitis in cattle from northern Paraná, Brazil." *Pesquisa Veterinária Brasileira* 35 (4): 329-336.

Headley, Selwyn A., Daniele Voltarelli, Victor H. S. Oliveira, Dalton E. Bronkhorst, Alice F. Alfieri, Luiz C. Negri, Werner Okano, and Amauri A. Alfieri. 2015b. "Association of *Histophilus somni* with spontaneous abortions in dairy cattle herds from Brazil." *Tropical Animal Health and Production* 47 (2): 403-413. https://doi.org/10.1007/s11250-014-0740-0.

Headley, Selwyn A., Luciana C. Balbo, Alice F. Alfieri, João Paulo Elsen Saut, and Amauri A. Alfieri. 2017. "Bovine respiratory disease associated with *Histophilus somni* and bovine respiratory syncytial virus in a beef cattle feedlot from Southeastern Brazil." *Semina Ciêncas Agrárias* 38 (1): 283-294.

Headley, Selwyn A., Werner Okano, Luciana C. Balbo, Rogério A. Marcasso, Thalita E. S. Oliveira, Alice F. Alfieri, Luiz C. Negri Filho, Mariana M. Z. Michelazzo, Silvio M. C Rodrigues, Anderson L. Baptista, João P. E. Saut, and Amauri A. Alfieri. 2018a. "Molecular survey of infectious agents associated with bovine respiratory disease in a beef cattle feedlot in southern Brazil." *Journal of Veterinary Diagnostic Investigation* 30 (2): 249-251. https://doi.org/10.1177/1040638717739945.

Headley, Selwyn Arlington, Juliana Torres Tomazi Fritzen, Vinícius Rodrigues Bon, Ana Aparecida Correa Xavier, Alais Maria Dall Agnol, Natália Zaparoli Zucoloto, Flávia Helena Pereira Silva, Julia Raisa Ximenes Figueiredo, Alice Fernandes Alfieri, Werner Okano, and Amauri Alcindo Alfieri. 2022. "Detection of bovine gammaherpesvirus 6 in tissues of aborted fetuses from dairy cows concomitantly infected by *Histophilus somni*." *Microbial Pathogenesis* https://doi.org/10.1016/j.micpath.2022.105621.

Headley, Selwyn Arlington, Melissa Cristina Müller, Thalita Evani Silva de Oliveira, Caroline Ambiel Barros Gil Duarte, Priscilla Fajardo Valente Pereira, Marcos Vinícius Vieira, Cristina Wetzel Cunha, Eduardo Furtado Flores, Júlio Augusto Naylor Lisbôa, and Lucienne Garcia Pretto-Giordano. 2020b. "Diphtheric aspergillosis tracheitis with gastrointestinal dissemination secondary to viral infections in a dairy calf." *Microbial Pathogenesis* 149: 104497-104497. https://doi.org/10.1016/j.micpath.2020.104497. https://pubmed.ncbi.nlm.nih.gov/32910985.

Humphrey, J. D., P. B. Little, D. A. Barnum, P. A. Doig, L. R. Stephens, and J. Thorsen. 1982. "Occurrence of "*Haemophilus somnus*" in bovine semen and in the prepuce of bulls and steers." *Canadian Journal of Comparative Medicine* 46 (2): 215-217. https://pubmed.ncbi.nlm.nih.gov/7093816.

Inzana, T. J. and L. Corbeil. 2004. "*Haemophilus*." In *Pathogenesis of bacterial infections in animals*, edited by C. L. Gyles, J. F. Prescott, G. Songer and C. O. Thoen, 243-258. Ames, Iowa, USA: Blackwell Publishing.

Ishikawa, Y., S. Tsukuda, Y. Nakajima, and K. Ohshima. 1984. "Atypical nervous lesion in *Haemophilus somnus* infection of cattle." *Cornell Veterinarian* 74 (4): 349-53.

Kennedy, P. C., E. L. Biberstein, J. A. Howarth, L. M. Frazier, and D. L. Dungworth. 1960. "Infectious meningo-encephalitis in cattle, caused by a *Haemophilus*-like organism." *American Journal of Veterinary Research* 21: 403-9.

Kessell, A. E., J. W. Finnie, and P. A. Windsor. 2011. "Neurological diseases of ruminant livestock in Australia. III: bacterial and protozoal infections." *Australian Veterinary Journal* 89 (8): 289-96. https://doi.org/10.1111/j.1751-0813.2011.00807.x.

Kwiecien, J. M., and P. B. Little. 1991. "*Haemophilus somnus* and reproductive disease in the cow: A review." *Canadian Veterinary Journal* 32 (10): 595-601.

Lancaster, M. J., D. J. McGillivery, R. M. Patterson, and S. Irwin. 1984. "Pneumonia associated with *Haemophilus somnus* in a calf." *Australian Veterinary Journal* 61 (8): 269.

López, Alfonso, and Shannon A. Martinson. 2017. "Respiratory system, mediastinum, and pleurae." In *Pathologic Basis of Veterinary Disease*, edited by James F Zachary, 471-560. St. Louis, Missouri: Elsevier.

MacDonald, D. W., R. G. Christian, and G. A. Chalmers. 1973. "Infectious thromboembolic meningoencephalitis: literature review and occurrence in Alberta, 1969-71." *Canadian Veterinary Journal* 14 (3): 57-61.

Magalhães, Layane Queiroz, Anderson Lopes Baptista, Pedro de Almeida Fonseca, Guilherme Lobato Menezes, Geison Morel Nogueira, Selwyn Arlington Headley, Juliana Torres Tomazi Fritzen, Amauri Alcindo Alfieri, and João Paulo Elsen Saut. 2017. "Use of metaphylactic protocols based on the risk to develop bovine respiratory diseases in feedlot cattle." *Ciência Rural* 47 (8). https://doi.org/https://doi.org/ 10.1590/0103-8478cr20161110. http://www.scielo.br/scielo.php?script=sci_arttext &pid=S0103-84782017000800454&nrm=iso.

Margineda, Carlos A., Donal O'Toole, Mónica Prieto, Francisco A. Uzal, and Gustavo C. Zielinski. 2019. "*Histophilus somni* myocarditis and leptomeningitis in feedlot cattle: case report and occurrence in South America." *Journal of Veterinary Diagnostic Investigation* 31 (6): 893-898. https://doi.org/10.1177/1040638719876302.

Moreira, A. R., H. R. Terzolo, E. Odriozola, A. G. Salamanco, A. P. Casaro, and J. Arnaude. 1987. "Bronconeumonía bovina asociada a *Haemophilus somnus* [*Bronchopneumonia asociated with* Haennphilus somnus]." *Revista de Medicina Veterinaria* 68: 36-38.

O'Toole, D., and K. S. Sondgeroth. 2016. "Histophilosis as a natural disease." *Current Topics in Microbiology and Immunology* 396: 15-48. https://doi.org/10.1007/82_ 2015_5008.

O'Toole, D., R. Hunter, T. Allen, B. Zekarias, J. Lehmann, K. S. Kim, D. Grab, and L. B. Corbeil. 2017. "Effect of *Histophilus somni* on heart and brain microvascular endothelial cells." *Veterinary Pathology* 54 (4): 629-639. https://doi.org/10.1177/ 0300985817691581. https://dx.doi.org/10.1177/0300985817691581.

Oliveira, Thalita Evani Silva, Gabriela Sanches Scuisato, Isadora Fernanda Pelaquim, Cristina Wetzel Cunha, Lucas Santana Cunha, Eduardo Furtado Flores, Lucienne Garcia Pretto-Giordano, Júlio Augusto Naylor Lisbôa, Amauri Alcindo Alfieri, João Paulo Elsen Saut, Paulo Henrique Jorge Cunha, and Selwyn Arlington Headley. 2021. "The participation of a virus within the malignant catarrhal fever virus group and *Mycoplasma bovis* in the development of single and mixed infections in beef and dairy cattle with bovine respiratory disease." *Frontiers in Veterinary Science* doi: 10.3389/fvets.2021.691448.

Oliveira, Victor H. S., Alais M. Dall Agnol, Juliana T. T. Fritzen, Elis Lorenzetti, Amauri A. Alfieri, and Alice F. Alfieri. 2020. "Microbial diversity involved in the etiology of a bovine respiratory disease outbreak in a dairy calf rearing unit." *Comparative Immunology, Microbiology and Infectious Diseases* 71: 101494-101494. https://doi. org/10.1016/j.cimid.2020.101494. https://pubmed.ncbi.nlm.nih.gov/32434101.

Palomares, G., F. Aguilar, L. Hernández, J. Acosta, E. Herrera, and V. Tenorio. 2005. "Isolation and characterization of *Histophilus somni* (*Haemophilus somnus*) in semen samples of rams with epididymitis." *Small Ruminant Research* 60 (3): 221-225. https://doi.org/http://dx.doi.org/10.1016/j.smallrumres.2004.12.010.

Panciera, R. J., R. R. Dahlgren, and H. B. Rinker. 1968. "Observations on septicemia of cattle caused by a *Haemophilus*-like organism." *Pathologia Veterinaria* 5 (3): 212-6. https://doi.org/10.1177/030098586800500303.

Pérez, D. S., F. A. Pérez, and G. Bretschneider. 2010. "*Histophilus somni*: pathogenecity in cattle an update." *Anales de Veterinaria de Murcia* 26: 5-21.

Perez-Romero, N., F. Aguilar-Romero, B. Arellano-Reynoso, E. Diaz-Aparicio, and R. Hernandez-Castro. 2011. "Isolation of *Histophilus somni* from the nasal exudates of a clinically healthy adult goat." *Tropical animal health and production* 43 (5): 901-3. https://doi.org/10.1007/s11250-011-9792-6.

Philbey, A. W., J. R. Glastonbury, J. T. Rothwell, I. J. Links, and J. E. Searson. 1991. "Meningoencephalitis and other conditions associated with *Histophilus ovis* infection in sheep." *Australian Veterinary Journal* 68 (12): 387-90.

Queiroz, Gustavo R., Rodrigo A. M. de Oliveira, Karina K. M. C. Flaiban, Giovana W. Di Santis, Ana Paula F. R. L. Bracarense, Selwyn A. Headley, Amauri A. Alfieri, and Júlio A. N. Lisbôa. 2018. "Diagnóstico diferencial das doenças neurológicas dos bovinos no estado do Paraná [*Differential diagnosis of neurologic diseases of cattle in the state of Paraná*]." *Pesquisa Veterinária Brasileira* 38: 1264-1277. http://www.scielo.br/scielo.php?script=sci_arttext&pid=S0100-736X2018000701264&nrm=iso.

Rizzo, H., L. Gregory, A. F. Carvalho, and E. S. Pinheiro. 2012. "*Histophilus somni* isolation on sheep with endometritis first case report on Brazil." *Revista Brasileira de Reprodução Animal* 36 (2): 136-138.

Romero, A., C. Quinteros, P. Marinho, D. O'Tool, and F. Dutra. 2013. "Thrombotic meningoencephalitis (TME) by *Histophilus somni* in sheep in Uruguay." *Veterinaria (Montevideo)* 49 (191): 38-47.

Romero, Agustín, Carolina Briano, Marcelo Pereira, and Fernando Dutra. 2020. "Síndrome de Leptomeningitis/Ventriculitis/Coroiditis (*Histophilus somni*) en bovinos: descripción de tres focos en el Este del Uruguay [*Leptomeningitis Ventriculitis/ Choroiditis Syndrome (*Histophilus somni*) in cattle: description of three outbreaks in Eastern Uruguay*]." *Veterinaria (Montevideo)* 56. http://www.scielo.edu.uy/scielo.php?script=sci_arttext&pid=S1688-48092020000201504&nrm=iso.

Sanches, Adrien Wilhelm Dilger, Ingeborg Maria Langohr, Adriana Lücke Stigger, and Claudio S. L. Barros. 2000. "Doenças do sistema nervoso central em bovinos no Sul do Brasil [*Diseases of the central nervous system in cattle of southern Brazil*]." *Pesquisa Veterinária Brasileira* 20 (3): 113-118.

Saunders, J. R., and E. D. Janzen. 1980. "*Haemophilus somnus* infections. II. A Canadian field trial of a commercial bacterin: clinical and serological results." *Canadian Veterinary Journal* 21 (8): 219-24.

Scarcelli, Eliana, Margareth Élide Genovez, Maristela Vasconcellos Cardoso, Fabíola Ribeiro Campos, Simone Miyashiro, Rosa Maria Piatti, Solange Rosa Teixeira, Eliana Stefano, Líria Hiromi Okuda, and Edwiges Maristela Pituco. 2004. "Abortamento e morte embrionária em receptoras bovinas por *Histophilus somni* (*Haemophilus somnus*) [*Abortion and embryonic death in bovine recipients due to* Histophilus somni (Haemophilus somnus)]." *Acta Scientiae Veterinariae* 32 (1): 59-64.

Smith, B. P., and E. L. Biberstein. 1977. "Septicemia and meningoencephalitis in pastured cattle caused by a *Haemophilus*-like organism ("*Haemophilus somnus*")." *Cornell Veterinarian* 67 (2): 300-5.

Snowder, G. D., L. D. Van Vleck, L. V. Cundiff, and G. L. Bennett. 2006. "Bovine respiratory disease in feedlot cattle: environmental, genetic, and economic factors." *Journal of Animal Science* 84 (8): 1999-2008. https://doi.org/10.2527/jas.2006-046.

Taylor, J. D., R. W. Fulton, T. W. Lehenbauer, D. L. Step, and A. W. Confer. 2010. "The epidemiology of bovine respiratory disease: What is the evidence for predisposing factors?" *Canadian Veterinary Journal* 51 (10): 1095-102.

Tegtmeier, C., A. Uttenthal, N. F. Friis, N. E. Jensen, and H. E. Jensen. 1999. "Pathological and microbiological studies on pneumonic lungs from Danish calves." *Journal of Veterinary Medicine. Series B* 46 (10): 693-700. http://www.ncbi.nlm.nih.gov/pubmed/10676147.

Terra, Juliano P., Guilherme R. Blume, Rogério E. Rabelo, Jussara T. Medeiros, Caio G. N. Rocha, Imara N. Chagas, Marília S. Aguiar, and Fabiano J. F. Sant'Ana. 2018. "Neurological diseases of cattle in the state of Goiás, Brazil (2010-2017)." *Pesquisa Veterinária Brasileira* 38 (9): 1752-1760.

USDA. 2011. *Cattle and Calves Nonpredator Death Loss in the United States 2010.* USDA-APHIS-VS-CEAH (Fort Collins, CO).

Van Donkersgoed, J., E. D. Janzen, and R. J. Harland. 1990. "Epidemiological features of calf mortality due to hemophilosis in a large feedlot." *Canadian Veterinary Journal* 31 (12): 821-825. https://pubmed.ncbi.nlm.nih.gov/17423705.

Van Dreumel, A. A., R. A. Curtis, and H. L. Ruhnke. 1970. "Infectious thromboembolic meningoencephalitis in Ontario feedlot cattle." *Canadian Veterinary Journal* 11 (7): 125-30.

Ward, A. C., N. W. Dyer, and L. B. Corbeil. 1999. "Characterization of putative *Haemophilus somnus* isolates from tonsils of American bison (*Bison bison*)." *Can J Vet Res* 63 (3): 166-9. http://www.ncbi.nlm.nih.gov/pubmed/10480457.

Wessels, J., and M. E. Wessels. 2005. "*Histophilus somni* myocarditis in a beef rearing calf in the United Kingdom." *Veterinary Record* 157 (14): 420-1.

Zhang, M., J. E. Hill, D. L. Godson, M. Ngeleka, C. Fernando, and Y. Huang. 2020. "The pulmonary virome, bacteriological and histopathological findings in bovine respiratory disease from western Canada." *Transboundary and Emerging Diseases* 67 (2): 924-934. https://doi.org/10.1111/tbed.13419.

Chapter 3

Swine Dysentery Caused by *Brachyspira hyodysenteriae* Infection

Amanda Gabrielle de Souza Daniel
Jose Paulo Hiroji Sato
and Roberto Maurício Carvalho Guedes*
School of Veterinary Medicine,
Federal University of Minas Gerais,
Belo Horizonte, Minas Ferausm, Brazil

Introduction

Enteric diseases affect pigs between neonatal and finishing stages and remain one of the biggest efficiency and profitability limiting factor of swine production worldwide (Thomson et al., 2019). These diseases are not only a welfare issue but also economically significant problem demonstrated by increase of feed conversion rate, costs with antimicrobial treatment and mortality (Stanton, 2006).

The genus *Brachyspira* is among the main bacterial agents causing diarrhea in growing and finishing pigs. Swine dysentery (SD), caused by *B. hyodysenteriae*, has a worldwide distribution in regions with highest density of production systems. The morbidity and mortality in herds is 90% and 50%, respectively (Hampson, 2012), however subclinical infections have also been reported (La et al., 2016).

Mucohemorrhagic diarrhea, occasionally with fibrin, associated with anorexia and the occurrence of mortalities few days after the onset of clinical

* Corresponding Author's Email: guedes@vet.ufmg.br.

In: Infectious and Parasitic Diseases of Animals in Developing Countries
Editor: Selwyn Arlington Headley
ISBN: 979-8-88697-504-8

signs in untreated animals are the most important clinical signals (Guedes, 2005). In Recently years, two new species of *Brachyspira* were characterized in the world also as primary agents of SD (Chander et al., 2012; Rasback et al., 2007).

Swine dysentery pathogenesis is complex and poorly understood, mainly due to multifactorial characteristics, such as virulence factors including chemotaxis, motility, adherence, hemolysin production and endotoxic lipooligosaccharide (LOS) activity (Guedes & Barcellos, 2012; Hampson et al., 2010).

Clinical data, macroscopic, and histological findings are important for directing the diagnosis of diseases caused by *Brachyspira* spp. (Barcellos et al., 2000). Swine dysentery is controlled by antimicrobial therapy associated with an eradication program, health monitoring, and management of infected farms (Hampson et al., 1997). Vaccines are other important control alternative, but effective commercial vaccines that work against diverse strains in diverse geographic regions are unfortunately not available for swine dysentery (Hampson & Burrough, 2019).

This article summarizes the available knowledge about swine dysentery and review aspects of DS transmission, diagnosis and control of diseases caused by *Brachyspira hyodysenteriae* in swine.

Brachyspira spp.

The genus *Brachyspira* is composed of anaerobic intestinal spirochetes that colonize the large intestine. In pigs, the main pathogenic species are *B. hyodysenteriae*, *B. pilosicoli* and *B. hampsonii* (Stanton et al., 1997; Taylor & Trott, 1997; Hampson et al., 2010; Chander et al., 2012).

In addition, the species *B. intermedia*, *B. innocens*, *B. murdochii*, *B. suanatina*, *B. alvinipulli* and *B. aalborgi* colonize the gastrointestinal tract of animals and humans. Some of them colonize the pig intestine except *B. alvinipulli* and *B. aalborgi* (Stanton, 2006; Rasback et al., 2007). Table 1 presents hemolysis characteristics, biochemical reactions, and sugars fermentation features of the main *Brachyspira* spp. found in swine.

B. pilosicoli is an important pathogen that colonize many species such as swine, birds, dogs, and humans. In swine, it is the etiologic agent of spirochetal colitis, characterized by increase of conversion rate, growth delay, moderate colitis, and diarrhea, mainly in growing and finishing pigs (Hampson et al.,

2010). *B. intermedia*, *B. innocens* and *B. murdochii* were associated with mild and sporadic diarrhea in pigs (Hampson & Burrough, 2019).

Table 1. Differentiation of *Brachyspira* species that infect swine by hemolysis patterns on blood-supplemented trypticase soy agar (TSA), biochemical reactions and sugars fermentation features (Adapted from Hampson, 2012 and Chander et al. al., 2012)

Species	Hemolysis	Indole	Hippurate	API-ZYM[d]	D-ribose
B. hyodysenteriae	Strong	+[a]	-	1	-
B. intermedia	Weak	+	-	1	-
B. innocens	Weak	-	-	2	-
B. murdochii	Weak	-	-	3	-
B. pilosicoli	Weak	+[a]	+[c]	4	+
B. suanatina	Strong	+[b]	-	5	-
B. hampsonii	Strong	-	-	3	

[a] Indole-negative isolates of *B. hyodysenteriae* and indole-positive strains of *B. pilosicoli* are described.
[b] Weak indole positive.
[c] Hippurate-negative isolates of *B. pilosicoli* are described.
[d] Reactions in commercial API-ZYM test:
1, alpha-glucosidase positive, alpha-galactosidase negative.
2, alpha-glucosidase positive or negative, alpha-galactosidase positive.
3, alpha-glucosidase negative, alpha-galactosidase negative.
4, variable reactions, including positive reactions for both enzymes, beta-glucosidase negative.
5, alpha-galactosidase negative, beta-glucosidase positive.
+, Positive reaction; -, negative reaction.

Etiology

Swine dysentery was first reported in 1920s (Whiting, 1937), but the causative agent was identified in 1971 as *Treponema hyodysenteriae*, now classified as *Brachyspira hyodysenteriae* (Taylor & Alexander, 1971; Harris, 1972; Ochiai et al., 1997).

B. hyodysenteriae is a Gram-negative anaerobic bacterium, motile, spiral morphology, 6-8.5 µm in length and 320-380 nm in diameter (Fellstrom et al., 1997; Hampson et al., 2010). It is the most common agent of swine dysentery, characterized by severe mucohemorrhagic diarrhea in growing and finishing pigs (Taylor & Alexander, 1971; Taylor et al., 1980; Hampson et al., 2010).

In addition to *B. hyodysenteriae*, in recent years, two new species of *Brachyspira* were described and characterized as primary agents of SD. *B. suanatina* was isolated from swine and wild ducks, with indistinguishable phenotypic and clinical characteristics as observed in *B. hyodysenteriae*, but genetically distinct. This specie has a smaller geographic distribution, with reports so far only in Sweden and Denmark (Råsbäck et al., 2007; Mushtaq et al., 2015).

In 2012, the spirochete named *B. hampsonii*, with strong hemolysis on blood agar and high pathogenicity, was initially described in North America and outbreaks of clinical disease identical to SD caused by *B. hyodysenteriae* has been detected in herds of United States of America, Canada, Belgium, Germany, and the Czech Republic (Chander et al., 2012; Harding et al., 2012; Mahu et al., 2014; Rohde et al., 2014). Experimental inoculations in pigs with this new species have been performed and clinical signs and lesions were identical to *B. hyodysenteriae* infection (Rubin et al., 2013; Costa et al., 2014). Initially, this species was divided into clades I and II (Chander et al., 2012). However, in more recent genetic analyses, using the genome typing of this species, classification into genomovars I, II and III was performed (Mirajkar et al., 2016).

Epidemiology

Transmission can occur by contact with fomites and mechanical vectors that are contaminated with feces of infected pigs. Fomites from transportation trucks, swine worker boots and clothing are important ways of transmission (Alvarez-Ordonez et al., 2013; Robertson et al., 1992). Further, infection and outbreaks can also occur due to introduction of infected or asymptomatic carrier pigs in a susceptible herd (La et al., 2016; Songer and Harris, 1978).

Swine dysentery is reported worldwide with 90% morbidity and 50% mortality in herds (Hampson, 2012). Subclinical infections have also been reported in some herds (La et al., 2016). Pigs of all ages are susceptible to infection by *B. hyodysenteriae*, but infection is more common in growing and finishing pigs (Hampson et al., 2012).

B. hyodysenteriae colonizes pigs (including the wild boar) and occasionally some bird species (Hampson & Burrough, 2019). Pathogenic *Brachyspira* sp. have been isolated from rodents (Backhans et al., 2013, 2011), domestic avian species (Feberwee et al., 2008; Glávits et al., 2011) and wild birds (Martinez-Lobo et al., 2013; Rubin et al., 2013b).

B. hampsonii and *B. suanatina* were isolated from swine and wild birds. The dissemination by biological vectors such as wild birds over long distances are extremely important. Strains of *B. hampsonii* obtained from different continents had homology in samples isolated from swine and migratory birds (Råsbäck et al., 2007; Martínez-Lobo et al., 2013; Mahu et al., 2014; Mushtaq et al., 2015; Mirajkar et al., 2015; Aller-Morán et al., 2016).

Swine dysentery has a worldwide distribution in regions with the highest density of pig farms (Muniappa et al., 1997; Boyc et al., 1998; Thomson et al., 1998; Calderaro et al., 2001). This disease was absent in North American swine herds for 20 years, however, since 2008, several cases have been reported in the United States, Canada (Chander et al., 2012), as well as European (Dors et al., 2015; Löbert et al., 2016) and Asian (Kajiwara et al., 2016) continents. In Brazil, the disease was described in the 1980s and 1990s, in sporadic reports (Barcellos et al., 2000). After 2010, there have been outbreaks in several Brazilian states located in regions with significant pig production (Daniel & Guedes, 2015; Daniel et al., 2017).

The Brazilian outbreaks were described in several states, including as Minas Gerais, Mato Grosso, São Paulo, Paraná, and Santa Catarina, but the epidemiological correlation among them was not confirmed (Daniel et al., 2013). However, in 2012, several outbreaks of SD were reported in piglet production units (PPUs) of different large integrator companies in many regions of the country, particularly in Southern Brazil (Daniel & Guedes, 2015). In subsequent years, most of these companies carried out eradication programs by partial depopulation and medication, eliminating the disease in almost all farms. However, some foci in western Santa Catarina and Paraná, São Paulo, Minas Gerais, and Mato Grosso do Sul remain, mainly in farrow-to-finish farms or rearing and finishing units (personal information, Roberto Guedes).

This recent re-emergence of SD could be associated with individual or combined factors related to the increased virulence of some strains, decreased antimicrobial susceptibility and emergence of new genotypes. Consequently, it is important to identify genotypic and phenotypic characteristics of these emerging pathogens and to develop diagnostic tests and potential vaccines to control this disease.

Brachyspira spp. Typification and Molecular Epidemiology

Identification and anatomopathological characterization are essential for controlling and understanding the dynamics of infectious diseases (MacCannell, 2013). Assessing the relationships between isolates by ancestry is important to determine the origin, possible routes of transmission, confirm outbreaks, assess cross-infection between associated pathogens, recognize particularly virulent strains, and evaluate the effectiveness of control measures (Tenover et al., 1997; MacCannell, 2013).

For *Brachyspira* genus, there are some techniques used for typing, including comparative methods of banding patterns and DNA sequencing (Li et al., 2009a). Restriction endonuclease analysis (REA: Restriction endonuclease analysis), random amplified DNA polymorphism (RAPD - Random Amplified Polymorphic DNA), pulsed-field gel electrophoresis (PFGE: Pulsed-field Gel Electrophoresis), restriction fragment length polymorphism (RFLP) and multilocus enzyme electrophoresis (MLEE) have already been described (Combs et al., 1992; Lee et al., 1993; Harel et al., 1994; Dugourd et al., 1996; Trott et al., 1996; Fisher et al., 1997; Hidalgo et al., 2010). The genetic relationships among the recognized *Brachyspira* spp., based on their 16S rRNA gene sequences, are shown in Figure 1.

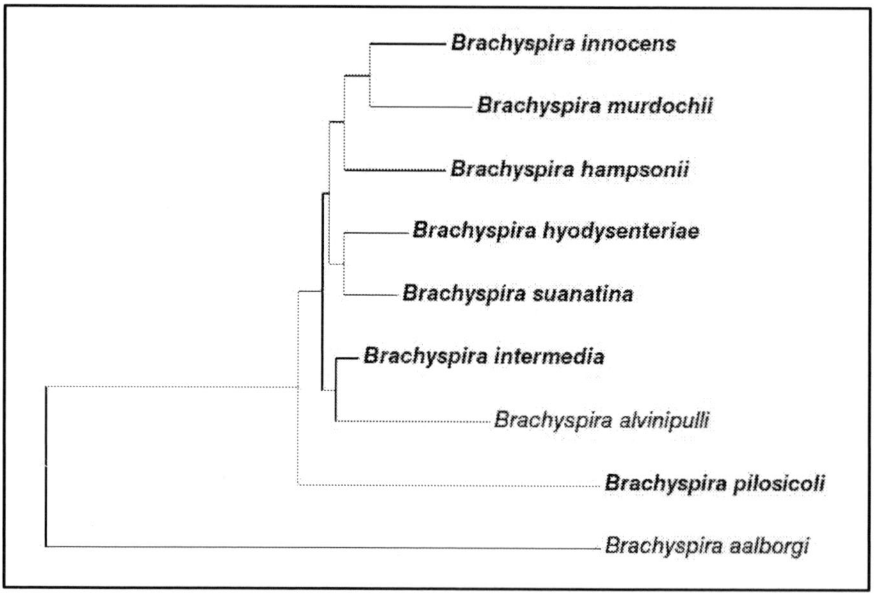

Figure 1. Relationships between the nine officially named *Brachyspira* species based on the 16S rRNA gene sequences of the type strains. The seven species that are known to colonize pigs are marked in bold. (David Hampson and Tom La in Hampson & Burrough, 2019).

Characterization of multilocus analysis of variable number tandem repeats (MLVA), multilocus sequence typing (MLST) and whole genome sequencing were also described for *Brachypira* spp (Råsbäck et al., 2007; Bellgard et al., 2009; La et al., 2009; Hidalgo et al., 2010; Phillips et al., 2010; Osorio et al., 2012; Neo et al., 2013; Mirajkar & Gebhart, 2014). MLST is the standard approach for similarity and ancestry analysis between *Brachyspira* strains (Råsbäck et al., 2007; Phillips et al., 2010; Neo et al., 2013, Mirajkar and Gebhart, 2014). This method analyzes allelic variation of specific genes, and it is used for epidemiological studies of numerous infectious agents (Urwin & Maiden, 2003).

The MLST has been used in local and global molecular epidemiological studies of *Brachyspira* spp. (Råsbäck et al., 2007), including *B. hyodysenteriae* (La et al., 2009; Osorio et al., 2012; Mirajkar & Gebhart, 2014), *B. pilosicoli* (Neo et al., 2013), *B. intermedia* (Phillips et al., 2010), *B. murdochii*, *B. innocens* (Osorio et al., 2013) and *B. hampsonii* (Mirajkar et al., 2015).

The MLST analysis using seven housekeeping genes (*adh*, *alp*, *est*, *gdh*, *glpK*, *pgm* and *thi*) in 46 Brazilian *Brachyspira hyodysenteriae* strains isolated from outbreaks of SD that occurred between 2011 – 2015 and historical isolates obtained in 1998 (Sato et al., 2022), demonstrated an independent international profile of the global sequences deposited in the *B. hyodysenteriae* database. The results indicated genetic relationships among the *B. hyodysenteriae* from different Brazilian states, among historical strains isolated in 1998 and from recent outbreaks, and relatedness with global isolates. The minimum spanning tree analysis of Brazilian isolates and the global database demonstrated the genetic close relation between Brazilian isolates and strains isolated from Italy, Canada, Australia, and the United States of America.

Pathogenesis

The pathogenesis of SD is complex and poorly understood, mainly because the infection is multifactorial (Guedes & Barcellos, 2012). The virulence factors described for *B. hyodysenteriae* include chemotaxis, motility, adherence, hemolysin production and endotoxic lipooligosaccharide (LOS) activity and are important to understand the pathogenesis of this bacteria (Hampson et al., 2010).

Infection occurs by ingestion of feces and contact with contaminated material. The mucus associated to dysenteric feces protects the agent from stomach acidity and oxygen toxicity (Guedes & Barcellos, 2012).

The chemotaxis by mucin is an important virulence factor (Milner & Sellwood, 1994). Using the bacterial whole genome information, several genes associated with chemotaxis and motility were identified (Bellgard et al., 2009; Quintana-Hayashi et al., 2015). The bacterium influences enterocytes cytoskeleton, increasing the number of goblet cells, and in consequence, increases mucus secretion associated to high expression of the MUC2 and MUC5AC genes (Quintana-Hayashi et al., 2015; Enns et al., 2019). Mucus is important for bacterial colonization because facilitates their motility and penetration into the intestinal crypts (Quintana-Hayashi et al., 2015; Enns et al. al., 2019). Thus, once established, the bacteria colonize the cecum and colon, at the base of the Liberkuhn crypts, invading goblet cells where there is multiplication and stimulation of mucus production.

Brachyspira spp. motility is provided through the activity of periplasmic flagella (Hampson et al., 2010) and the importance of motility was demonstrated by experimentally synthesized *flaA* and *flaB* genes mutants. These mutants had reduced motility and decrease the colonization of the microorganism (Kennedy et al., 1997).

The NADH oxidase activity is important for mucosal surface colonization, since the enzyme consumes oxygen, reduces potential toxicity (Hampson et al., 2010). NADH oxidase negative mutants have been shown reduced ability to colonize swine (Stanton et al., 1999).

Hemolysis is considered one of the main virulence factors (Hsu et al., 2001) and the phenotypic laboratory characteristic is often used to determine the pathogenic potential of isolates (Burrough et al., 2012b). Bellgard et al. (2009) sequenced the genome of *B. hyodysenteriae* and identified seven potential hemolysin genes, including four previously described. Some genes were reported *in vivo* experiments using mice and swine (ter Huurne et al., 1992; Hyatt et al., 1994). However, despite the studies described above, the pathogenic activity of each hemolysin has not yet been elucidated (Burrough, 2016).

The bacteria can be observed at lamina propria in affected areas. Lipoolygosaccharides (LOS) is an important virulence factor related to protein bacterial surface, which have similar properties to the lipopolysaccharides (LPS) (Guedes & Barcellos, 2012; Hampson, 2012). These toxic substances apparently break cell junctions (Guedes & Barcellos, 2012), forming lesions in the intestinal epithelium, enhancing colonization (Hampson et al., 2010; Hampson & Burrough, 2019).

There is an increase of mucus, associated to inflammatory process with leukocyte infiltration and severe local circulatory changes, mesocolon edema, hemorrhage, and superficial necrosis with fibrin (Guedes & Barcellos, 2012). Electrolytes malabsoprtion is one of mechanism of diarrhea (Hampson et al., 2010). Inflammation foci can persist for 40 to 50 days after clinical recovery and the mucosa remains infected (Guedes & Barcellos, 2012). Spirochetes are found in feces between one and four days before started diarrhea (Kinyon et al., 1977).

The SD diarrhea is consequence of malabsorption while effusive diarrhea is due to inflammation of the lamina propria, lymphangiectasis, increased vascular permeability, edema, loss of enteric plasma proteins, fibrin exudation, and hemorrhage (Argenzio et al., 1980; Enns et al., 2019; Zlotowski et al., 2008). Chronic lesions result in lower serum bicarbonate concentrations and increase of plasma potassium levels, which can lead to metabolic acidosis and hyperkalemia (Argenzio, et al., 1980; Hampson, 2012).

There are several studies describing low pathogenic strains of *B. hyodysenteriae* which can colonize but do not induce clinical disease (Lysons et al., 1982; Lee et al., 1993; Thomson et al., 2001). Daniel et al. (2017) described the first Brazilian low pathogenic *B. hyodysenteriae* strains, which showed characteristic strong beta hemolysis on blood agar and positive PCR for *B. hyodysenteriae,* isolated from animals without apparent macroscopic lesions or clinical presentation suggestive of SD.

Clinical and Pathological Aspects

SD is characterized by mucohemorrhagic fibrinous diarrhea associated to anorexia and death in untreated animals (Guedes, 2005). The incubation period for SD varies between 2 days to 3 months, but the disease usually occurs within 10 to 14 days in naturally infected animals (Hampson & Burrough, 2019). The clinical signs include soft, yellowish feces, anorexia, fever, dehydration, metabolic acidosis, and hyperkalemia (Hampson, 2012).

Macro and microscopic lesions of SD are restricted to the large intestine. Macroscopically, mucohemorrhagic or fibrinohemorrhagic enteritis and foci of superficial necrosis are observed, forming a pseudomembrane. Marked mucosal hyperemia, mesocolon edema, reactive and enlarged mesenteric lymph nodes are observed in the acute phase (Hampson et al., 2012). Microscopic lesions include mucosal and submucosal thickening due to vascular congestion and fluid leakage, goblet cell hyperplasia, loss cohesion cell junctions, hemorrhage, lamina propria marked to neutrophilic inflammatory infiltrate, associated with necrosis and detachment of the epithelium. Spirochetes can be seen attached to the surface of the lumen and within the disrupted epithelial cells (Hampson & Burrough, 2019).

Diagnosis

Swine dysentery cases must be differentiated from other enteric diseases of growing and finishing pigs (Thomson et al., 1998). The differential diagnosis includes proliferative enteropathy, salmonellosis, and *Trichuris* sp. infections (Hampson, 2012). Differential diagnosis of mild SD from porcine intestinal spirochetosis requires laboratory confirmation.

Clinical data, macroscopic changes and histological findings are important for suggesting the diagnosis of diseases caused by *Brachyspira* spp. (Barcellos et al., 2000).

Isolation compared to other detection techniques is considered the gold standard for *B. hyodysenteriae* diagnosis (Råsbäck et al., 2006). However, bacteria of the genus *Brachyspira* have fastidious growth at 37° – 42°C, need selective media and anaerobic incubation (Lemcke et al., 1979). In general, colonies can be visualized after 72 hours, but in certain cases, incubation for up to 10 days on selective media may be necessary (Duhamel & Joens, 1994).

The observation of *Brachyspira* spp. in histological section can be performed by the Warthin Starry staining, immunohistochemistry and/or fluorescent *in situ* hybridization (FISH). The Warthin Starry staining is a technique that allows the visualization of the morphology of the bacteria. Immunohistochemistry allows the detection of the genus *Brachyspira*, without differentiating between pathogenic and non-pathogenic species (Paulovich et al., 2004; Hampson et al., 2012). The FISH technique is an effective alternative for specific and conclusive detection in histological sections using specific probes labeled with fluorochrome to identify different species of *Brachyspira* (Jensen et al., 1998 and 2000).

Techniques based on nucleic acid analysis have facilitated and dynamized the diagnosis of *Brachyspira* spp. infections, especially in *ante-mortem* diagnosis. Polymerase chain reaction (PCR) specific for segments of 16S or 23S of ribosomal RNA genes (16S rRNA and 23S rRNA) and NAD oxidase (*Nox*) has been widely used in the diagnosis of SD (Elder et al., 1994; La et al. al., 2006; Phillips et al., 2009). Stanton & Sellwood (1999), sequencing the *Nox* gene from strains of *B. hyodysenteriae* from different hosts and different geographic locations, found identical highly conservation among *Brachyspira* species.

The matrix-assisted laser desorption ionization time-of-flight mass spectrometry (MALDI-TOF MS) is described as a useful tool for the identification of several bacterial species, including *Brachyspira* spp. (Calderaro et al., 2013).

Bacterial isolation and biochemical tests are the routine procedure, often confirmed by molecular tests such as PCR (Lee et al., 1993; Fellstrom et al., 1997). These techniques form a reliable combination clinical and subclinical for diagnostic (Råsbäck et al., 2007; La et al., 2016ab).

Serological tests were performed to identify herds with SD, but there are no commercial kits that can be used. Based on lipooligosaccharides (LOS), *B. hyodysenteriae* has 11 serotypes widely distributed in different geographic regions. Genetic variation and marked differences in antigenic proteins are significant limitations for development of a globally applicable serological test (Herbst et al., 2017). Some studies using recombinant proteins have been carried out to develop a serological test that would be an important tool for detecting *B. hyodysenteriae* positive herds without clinical signs of SD (Song et al., 2015; Hampson et al., 2016).

Treatment and Control

The treatment and control of swine dysentery is usually based on antimicrobials, which can be added to the feed or water (Hampson & Burrough, 2019). The most used drugs are the pleuromutilins (tiamulin and valnemulin) (Novotna and Skardova, 2002). In general, Brachyspira species showed high susceptibility to tiamulin, valnemulin, with heterogeneous susceptibility to doxycycline and low susceptibility to lincomycin and tylosin being observed (Mirajkar et al., 2016; Daniel et al., 2017).

SD is generally controlled by antimicrobial therapy associated with an eradication program, health monitoring and management of infected farms (Hampson et al., 1997). The complete elimination is a challenge mainly due the intermittent shedding associated to asymptomatic animals. The recurrence of outbreaks is frequent, as a result, the best alternative for eliminating the disease is based on eradication program development with total and partial depopulation associated with disinfection, use of antimicrobials during the process and changes in management (Neirynck et al., 2020; Speiser et al., 2011). It is recommended to conduct eradication programs during the summer when the environmental bacterial resistance is reduced. In addition, rodent and insect control are essential. After the eradication program it is important to sample a large number of pigs in susceptible age groups on repeated occasions, combined with the analysis of pooled samples through bacterial isolation, biochemical tests and PCR for monitoring during six months until confirmation that the program was successful (Fellstrom et al., 2001; Neirynck et al., 2020).

Other important control alternative would be the use of vaccines. However, effective commercial vaccines that work against diverse strains in diverse geographic regions are unfortunately not available for SD (Hampson, 2012).

There are currently 11 recognized serotypes of *B. hyodysenteriae* and the problems related to this are difficulties in designing a vaccine able to induce cross-protection against a range of serotypes. In contrast, when pigs have been vaccinated and challenged with homologous serotypes the vaccine was highly effective (Olson, 1974; Joens et al., 1979; Fernie et al., 1983; Diego et al., 1995; Waters et al., 1999ab). One alternative is the use of autogenous or multivalent bacterins, but *B. hyodysenteriae* bacterins are difficult to produce in large-scale as this microorganism is a fastidious to grow.

Several attempts have been made to use live attenuated or genetically modified avirulent vaccines for SD (Hudson et al., 1976; Hyatt et al., 1994; Rosey et al., 1996; Kennedy et al., 1997; Stanton et al., 1999). This approach has the disadvantage that modified strains show reduced immune stimulation due to decrease of colonization.

The use of recombinant vaccines is attractive, and many studies tried to identify immunogenic proteins (Chatfield et al., 1988; Joens et al., 1993), but to date the reported use of a recombinant protein as a vaccine failed to prevent colonization in pigs (Gabe et al., 1995; La et al., 2004; Song et al., 2009).

One research evaluating exoproteins in *B. hyodysenteriae* detected 42 of 307 surface proteins commonly observed in *B. hyodysenteriae* strains, including McpA, McpC and Vsp. Vsp is considered the most frequently expressed protein by *B. hyodysenteriae* (Witchell et al., 2011; Casas et., 2016). These newly detected proteins are an important device for obtaining new recombinant proteins.

Antimicrobial Resistance

Antimicrobials have been used in animal production since the 1960s. The exhaustive use, combined to underdosage, induced an increased antimicrobial resistance for many bacterial strains. It is believed that alternatives such as surveillance and diagnosis in animal production can reduce the pressure of selection for resistant isolates and the incidence of resistance genes.

Emergence of antimicrobial resistant *B. hyodysenteriae* strains has been reported across Europe, Asia and Australia (Buller and Hampson, 1994; Hidalgo et al., 2009; Karlsson et al., 2001; Lobová et al., 2004; Novotná and Škardová, 2002; Ohya and Sueyoshi, 2010; Rohde et al., 2004; Uezato et al., 2004). Multidrug-resistant isolates have been described for macrolides, lincosamides, pleuromutilins, doxycycline, chloramphenicol and florfenicol (Molnar 1996; Karlsson et al., 2002, 2003, 2004; Lobova et al., 2004; Pringle et al., 2004; Rohde et al., 2004; Pringle et al., 2007; Duinhof et al., 2008; Hidalgo et al., 2011; Verlinden et al., 2011; Sperling et al., 2011; Pringle et al., 2012; van Duijkeren et al., 2014; Hillen et al. 2014; Rugna et al., 2015; Mirajkar et al., 2016; Daniel et al., 2017).

Resistance have been demonstrated for commonly used antimicrobials such as macrolides (Karlsson et al., 1999), lincosamides (Karlsson et al., 1999), doxycycline (Pringle et al., 2007) and tiamulin (Hidalgo et al., 2011; Pringle et al., 2004). For this reason, in recent decades, countries and international organizations in the United States and the European Union have initiated policies to control and regulate the use of antimicrobials as growth promoters and prophylactics (USA FDA, 2012; 2013; 2019; Union, 2019). Initially, the European Union controlled the commercialization of these products, demanding that they could only be sold under the prescription of a veterinarian (Union, 2003). The same events began in other countries around the world, such as the United States, which since 2015 have required the control of medicated animal feed through prescriptions from registered and accredited veterinarians. In Brazil, the control and use of antimicrobials is subject to approval by the Ministério da Agricultura, Pecuária e Abastecimento (MAPA), which regulates this use through normative instructions (IN). The INs 65/2006 and 14/2016 are related to medicated feed usage control, which addresses the measures necessary for the manufacture of these feeds, employing actions aimed mainly at identifying these feeds and applying cleaning programs to avoid contamination of non-medicated feed (Brasil, 2006 2016a). Other measures adopted by MAPA include banning the use of colistin sulfate as a growth promoter throughout the national territory (Brasil, 2016b), as well as erythromycin and spiramycin (BRASIL, 2012).

This fact demonstrates the need for new alternatives for the prevention and control of the disease on farms, in addition to the great international pressure to reduce the use of antimicrobials in animal production (Mahu, et al., 2017).

Additives

Among the alternatives for antimicrobials, we can highlight the use of probiotics, prebiotics, organic acids, and essential oils. These alternative compounds have a widespread use in animal feed for their role as antibacterial, antiviral, antifungal, antioxidant, digestive stimulant, immunomodulator (Dhama et al., 2014; Filazi and Yurdakok-Dikmen, 2019; Mazzeranghi et al., 2017; Yadav et al., 2016).

A recently used alternative for SD control has been essential oils. Nutraceuticals are functional food that improve health by changing the nutritional, immunological and physiological parameters of the host with modulation of the intestinal microbiota (Al-Khalaifah, 2018, Cencic and Chingwaru, 2010, Dhama et al., 2008). Essential oils are believed to cause a change in bacterial cell membrane permeability, which in turn would alter several cellular activities, including energy production and transport, cytoplasmic protein assembly, and other regulatory functions (Swamy et al., 2016). In addition, essential oils could chelate metals, reducing their availability for bacterial growth, inhibit bacterial enzymes and the uptake and use of glucose as a means of obtaining energy, biofilm formation, capsule production or even acting synergistically with antimicrobials and other essential oils. There are some studies evaluating nutraceutical responses but more "*in vivo* efficacy" studies are necessary (Gill &; Holley, 2004; Upadhyay et al., 2014; Omonijo et al., 2018).

Conclusion

Swine dysentery is a reemerging disease in Brazil and an endemic infectious disease in many swine farming countries with limited control by the lack of effective vaccines and the emergence of strains of *B. hyodysenteriae* with reduced susceptibility to common antimicrobials.

Despite the great impact of SD, much remains unknown about the virulence traits of its etiologic agent and the modes of disease transmission. Carrying out studies that predict the functions of different genes and macromolecules in the "genomic era" will allow the identification of new virulence factors and regulatory systems important for host colonization by *B. hyodysenteriae*.

SD eradication programs have traditionally been based on the use of antimicrobials associated proper cleaning and disinfection, followed by down time and health monitoring in farms with adequate biosecurity conditions.

The increasing restrictions for antimicrobial usage, associated to the emergence of multiresistant strains have demonstrated the need to develop alternatives in the treatment and prevention of SD. The activity of nutraceuticals compounds also represents an attractive alternative for conventional antimicrobials.

The characterization of the *B. hyodysenteriae* strain isolated from a herd without clinical signs increased the concern related to the risk of entry of this microorganism in some farms.

Future challenge studies using whole genome sequencing and fecal microbiome are needed to elucidate possible differences between these isolates and host response during *Brachyspira* strains colonization and lack of clinical signals.

References

Al-Khalaifah, H. S. (2018). "Benefits of probiotics and/or prebiotics for antibiotic-reduced poultry." *Poultry Science*, 97, no. 11, 3807-3815.

Aller-Morán, Luis Miguel, Francisco Javier Martínez-Lobo, Pedro Rubio, and Ana Carvajal. (2016). "Experimental infection of conventional pigs with a '*Brachyspira hampsonii*' isolate recovered from a migrating waterfowl in Spain." *The Veterinary Journal*, 214, 10-13.

Barcellos, David, E. S. N., de Uzeda, M., Mathiesen, M. R., Duhamel, G. E., and Kader, I. I. T. A. (2000). "Prevalence of Brachyspira species isolated from diarrhoeic pigs in Brazil." *Veterinary Record*, 146, no. 14, 398-403.

Bellgard, Matthew, I., Phatthanaphong Wanchanthuek, Tom La, Karon Ryan, Paula Moolhuijzen, Zayed Albertyn, Babak Shaban, Yair Motro, David S. Dunn, David Schibeci, Adam Hunter, Roberto Barrero, Nyree D. Philips, David J. Hampson. (2009). "Genome sequence of the pathogenic intestinal spirochete *Brachyspira hyodysenteriae* reveals adaptations to its lifestyle in the porcine large intestine." *PLoS One*, 4, no. 3, e4641.

Boye, M., Jensen, T. K., Møller, K., Leser, T. D., and Jorsal, S. E. (1998). "Specific detection of the genus Serpulina, Serpulina hyodysenteriae and *Serpulina pilosicoli* in porcine intestines by rRNA *in situ* hybridization." *Molec Cell Probes*, 12, 323-330.

Brasil. Ministério da Agricultura Pecuária e Abastecimento: INSTRUÇÃO NORMATIVA No 17, DE 17 de julho de 2019. *Diário Oficial da União*, (2019) [*Ministry of Agriculture, Livestock and Supply: Normative Instruction No 17, of July 17, 2019. Official Gazette of the Union (2019)*.]

Brasil. Ministério da Agricultura Pecuária e Abastecimento: INSTRUÇÃO 43 NORMATIVA No 14, DE 17 de maio de 2012. *Diário Oficial da União*, (2012) [*Ministry of Agriculture, Livestock and Supply: Normative Instruction No 43, of May 17, 2012. Oficial Gazette of the Union (2012).*]

Brasil. Ministério da Agricultura Pecuária e Abastecimento: INSTRUÇÃO NORMATIVA No 45, DE 22 de novembro de 2016. *Diário Oficial da União*, v. 229, (2016) [*Ministry of Agriculture, Livestock and Supply: Normative Instruction No 45, of November 22, 2016. Official Gazette of the Union (2016).*]

Brasil. Ministério da Agricultura Pecuária e Abastecimento: INSTRUÇÃO NORMATIVA No 65, de 21 de novembro de 2006. *Diário Oficial da União*, (2006) [*Ministry of Agriculture, Livestock and Supply: Normative Instruction No 65, of November 6, 2006. Official Gazette of the Union, v. 229 (2006).*]

Burrough, and Eric, R. (2017). "Swine dysentery: etiopathogenesis and diagnosis of a reemerging disease." *Veterinary Pathology*, 54, no. 1, 22-31.

Burrough, Eric, R., Erin L. Strait, Joann M. Kinyon, Leslie P. Bower, Darin M. Madson, Bailey L. Wilberts, Kent J. Schwartz, Timothy S. Frana, and Glenn Songer, J. (2012). "Comparative virulence of clinical *Brachyspir*a spp. isolates in inoculated pigs." *Journal of Veterinary Diagnostic Investigation*, 24, no. 6, 1025-1034.

Calderaro, A., Merialdi, G., Perini, S., Ragni, P., Guégan, R., Dettori, G., and Chezzi, C. (2001). "A novel method for isolation of *Brachyspira* (Serpulina*) hyodysenteriae* from pigs with swine dysentery in Italy." *Veterinary Microbiology*, 80, no. 1, 47-52.

Calderaro, Adriana, Giovanna Piccolo, Sara Montecchini, Mirko Buttrini, Chiara Gorrini, Sabina Rossi, Maria Cristina Arcangeletti, Flora De Conto, Maria Cristina Medici, and Carlo Chezzi. (2013). "MALDI-TOF MS analysis of human and animal Brachyspira species and benefits of database extension." *Journal of Proteomics*, 78, 273-280.

Cencic, Avrelija, and Walter Chingwaru. (2010). "The role of functional foods, nutraceuticals, and food supplements in intestinal health." *Nutrients*, 2, no. 6, 611-625.

Chander, Yogesh, Alexander Primus, Simone Oliveira, and Connie J. Gebhart. (2012). "Phenotypic and molecular characterization of a novel strongly hemolytic Brachyspira species, provisionally designated "*Brachyspira hampsonii*"." *Journal of Veterinary Diagnostic Investigation*, 24, no. 5, 903-910.

Chatfield, Steven, N., Fernie, D. S., Penn, C., and Dougan, G. (1988). "Identification of the major antigens of *Treponema hyodysenteriae* and comparison with those of *Treponema innocens*." *Infection and Immunity*, 56, no. 5, 1070-1075.

Combs, B. G., Hampson, D. J., and Harders, S. J. (1992). "Typing of Australian isolates of *Treponema hyodysenteriae* by serology and by DNA restriction endonuclease analysis." *Veterinary Microbiology*, 31, no. 2-3, 273-285.

Costa, Matheus, O., Bonnie Chaban, John C. S. Harding, and Janet E. Hill. (2014). "Characterization of the fecal microbiota of pigs before and after inoculation with "*Brachyspira hampsonii*"." *PLoS One*, 9, no. 8, e106399.

Daniel, Amanda, G. S., Guedes, and Roberto M. Carvalho. (2015). Evolution of *Brachyspira hyodysenteriae* infection in the last few years in Brazil and adopted control measures. In: *IX SINSUI - Simpósio Internacional de Suinocultura, Anais*.

Daniel, Amanda, G. S., José P. H. Sato, Michelle P. Gabardo, Talita P. Resende, David ESN de Barcellos, Carlos ER Pereira, Fábio A. Vannucci, and Roberto Guedes.

(2017). "Minimum inhibitory concentration of Brazilian *Brachyspira hyodysenteriae* strains." *Pesquisa Veterinária Brasileira*, 37, 331-338.

Daniel, Amanda, G. S., Talita P. Resende, Sato, J. P. H., and Guedes, R. M. C. (2013). "Infection by Brachyspira spp in swine in Brazil." *VIII Simpósio Internacional de Suinocultura (SINSUI), Porto Alegre, RS*, 131-140.

Dhama, K., Mahendran, M., Tomar, S., and Chauhan, R. S. (2008). "Beneficial effects of probiotics and prebiotics in livestock and poultry: the current perspectives." *Intas Polivet*, 9, no. 1, 1-12.

Dhama, Kuldeep, Sandip Chakraborty, Ruchi Tiwari, Amit Kumar Verma, Mani Saminathan, Malik YS Amarpal, Zahra Nikousefat, Moosa Javdani, and Rifat Ullah Khan. (2014). "A concept paper on novel technologies boosting production and safeguarding health of humans and animals." *Research Opinion in Animal Veteterinary Science*, 4, no. 7, 353-370.

Di Cerbo, Alessandro, and Beniamino Palmieri. (2015). "The market of probiotics." *Pakistan Journal of Pharmaceutical Sciences*, 28, no. 6.

Diego, Rafael, Ignacio Lanza, Ana Carvajal, Pedro Rubio, and Pedro Cármenes. (1995). "*Serpulina hyodysenteriae* challenge of fattening pigs vaccinated with an adjuvanted bivalent bacterin against swine dysentery." *Vaccine*, 13, no. 7, 663-667.

Dors, A., Pomorska-Mól, M., Czyżewska, E., Wasyl, D., and Pejsak, Z. (2015). "Prevalence and risk factors for *Lawsonia intracellularis, Brachyspira hyodysenteriae* and Salmonella spp. in finishing pigs in Polish farrow-to-finish swine herds." *Polish Journal of Veterinary Sciences*, 4.

Dugourd, Dominique, Mario Jacques, Michel Bigras-Poulin, and Josée Harel. (1996). "Characterization of *Serpulina hyodysenteriae* isolates of serotypes 8 and 9 by random amplification of polymorphic DNA analysis." *Veterinary Microbiology*, 48, no. 3-4, 305-314.

Duhamel, Gerald Ernest, and Lynn A. Joens. (1994). "Laboratory procedures for diagnosis of swine dysentery." *American Association of Veterinary Laboratory Diagnosticians*.

Elder, R. O., Duhamel, G. E., Schafer, R. W., Mathiesen, M. R., and Ramanathan, M. (1994). "Rapid detection of *Serpulina hyodysenteriae* in diagnostic specimens by PCR." *Journal of Clinical Microbiology*, 32, no. 6, 1497-1502.

Enns, Cole, B., John C. S. Harding, and Matthew E. Loewen. (2019). "Decreased electrogenic anionic secretory response in the porcine colon following *in vivo* challenge with *Brachyspira* spp. supports an altered mucin environment." *American Journal of Physiology-Gastrointestinal and Liver Physiology*, 316, no. 4, G495-G508.

European Commission. Council and Parliament prohibit antibiotics as growth promoters: Commissioner Byrne welcomes adoption of Regulation on feed additives. Press release IP/03/1058, 22 July 2003. http://europa.eu.int/rapid/start/cgi/ guesten.ksh?p_action.gettxt=gt&doc=IP/03/1058|0|RAPID&lg=EN&display= (Accessed Jan 5, 2022).

Fellström, Claes, Ulla Zimmerman, Anna Aspan, and Anders Gunnarsson. (2001). "The use of culture, pooled samples and PCR for identification of herds infected with *Brachyspira hyodysenteriae*." *Animal Health Research Reviews*, 2, no. 1, 37-43.

Fernie, D. S., Ripley, P. H., and Walker, P. D. (1983). "Swine dysentery: protection against experimental challenge following single dose parenteral immunisation with inactivated *Treponema hyodysenteriae*." *Research in Veterinary Science*, 35, no. 2, 217-221.

Filazi, Ayhan, and Begüm Yurdakok-Dikmen. (2019). "Nutraceuticals in poultry health and disease." In *Nutraceuticals in Veterinary Medicine*, pp. 661-672. Springer, Cham.

Fisher, Laurie, N., Michelle R. Mathiesen, and Gerald E. Duhamel. (1997). "Restriction fragment length polymorphism of the periplasmic flagellar flaA1 gene of Serpulina species." *Clinical Diagnostic Laboratory Immunology*, 4, no. 6, 681-686.

Food and Drug Association. Guidance for Industry. In: Medicine CfV, ed. *Evaluating the Safety of Antimicrobial New Animal Drugs with Regard to their Microbiological Effects on Bacteria of Human Health Concern*. Rockville, MD: US Food and Drug Administration; (2003): 1– 35.

Gill Alexander, O., and Richard A. Holley. (2004). "Mechanisms of bactericidal action of cinnamaldehyde against Listeria monocytogenes and of eugenol against L. monocytogenes and Lactobacillus sakei." *Applied and Environmental Microbiology*, 70, no. 10, 5750-5755.

Guedes, R. M. C. (2005). Diarrhea in growing-finishing pigs: main diseases. *Suíno & cia*, v. 11, 11-18.

Guedes, R. M. C. and Barcellos, D. (2012). Spiroquetal colitis. In: SobestianskY, J.; Barcellos, D.E.S.N. (Eds.). *Diseases of Swine*. 2.ed., Goiânia: Cânone editorial, p. 128-134.

Guedes, R. M. C., and Daniel, A. G. S. (2013). Outbreak of swine dysentery (SD) in pig herds in south Brazil. *Spirochaete conference Proceedings*., University of Surrey, Guildford, UK, 37.

Gyles, Carlton, L., John F. Prescott, Glenn Songer, J., and Charles O. Thoen, eds. *Pathogenesis of Bacterial Infections in Animals*., John Wiley & Sons, 2008.

Hampson, and David, J. (2012). "Brachyspiral colitis." *Diseases of Swine*, 10, 680-696.

Hampson, David, J., and Eric R. Burrough. (2019). "Swine dysentery and Brachyspiral colitis." *Diseases of Swine*, 951-970.

Hampson, David, J., Nagaraja, T. G., Kennan, R. M., and Julian I. Rood. (2010). "Gram-negative anaerobes." *Pathogenesis of Bacterial Infections in Animals*, 373.

Hampson, David, J., Tom La, Nyree D. Phillips, and Patricia K. Holyoake. (2016). "*Brachyspira hyodysenteriae* isolated from apparently healthy pig herds following an evaluation of a prototype commercial serological ELISA." *Veterinary Microbiology*, 191, 15-19.4.

Harding, J., Fernando, C., Rubin, J., and Hill, J. (2012). "Swine dysentery and other emerging Brachyspiras." *Advances in Pork Production*, 127-132.

Harel, Josee, Myriam Belanger, Celine Forget, and Mario Jacques. (1994). "Characterization of *Serpulina hyodysenteriae* isolates of serotypes 8 and 9 from Quebec by restriction endonuclease fingerprinting and ribotyping." *Canadian Journal of Veterinary Research*, 58, no. 4, 302.

Harris, D. L. (1972). "Swine dysentery. I. Inoculation of pigs with *Treponema hyodysenteriae* (new species) and reproduction of the disease." *Vet. Med. Small. Anim. Clin.*, 67, 61-64.

Herbst, Werner, Simone Schneider, Georg Baljer, and Stefanie A. Barth. (2017). "An update of *Brachyspira hyodysenteriae* serotyping." *Research in Veterinary Science*, 111, 135-139.

Hidalgo, A., Carvajal, A., Pringle, M., Rubio, P., and Fellström, C. (2010). "Characterization and epidemiological relationships of Spanish *Brachyspira hyodysenteriae* field isolates." *Epidemiology & Infection*, 138, no. 1, 76-85.

Hsu, Tsungda, David L. Hutto, Chris Minion, F., Richard L. Zuerner, and Michael, J. Wannemuehler. (2001). "Cloning of a beta-hemolysin gene of *Brachyspira* (Serpulina) *hyodysenteriae* and its expression in *Escherichia coli.*" *Infection and Immunity*, 69, no. 2, 706-711.

Hudson, M. J., Alexander, T. J., Lysons, R. J., and Prescott, J. F. (1976). "Swine dysentery: protection of pigs by oral and parenteral immunisation with attenuated *Treponema hyodysenteriae.*" *Research in Veterinary Science*, 21, no. 3, 366-367.

Hyatt, Doreene, R., Ter Huurne, A. A., Van Der Zeijst, B. A., and Lynn A. Joens. (1994). "Reduced virulence of *Serpulina hyodysenteriae* hemolysin-negative mutants in pigs and their potential to protect pigs against challenge with a virulent strain." *Infection and Immunity*, 62, no. 6, 2244-2248.

Jensen, T. K., Mette Boye, Møller, K., Leser, T. D., and Jorsal, S. E. (1998). "Association of *Serpulina hyodysenteriae* with the colonic mucosa in experimental swine dysentery studied by fluorescent *in situ* hybridization." *Apmis*, 106, no. 7-12, 1061-1068.

Jensen, Tim Kåre, Kristian Møller, Mette Boye, Thomas D. Leser, and Jorsal, S. E. (2000). "Scanning electron microscopy and fluorescent *in situ* hybridization of experimental *Brachyspira* (Serpulina) *pilosicoli* infection in growing pigs." *Veterinary Pathology*, 37, no. 1, 22-32.

Joens, L. A., Harris, D. L., and Baum, D. H. (1979). "Immunity to Swine dysentery in recovered pigs." *American Journal of Veterinary Research*, 40, no. 10, 1352-1354.

Joens, Lynn, A., Rodolfo Marquez, and Mitchell Halter. (1993). "Comparison of outer-membrane fractions of *Serpulina* (Treponema) *hyodysenteriae.*" *Veterinary Microbiology*, 35, no. 1-2, 119-132.

Kajiwara, Keita, Midori Kozawa, Takuya Kanazawa, Kouji Uetsuka, Hiromi Nakajima, and Yoshikazu Adachi. (2015). "Drug-susceptibility of isolates of *Brachyspira hyodysenteriae* isolated from colonic mucosal specimens of pigs collected from slaughterhouses in Japan in 2009." *Journal of Veterinary Medical Science*, 15-0608.

Karlsson, M., Aspán, A., Landén, A., and Franklin, A. (2003). "Further characterization of porcine *Brachyspira hyodysenteriae* isolates with decreased susceptibility to tiamulin." *Journal of Medical Microbiology*, 53, no. 4, 281-285.

Karlsson, Märit, Claes Fellström, Malin UK Heldtander, Karl-Erik Johansson, and Anders Franklin. (1999). "Genetic basis of macrolide and lincosamide resistance in *Brachyspira* (Serpulina) *hyodysenteriae.*" *FEMS Microbiology Letters*, 172, no. 2, 255-260.

Kennedy, Michael, J., Everett L. Rosey, and Robert J. Yancey Jr. (1997). "Characterization of flaA− and flaB− mutants of *Serpulina hyodysenteriae*: both flagellin subunits, FlaA and FlaB, are necessary for full motility and intestinal colonization." *FEMS Microbiology Letters*, 153, no. 1, 119-128.

Kinyon, Joann, M., Harris, D. L., and Glock, R. D. (1977). "Enteropathogenicity of various isolates of *Treponema hyodysenteriae*." *Infection and Immunity*, 15, no. 2, 638-646.

La, T., Collins, A. M., Phillips, Oksa, A., and Hampson, D. J. (2006). "Development of a multiplex-PCR for rapid detection of the enteric pathogens *Lawsonia intracellularis*, *Brachyspira hyodysenteriae*, and *Brachyspira pilosicoli* in porcine faeces." *Letters in Applied Microbiology*, 42, no. 3, 284-288.

La, Tom, Judith Rohde, Nyree Dale Phillips, and David J. Hampson. (2016b). "Comparison of *Brachyspira hyodysenteriae* isolates recovered from pigs in apparently healthy multiplier herds with isolates from herds with swine dysentery." *PLoS One*, 11, no. 8, e0160362.

La, Tom, Nyree D. Phillips, and David J. Hampson. (2016a). "An investigation into the etiological agents of swine dysentery in Australian pig herds." *PLoS One*, 11, no. 12, e0167424.

Lee, J. I., Hampson, D. J., Combs, B. G., and Lymbery, A. J. (1993). "Genetic relationships between isolates of *Serpulina* (Treponema) *hyodysenteriae*, and comparison of methods for their subspecific differentiation." *Veterinary Microbiology*, 34, no. 1, 35-46.

Lemcke, R. M., and Burrows, M. R. (1979). "A disc growth-inhibition test for differentiating *Treponema hyodysenteriae* from other intestinal spirochaetes." *The Veterinary Record*, 104, no. 24, 548-551.

Li, Wenjun, Didier Raoult, and Pierre-Edouard Fournier. (2009). "Bacterial strain typing in the genomic era." *FEMS Microbiology Reviews*, 33, no. 5, 892-916.

Löbert, S., Werner Zimmermann, Sibylle Bürki, Joachim Frey, Heiko Nathues, Scheer, P., Doherr, M. G., Ueli Stalder, and Friederike Zeeh. (2016). "Occurrence of *Brachyspira hyodysenteriae* in multiplier pig herds in Switzerland." *Tierärztliche Praxis Ausgabe G: Großtiere/Nutztiere*, 44, no. 01, 13-18.

Lysons, R. J., Lemcke, R. M., Bew, J., Burrows, M. R., and Alexander, T. J. L. (1982). "An avirulent strain of *Treponema hyodysenteriae* isolated from herds free of swine dysentery." In *Proceedings of the 7th International Pig Veterinary Society Congress*, vol. 1982, p. 40.

MacCannell, Duncan. (2013). "Bacterial strain typing." *Clinics in Laboratory Medicine*, 33, no. 3, 629-650.

Mahu, Maxime, Ellen de Jong, Nele De Pauw, Lien Vande Maele, Virginie Vandenbroucke, Tamara Vandersmissen, Miry, Cora, Pasmans, F., Haesebrouck, F., Martel, A., and Boyen, F. (2014). "First isolation of' *Brachyspira hampsonii*' from pigs in Europe." *Veterinary Record*, 174, no. 2.

Mahu, Maxime, Frank Pasmans, Katleen Vranckx, Nele De Pauw, L. Vande Maele, Philip Vyt, Tamara Vandersmissen, An Martel, Freddy Haesebrouck, and Filip Boyen. (2017). "Presence and mechanisms of acquired antimicrobial resistance in Belgian *Brachyspira hyodysenteriae* isolates belonging to different clonal complexes." *Veterinary Microbiology*, 207, 125-132.

Martínez-Lobo, Francisco Javier, Álvaro Hidalgo, Marta García, Héctor Argüello, Germán Naharro, Ana Carvajal, and Pedro Rubio. (2013). "First identification of "*Brachyspira hampsonii*" in wild European waterfowl." *PLoS One*, 8, no. 12, e82626.

Mazzeranghi, F., Zanotti, C., Di Cerbo, A., Verstegen, J. P., Coccoa, R., Guidetti, G., and Canello, S. (2017). "Clinical efficacy of nutraceutical diet for cats with clinical signs of cutaneus adverse food reaction (CAFR)." *Polish Journal of Veterinary Sciences*, 20, no. 2.

Mirajkar, Nandita, S., and Connie, J. Gebhart. (2014). "Understanding the molecular epidemiology and global relationships of *Brachyspira hyodysenteriae* from swine herds in the United States: a multi-locus sequence typing approach." *PLoS One*, 9, no. 9, e107176.

Mirajkar, Nandita, S., Aschalew Z. Bekele, Yogesh Y. Chander, and Connie J. Gebhart. (2015). "Molecular epidemiology of novel pathogen "*Brachyspira hampsonii*" reveals relationships between diverse genetic groups, regions, host species, and other pathogenic and commensal Brachyspira species." *Journal of Clinical Microbiology*, 53, no. 9, 2908-2918.

Mirajkar, Nandita, S., Nyree D. Phillips, Tom La, David J. Hampson, and Connie J. Gebhart. (2016). "Characterization and recognition of *Brachyspira hampsonii* sp. nov., a novel intestinal spirochete that is pathogenic to pigs." *Journal of Clinical Microbiology*, 54, no. 12, 2942-2949.

Molnar, L. (1996). "Sensitivity of strains of *Serpulina hyodysenteriae* isolated in Hungary to chemotherapeutic drugs." *Veterinary Record*, 138, no. 7, 158-160.

Muniappa, Nagaraja, Michelle R. Mathiesen, and Gerald E. Duhamel. (1997). "Laboratory identification and enteropathogenicity testing of *Serpulina pilosicoli* associated with porcine colonic spirochetosis." *Journal of Veterinary Diagnostic Investigation*, 9, no. 2, 165-171.

Mushtaq, Mamoona, Saima Zubair, Therese Råsbäck, Erik Bongcam-Rudloff, and Désirée S. Jansson. (2015). "*Brachyspira suanatina* sp. nov., an enteropathogenic intestinal spirochaete isolated from pigs and mallards: genomic and phenotypic characteristics." *BMC Microbiology*, 15, no. 1, 1-13.

Neirynck, Willem, Filip Boyen, Ilias Chantziaras, Tamara Vandersmissen, Philip Vyt, Freddy Haesebrouck, Jeroen Dewulf, and Dominiek Maes. (2020). "Implementation and evaluation of different eradication strategies for *Brachyspira hyodysenteriae*." *Porcine Health Management*, 6, no. 1, 1-11.

Neo, Eugene, Tom La, Nyree Dale Phillips, Mohammad Yousef Alikani, and David J. Hampson. (2013). "The pathogenic intestinal spirochaete *Brachyspira pilosicoli* forms a diverse recombinant species demonstrating some local clustering of related strains and potential for zoonotic spread." *Gut Pathogens*, 5, no. 1, 1-8.

Ohya, T., and Sueyoshi, M. (2010). *In vitro* antimicrobial susceptibility of *Brachyspira hyodysenteriae* strains isolated in Japan from 1985 to 2009. *Journal of Veterinary Medical Science*, pp. 1007300298-1007300298.

Olson, L. D. (1974). "Clinical and pathological observations on the experimental passage of swine dysentery." *Canadian Journal of Comparative Medicine*, 38, no. 1, 7.

Omonijo, Faith, A., Liju Ni, Joshua Gong, Qi Wang, Ludovic Lahaye, and Chengbo Yang. (2018). "Essential oils as alternatives to antibiotics in swine production." *Animal Nutrition*, 4, no. 2, 126-136.

Osorio, J., Carvajal, A., Naharro, G., Rubio, P., La, T., Phillips, N. D., and Hampson, D. J. (2013). "Identification of weakly haemolytic Brachyspira isolates recovered from pigs with diarrhoea in Spain and Portugal and comparison with results from other countries." *Research in Veterinary Science*, 95, no. 3, 861-869.

Osorio, Jesús, Ana Carvajal, Germán Naharro, Tom La, Nyree D. Phillips, Pedro Rubio, and David J. Hampson. (2012). "Dissemination of clonal groups of *Brachyspira hyodysenteriae* amongst pig farms in Spain, and their relationships to isolates from other countries." *PLoS One*, 7, no. 6, e39082.

Paulovich, Fabiana Beatriz, Sandra Maria Borowski, David Driemeier, Luis Eduardo Razia, Tania Allen Coutinho, Aline Beatriz Heinen Prates, Caroline Pescador, André Correa, and David Emilio SN de Barcellos. (2004). "Avaliação da patogenicidade de amostras de *Brachyspira pilosicoli* através de técnicas histopatológicas convencionais e por imuno-histoquímica [*Evaluation of the pathogenicity of* Brachyspira pilosicoli *samples by conventional histopathological techniques and by immuno-histochemistry*]." *Pesquisa Veterinária Brasileira*, 24, no. 3, 144-148.

Phillips, Nyree, D., Tom La, Peter J. Adams, Belinda L. Harland, Stanley G. Fenwick, and David J. Hampson. (2009). "Detection of *Brachyspira hyodysenteriae*, *Lawsonia intracellularis* and *Brachyspira pilosicoli* in feral pigs." *Veterinary Microbiology*, 134, no. 3-4, 294-299.

Quintana-Hayashi, Macarena, P., Maxime Mahu, Nele De Pauw, Filip Boyen, Frank Pasmans, An Martel, Pushpa Premaratne, Fernandez, Harvey R, Teymournejad, Omid, Maele, Lien Vande, Haesebrouck, Freddy, Linden, and Sara K. (2015). "The levels of *Brachyspira hyodysenteriae* binding to porcine colonic mucins differ between individuals, and binding is increased to mucins from infected pigs with de novo MUC5AC synthesis." *Infection and Immunity*, 83, no. 4, 1610-1619.

Råsbäck, T., Fellström, C., Gunnarsson, A., and Aspán, A. (2006). Comparison of culture and biochemical tests with PCR for detection of *Brachyspira hyodysenteriae* and *Brachyspira pilosicoli*. *Journal of Microbiological Methods*, 66(2), pp. 347-353.

Rohde, Judith, Kerstin Habighorst-Blome, and Frauke Seehusen. (2014). """*Brachyspira hampsonii*" clade I isolated from Belgian pigs imported to Germany." *Veterinary Microbiology*, 168, no. 2-4, 432-435.

Rubin, Joseph, E., Matheus O. Costa, Janet E. Hill, Heather E. Kittrell, Champika Fernando, Yanyun Huang, Brendan O'Connor, and John C. S. Harding. (2013). "Reproduction of mucohaemorrhagic diarrhea and colitis indistinguishable from swine dysentery following experimental inoculation with "*Brachyspira hampsonii*" strain 30446." *PloS one*, 8, no. 2, e57146.

Song, Yong, and David J. Hampson. (2009). "Development of a multiplex qPCR for detection and quantitation of pathogenic intestinal spirochaetes in the faeces of pigs and chickens." *Veterinary Microbiology*, 137, no. 1-2, 129-136.

Song, Yong, Tom La, Nyree D. Phillips, and David J. Hampson. (2015). "Development of a serological ELISA using a recombinant protein to identify pig herds infected with *Brachyspira hyodysenteriae*." *The Veterinary Journal*, 206, no. 3, 365-370.

Speiser, S. A., Friederike Zeeh, Goy, N., Albini, S., Werner Zimmermann, and Luginbühl, A. (2011). "Swine dysentery eradication in a grower-finisher farm in Switzerland." *Schweizer Archiv fur*, 153, no. 1, 14-18.

Stanton, T. B. (1997). "Physiology of ruminal and intestinal spirochaetes."

Stanton, T. B. (2006). "The genus Brachyspira. Falkow S Rosenberg SE Schleifer KH Stackebrant E The Prokaryotes (Volume 7)."

Stanton, Thad, B., and Richard Sellwood. (1999). "Cloning and characteristics of a gene encoding NADH oxidase, a major mechanism for oxygen metabolism by the anaerobic spirochete, Brachyspira (Serpulina) hyodysenteriae." *Anaerobe*, 5, no. 5, 539-546.

Stanton, Thad, B., Everett L. Rosey, Michael J. Kennedy, Neil S. Jensen, and Brad, T. (1999). Bosworth. "Isolation, oxygen sensitivity, and virulence of NADH oxidase mutants of the anaerobic spirochete *Brachyspira* (Serpulina) *hyodysenteriae*, etiologic agent of swine dysentery." *Applied and Environmental Microbiology*, 65, no. 11, 5028-5034.

Swamy, Mallappa Kumara, Mohd Sayeed Akhtar, and Uma Rani Sinniah. (2016). "Antimicrobial properties of plant essential oils against human pathogens and their mode of action: an updated review." *Evidence-based complementary and alternative medicine*.

Taylor, D. J. (1997). "Porcine intestinal spirochaetosis and spirochaetal colitis." *Intestinal Spirochetes in Domestic Animals and Humans*, 211-242.

Taylor, D. J., and Alexander, T. J. L. (1971). "The production of dysentery in swine by feeding cultures containing a spirochaete." *British Veterinary Journal*, 127, no. 11, lviii-lxi.

Taylor, D. J., Simmons, J. R., and Laird, H. M. (1980). "Production of diarrhoea and dysentery in pigs by feeding pure cultures of a spirochaete differing from *Treponema hyodysenteriae*." *The Veterinary Record*, 106, no. 15, 326-332.

Tenover, Fred, C., Robert D. Arbeit, and Richard V. Goering. (1997). "How to select and interpret molecular strain typing methods for epidemiological studies of bacterial infections a review for healthcare epidemiologists." *Infection Control & Hospital Epidemiology*, 18, no. 6, 426-439.

ter Huurne, Agnes A. H. M., Marina van Houten, Susie Muir, Johannes G. Kusters, Bernard AM van der Zeijst, and Wim Gaastra. (1992). "Inactivation of a *Serpula* (Treponema) *hyodysenteriae* hemolysin gene by homologous recombination: importance of this hemolysin in pathogenesis of *S. hyodysenteriae* in mice." *FEMS Microbiology Letters*, 92, no. 1, 109-113.

Thomson, J. R., Smith, W. J., Murray, B. P., Murray, D., Dic, J. E., and Sumption, K. J. (2001). "Porcine enteric spirochete infections in the UK: surveillance data and preliminary investigation of atypical isolates." *Animal Health Research Reviews*, 2, no. 1, 31-36.

Thomson, Jill, R., and Robert M. Friendship. (2019). "Digestive system." *Diseases of Swine*, 234-263.

Trott, D. J., Atyeo, R. F., Lee, J. I., Swayne, D. A., Stoutenbgurg, J. W., and Hampson, D. J. (1996). "Genetic relatedness amongst intestinal spirochaetes isolated from rate and brids." *Letters in Applied Microbiology*, 23, no. 6, 431-436.

U.S. Department of Agriculture Economic Research Service (USDA ERS). 2019. Livestock & Meat Domestic Data. https://www.ers.usda.gov/data-products/ livestock-meat-domestic-data/ (Accessed Jan 5, 2022).

U.S. Food and Drug Administration (FDA). 2012. Guidance for Industry: The Judicious Use of Medically Important Antimicrobial Drugs in Food-Producing Animals.

Department of Health and Human Services Center for Veterinary Medicine. #209. https://www.fda.gov/regulatory-information/search-fda-guidance-documents/cvm-gfi-209-judicious-use-medically-important-antimicrobial-drugs-food-producing-animals (Accessed Jan 5, 2022).

U.S. Food and Drug Administration (FDA). 2013. *Guidance for Industry: New Animal Drugs and New Animal Drug Combination Products Administered in or on Medicated Feed or Drinking Water of Food-Producing Animals: Recommendations for Drug Sponsors for Voluntarily Aligning Product Use Conditions with GFI #209*. #213. https://www.fda.gov/regulatory-information/search-fda-guidance-documents/cvm-gfi-213-newanimal-drugs-and-new-animal-drug-combination-products-administered-ormedicated-feed (Accessed Jan 5, 2022).

UNION, T. E. P. A. T. C. O. T. E. I (Legislative acts) REGULATIONS REGULATION (EU) 2019/4 OF THE EUROPEAN PARLIAMENT AND OF THE COUNCIL of 11 December 2018 on the manufacture, placing on the market and use of medicated feed, amending Regulation (EC) No 183/2005 of the European Parliament. (2019); 1-23.

Upadhyay, Abhinav, Indu Upadhyaya, Anup Kollanoor-Johny, and Kumar Venkitanarayanan. (2014). "Combating pathogenic microorganisms using plant-derived antimicrobials: a minireview of the mechanistic basis." *BioMed Research International*, 2014.

Urwin, Rachel, and Martin CJ Maiden. (2003). "Multi-locus sequence typing: a tool for global epidemiology." *Trends in Microbiology*, 11, no. 10, 479-487.

van Duijkeren, E., Greko, C., Pringle, M., Baptiste, K. E., Catry, B., Jukes, H., Moreno, M. A., Pomba, M. C., Pyörälä, S., Rantala, M., Ružauskas, M., Sanders, P., Teale, C., Threlfall, E. J., Torren-Edo, J., and Törneke, K. (2014). Pleuromutilins: use in food-producing animals in the European Union, development of resistance and impact on human and animal health. *Journal of Antimicrobial Chemotherapy*, 69, no. 8, 2022-2031.

Verlinden, Marc, Filip Boyen, Frank Pasmans, An Garmyn, Freddy Haesebrouck, and An Martel. (2011). "Antimicrobial susceptibility pattern of Brachyspira intermedia isolates from European layers." *Microbial Drug Resistance*, 17, no. 3, 485-488.

Waters, W. R., Pesch, B. A., Hontecillas, R., Sacco, R. E., Zuckermann, F. A. and Wannemuehler, M. J. (1999). Cellular immune responses of pigs induced by vaccination with either a whole cell sonicate or pepsin-digested *Brachyspira* (Serpulina) *hyodysenteriae* bacterin. *Vaccine*, 18(7-8), pp. 711-719.

Waters, W. R., Sacco, R. E., Dorn, A. D., Hontecillas, R., Zuckermann, F. A., and Wannemuehler, M. J. (1999). "Systemic and mucosal immune responses of pigs to parenteral immunization with a pepsin-digested *Serpulina hyodysenteriae* bacterin." *Veterinary Immunology and Immunopathology*, 69, no. 1, 75-87.

Yadav, Ajit Singh, Gautham Kolluri, Marappan Gopi, Kumaragurubaran Karthik, and Yashpal Singh. (2016). "Exploring alternatives to antibiotics as health promoting agents in poultry-a review." *J Exp Biol*, 4, no. 3s, 368-383.

Zlotowski, Priscila, David Driemeier, and David Emilio Santos Neves de Barcellos. (2008). "Pathogenia of swine diarrheas: models and examples." *Acta Scientiae Veterinariae*, 36, no. 1, s81-s86.

Chapter 4

Lumpy Skin Disease in the Cattle of Northern Nigeria, West Africa

Samaila Danbirni*, DVM, MSc, PhD, FCVSN

Department of Veterinary Medicine,
Ahmadu Bello University, Zaria, Nigeria

Introduction

Lumpy skin disease (LSD) is a highly infectious, viral, nodular cutaneous disease of cattle transmitted by certain arthropod vectors, such as Culicoides, Glossina, Stomoxys, etc., and an economically important transboundary disease affecting cattle of all ages (Idris, 1989; Otto et al., 2003). The disease was first reported in northern Rhodesia, now known as Zambia, in 1929 (MacDonald, 1930). The first report of this disease in Nigeria was in 1974 (Wood, 1974; Wood, 1988) with later reports by Bida et al., (1976); Nawathe et al., (1978); Nawathe et al., (1982); OIE, (2012); Adedeji et al., (2017); Danbirni et al., (2020) and Atai et al., (2021).

The disease has also been reported in other African countries such as Zambia, Kenya, and Egypt, as well as in the Middle East, in countries such as Israel and Oman (Brenner et al., 2009; Somasundaram, 2011). There are also reports of LSD sporadic outbreaks in Europe and Australia (Sevik and Dogan, 2017; Tuppurainen and Oura, 2012), where the disease was reported to have spread from Africa through the Middle East to Turkey and many other countries through mosquitoes and maintained by wildlife. This disease

* Corresponding Author's Email: sdanbirni@abu.edu.ng.

In: Infectious and Parasitic Diseases of Animals in Developing Countries
Editor: Selwyn Arlington Headley
ISBN: 979-8-88697-504-8

therefore has the potential for global emergence (Tuppurainen and Oura, 2012).

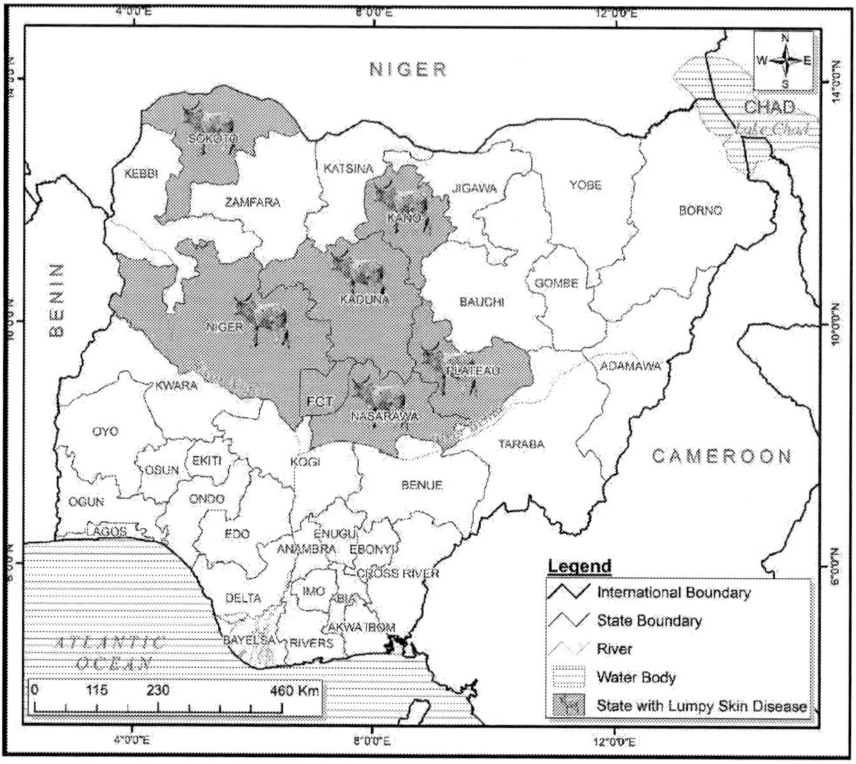

Source: Nawathe et al., (1978); Adedeji et al., (2018) and Atai et al., (2021).

Figure 1. Geographical distribution of cattle herds with Lumpy Skin Disease in Northern Nigeria from 1974 to 2021.

The morbidity of LSD in Nigeria ranged from 6.0% to 51.0% in 1974, and the states most affected were those near the river Niger, which included the Federal Capital Territory (FCT), Niger, Nasarawa, Kaduna, Plateau States, and those sharing a border with the Niger Republic (Sokoto and Kano), where the weather is wet and humid, favorable for the proliferation of the arthropod vectors of LSD, as shown in Figure 1. (Nawathe et al., 1978). However, from 2010–2021, the morbidity ranged from 5.0%–16.0% while the mortality is as low as 0.5%–5.6% in only Plateau and Nasarawa States (Adedeji et al., 2017; Adedeji et al., 2018; Atai et al., 2021) depending on the risk factors as well as the susceptibility of the host. Suspected outbreaks of LSD occur annually in

Nigeria, especially during the wet season, which corresponds to the breeding season of the arthropod vectors of the disease, but farmers are reluctant to report while laboratory diagnosis as well as assessment of its economic impacts are seldom carried out (Adedeji et al., 2017). This is probably due to the low mortality rate associated with LSD outbreaks, particularly in the local breeds of cattle (Gari et al., 2011). Another constraint with laboratory diagnosis of LSD in Nigeria is that farmers are reluctant to allow skin biopsies to be taken from their cattle because of the wound that will be created (Adedeji et al., 2017). Treatment of LSD in Nigeria is always symptomatic and often based on a tentative diagnosis.

Etiology

Lumpy skin disease is caused by a Neethling pox virus, a species of the genus Capri poxvirus in the subfamily *Chordopoxvirinae* and the family *Poxviridae*. It is a double stranded DNA containing around 150 kilobase pairs (kbp) with relatively large sizes (230–260 nm), enclosed in a lipid envelope, and it belongs to the family *Poxviridae* (Wood, 1988; Davies, 1982; Tulman et al., 2001; Buller et al., 2005; Bhanuprakash et al., 2006; Givens, 2018). The virus is closely related genetically to sheep and goat pox viruses in the genus *Capripoxvirus* (OIE, 2012). These viruses cannot be differentiated using routine serological testing and are resistant to environmental influence, surviving in desiccated crusts for up to 35 days. However, it is susceptible to ether (20%), chloroform, formalin (1%) and some detergents (sodium dodecyl sulphate), as well as phenol (2%).

Host Range

Lumpy skin disease virus affects cattle of all ages (calves and adults), breeds (local and exotic) and sexes (males and females) (Tuppurainen et al., 2011) and it has been reported that it is more severe in exotic breeds than in local breeds of cattle (Adedeji et al., 2018).

Transmission

Transmission of LSDV is primarily by mechanical means, by several probable arthropod vectors such as biting flies, mosquitoes (*Aedes aegypti*) (Chihota et al., 2001) and three tick species of the family Ixodidae, namely *Rhipicephalus appendiculatus, Rhipicephalus decoloratus* and *Amblyomma hebraeum* (Lubinga et al., 2019). These tick vectors have been shown to transmit LSDV under experimental conditions, but their capacity to transmit disease under natural field conditions is still unknown. The stable fly (*Stomoxys calcitrans*) is considered as the most probable vector for LSDV due to its abundance and association with several outbreaks (Yeruham et al., 1995). Veterinary equipment specifically needles (OIE, 2012; Carn and Kitching, 1995), has also been reported to transmit the virus. Other biting insects incriminated in the transmission of LSDV include Culicoides and Glossina, especially during their breeding season.

There is some variation in the susceptibility of the LSD virus in cattle. For instance, in Africa, imported cattle breeds from Europe or Australia have shown high susceptibility (Davies, 1991; Gari et al., 2011; Abera et al., 2015) when compared to local breeds (Adedeji et al., 2018).

Incubation Period

The incubation period varies from 2 to 4 weeks (Tuppurainen and Oura, 2012). Although the OIE report indicated that there have been no reports on the incubation period of LSDV infection under field conditions (OIE, 2018). Clinical signs can range from mild to severe. Host susceptibility, dose, and route of virus inoculation affect the severity of the disease.

Risk Factors of Lumpy Skin Disease

There are several significant factors that enhance the transmission and spread of LSDV in Nigeria, which, when well-managed, may lead to the control and possible eradication of the disease. These risk factors include management of cattle type, sex, age, mean annual rainfall, lack of vaccination, and lack of implementation of adequate government policies on animal health. Cattle maintained in fenced farms tend to show a higher risk of LSD infection than those grazed communally or in a pastoral husbandry system. In fenced farms, cattle are maintained in a confined grazing area and are potential prey for biting flies to easily bite and transmit the LSDV. The wet environment encourages farmers to adopt fenced farm management systems, thus providing a conducive environment for both higher densities of arthropod vectors as well as fenced farming practices. Female animals as well as older ones are usually kept longer by farmers for the purposes of production and replacement stock, while males are sold off at a younger age, so the effect of sex may be directly related to the duration of exposure of more females to LSDV. Calves have a lower frequency of exposure than adults, because calves are maintained in small, enclosed spaces away from biting insects and infected adults (Magori-Cohen et al., 2012; Abera et al., 2015; Molla et al., 2018).

High rainfall is associated with increased arthropod density because it corresponds to the breeding season as opposed to the dry season. The increased populations of insect vectors responsible for mechanical transmission of LSDV correspond with the detection of clinical cases of LSD in many herds (Tageldin et al., 2014). Cattle drinking from a communal water source were at a higher risk of contracting LSDV than those drinking from a non-communal water source. This is because studies have shown that animals having frequent contact with other animals at communal grazing and watering points are more at risk of acquiring LSDV than sedentary herds (Hailu et al., 2014; Gari et al., 2010).

Lumpy Skin Disease Morbidity and Mortality Pattern in Northern Nigeria from 2010 - 2021

The scanty reports of sporadic outbreaks of LSD in cattle in Nigeria do not represent the true prevalence of the disease in Nigeria, largely due to under reporting of the disease by farmers. The few reported cases of LSD outbreaks were either confirmed using histopathology, molecular (PCR) or based on the clinical signs observed in the field. For instance, Adedeji et al., (2017) reported a three-year outbreak of LSD in a farm in the Jos region of Plateau State where the morbidity and mortality rates were: 13.8% and 2.6% (2010), respectively; 14.8% and 5.3% (2013), respectively; and 11.5% and 1.5% (2014), respectively. Adedeji and his colleagues (2018) also reported similar LSD outbreaks in the Keffi region of Nasarawa State where morbidity and mortality rates of 6.25% and 2.5% (2014), respectively, as well as 5.0% and 0.5%

(2016), respectively, were observed. Atai et al., (2021) in Bokkos, Plateau State, reported a morbidity of 16.0% and a mortality of 2.0%. Based on the foregoing, all the reports occurred during the wet season and LSD seemed to be endemic in Nigeria, requiring more surveillance and reporting efforts (Figure 2).

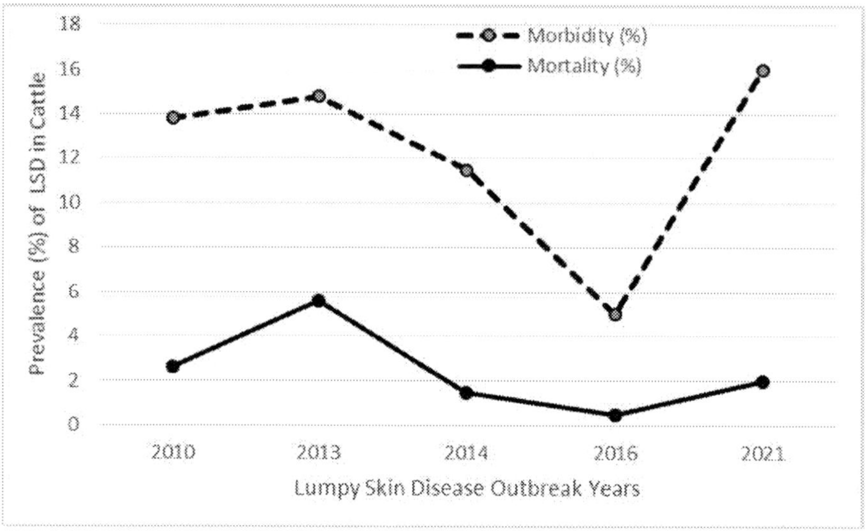

Figure 2. Lumpy skin disease morbidity and mortality pattern in northern Nigeria from 2010 – 2021 (Adedeji et al., 2018; Atai et al., 2021).

Seasonal Pattern of Lumpy Skin Disease in Northern Nigeria

The wet or rainy season in Northern Nigeria begins in the month of May, marking the end of the dry season. This early rainy season also marked the beginning of arthropod multiplication, some of which needed animal blood for their breeding (hematophagous). The insect population increases at the peak of the rainy season between August and September, when the wet season is coming to an end, and many vulnerable cattle at this time might have been infected with LSDV already through the bites of these hematophagous arthropods. This peak of the wet season corresponded with the high prevalence of LSD in cattle (Figure 2). For instance, Adedeji et al., (2018) in July and September of 2014 and 2016 respectively reported prevalence of 6.25% and 5.0%, while between October and November of 2021, Atai et al., (2021) reported a 16.0% prevalence (Figure 3).

The month of December marked the beginning of the dry season up to the end of April, corresponding with a decline in arthropod population and reported cases of LSD. However, LSD in cattle in northern Nigeria in both wet and dry seasons is underreported, hence the scanty data regarding the prevalence of LSD in northern Nigeria, where the cattle population is highest. However, it is so obvious that the LSDV infection is more prevalent due to an increase in the insect population, which peaks during the rainy season between August and September (Figure 3). The absence of cases in the months of November to April does not necessarily indicate that there was indeed no infection of LSDV but could have been a case of under reporting or/and a decrease in arthropod vector population.

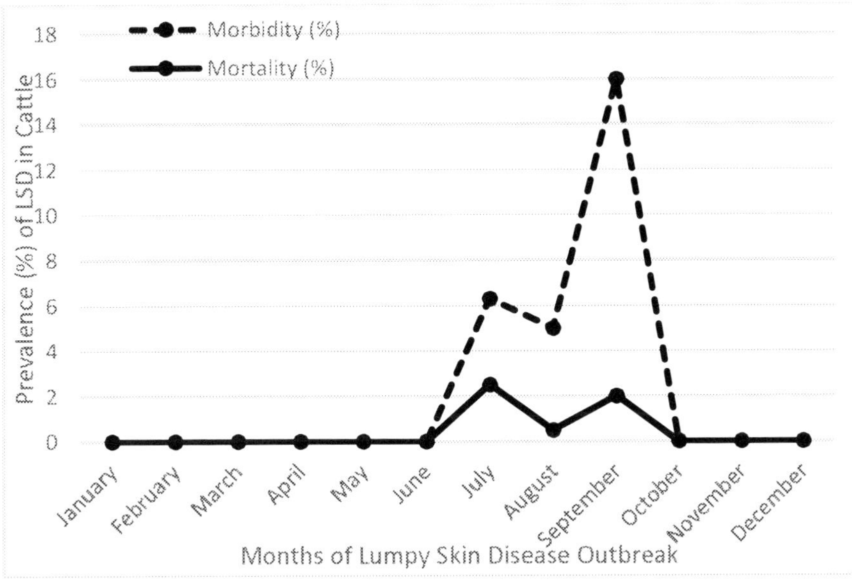

Figure 3. Seasonal pattern of lumpy skin disease in northern Nigeria from 2010 – 2021 (Adedeji et al., 2018; Atai et al., 2021).

Clinical Signs

The initial signs of LSD are pyrexia (39.9°C–41°C), lacrimation (Figure 5), nasal discharge (Figure 6), salivation, and lameness, and a week later, painful and multiple intradermal nodules of varying sizes appear (Abutarbush et al., 2013; Annandale et al., 2014; Babiuk et al., 2008; Tasioudi et al., 2016;

Adedeji et al., 2017; Danbirni et al., 2020). The characteristic nodules associated with LSD are round and firm, which may persist as hard lumps (Figure 7) or become moist, necrotic, and slough (Figure 8).

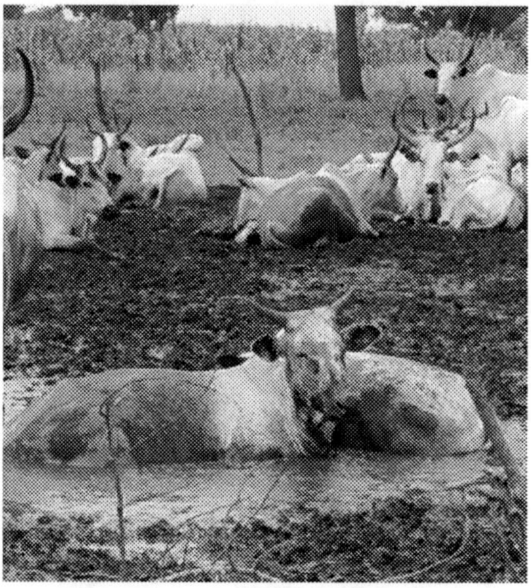

Figure 4. Cattle kept in a swampy area habited by Arthropod vectors of lumpy skin disease.

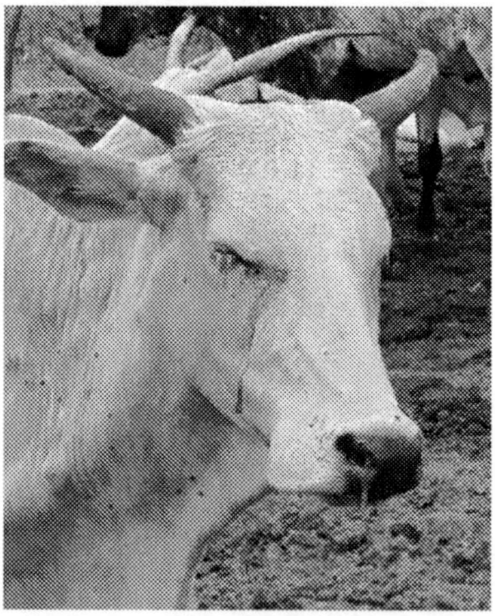

Figure 5. Bunaji cow with lumpy skin disease (cutaneous lumps, lacrimation and mucopurulent discharge).

In severe cases, lesions may appear at the nostrils and on the turbinates, causing mucopurulent nasal discharge (Figure 7) and dyspnea. Oral ulcers may result in salivation, and nodules on the conjunctiva can induce severe lacrimation (Figure 5). Lymph nodes draining the affected areas become enlarged, causing edema, and the limbs become grossly edematous due to lymphatic obstruction (Tuppurainen and Oura, 2012). Death is usually due to pneumonia or a secondary infection. Pregnant cows may abort (Radostits et al., 2006). An apparent recovery from LSD is manifested with a convalescence period of 4–12 weeks following high morbidity (up to 80%) and low case fatality (2%) in a susceptible population. Generally, the course of the disease is usually 4-5 weeks (Idris, 1989).

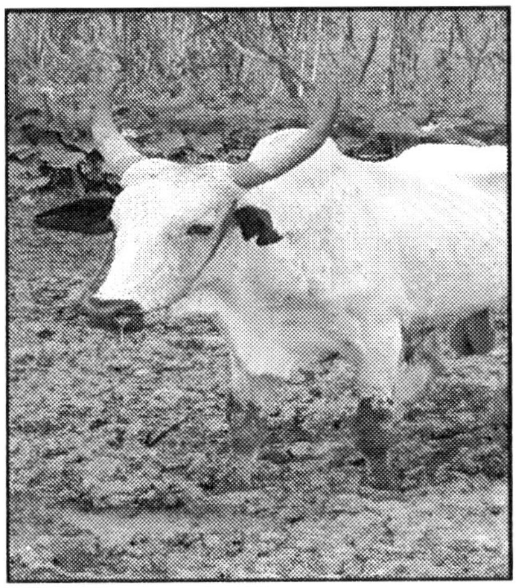

Figure 6. Bunaji draft bull with lumpy skin disease (cutaneous lumps and mucopurulent discharge).

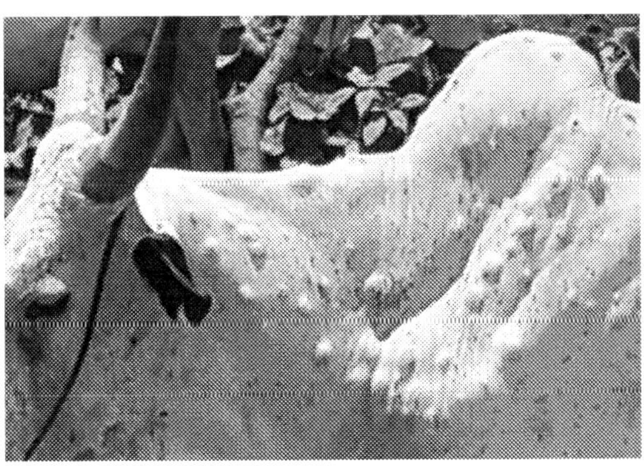

Figure 7. Bunaji draft bull with lumpy skin disease (cutaneous lumps about to rupture).

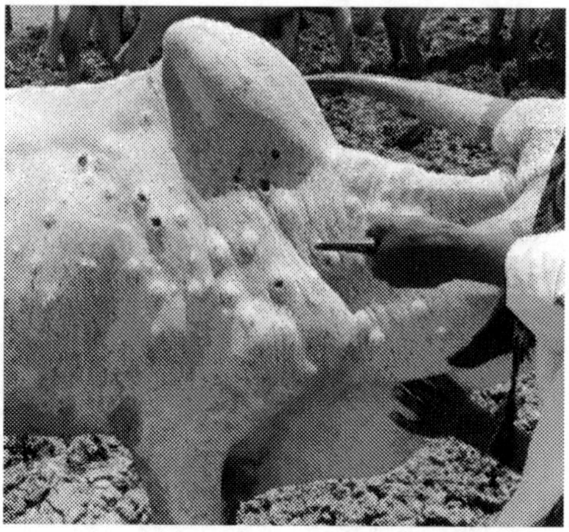

Figure 8. Bunaji draft bull with lumpy skin disease (cutaneous lumps beginning to rupture and coalesce, leaving ulcers).

Post-Mortem Lesions

Generalized lymphadenitis, nodules involving all cutaneous layers. Erosions and ulcers including those in the mouth, pharynx, trachea, bronchi, stomach, skeletal muscles, and pneumonia.

Diagnosis

Lumpy skin disease can be suspected when characteristic skin nodules transit into lumps and the manner of spread, fever, swollen lymph nodes, and edema of the limbs are observed in field cattle. Confirmation of lumpy skin disease in a new area requires virus isolation and identification from lymph nodes and skin lesions collected in 50% glycerine. Serology can be done using serum neutralization tests (SNT), immune peroxidase monolayer assays, and indirect fluorescent antibody tests, which are specific but low in sensitivity, and are costly for screening large numbers of serum samples. Furthermore, commercially available ELISAs for detecting LSD antibodies in naturally infected and vaccinated animals have recently become available.

This ELISA, ID Screen® Capripox double antigen multi-species ELISA, is able to detect antibodies against Capripox viruses including lumpy skin disease virus (LSDV), sheeppox virus and goatpox virus in serum and plasma.

It has demonstrated very high specificity (> 99.7%) and does not cross-react with parapox viruses. It also has equivalent sensitivity to IPMA (Grabels, 2018) when compared to SNT and IFAT, respectively. This ELISA is easy to perform and allows for high throughput screening without requiring high-level containment facilities (Tuppurainen, 2017). However, molecular methods such as polymerase chain reaction (PCR) have been reported to be more precise, reliable, and rapid compared with other methods (Stubbs et al., 2012). In Nigeria, two sets of published specific primers were used for the detection of LSDV genes using PCR (Adedeji et al., 2018). The primers targeted two genes [G-protein-coupled chemokine receptor (GPCR) gene and RNA polymerase subunit gene (RPO30)] of the LSDV, which are conserved regions of the LSDV and can differentiate the virus from other members of the genus *Capripox* (Lamien et al., 2011).

Differential Diagnosis

Field reports of suspected cases of LSD without laboratory confirmation are common in Nigeria. This results in limited reports about the disease because suspected cases cannot be easily confirmed to be LSD, as such cannot be reliable as LSD since it can be confused with other skin diseases such as Pseudo-lumpy skin disease (Allerton virus infection). Lesions are not granulomatous but superficial, ring-like lesions with an intact central skin area and raised edges. Urticaria – wheals without skin discontinuity and itching after contact with an insect or plant – which may suddenly disappear within hours or days when an antihistamine is used. Other differentials include demodicosis, dermatophilosis, and insect bites (Tuppuraine et al., 2017). The lesions in demodicosis are seen as tiny nodules of about 3 mm in diameter or as pustules with a cheesy white content or fluid in large abscesses. The hairs over the pustules in dermatophilosis are erected and matted in tufts, giving them a paintbrush appearance. The lesions are greasy with exudate, forming crumbly crusts of 2–5 cm in diameter that are hard to remove. The crusts later develop into scabs (Blood, 2000; Radostits et al., 2006).

Treatment

There is no known effective treatment for lumpy-skin disease. However, nonspecific treatments such as antibiotics or antimicrobial, anti-inflammatory drugs and vitamin injections are usually directed at treating the secondary bacterial infections, inflammation, fever, as well as improving the appetite of the affected cattle. Animals infected with the LSD virus generally recover. Complete recovery may take several months and may be prolonged when secondary bacterial infections are involved. It may take up to 6 months for animals that were severely affected by the LSD virus to recover fully.

Cattle that have recovered from natural infection by the LSDV have shown lifelong immunity. Calves from infected dams were reported to be resistant to clinical disease for approximately 6 months because of the acquired maternal antibodies (Tuppurainen et al., 2005). This means calves less than 6 months old should not be vaccinated against LSD, otherwise the maternal antibodies will neutralize the vaccine. Affected animals that have cleared the infection have not yet been reported to enter into a carrier state that may serve as an infection source to other members of the herd that are not infected (Tuppurainen et al., 2017).

Economic Impact of Lumpy Skin Disease

Lumpy skin disease is a reportable disease of economic importance in Nigeria (Idris, 1989). Although the mortality rate is usually low, the disease has a devastating effect on the livestock sector due to production losses resulting from severe emaciation, lowered milk production, abortion, secondary mastitis, loss of fertility, extensive damage to hides, loss of draft from lameness, and cost of supportive therapy. The disease tends to limit international trade, thereby depriving the country of its most needed foreign exchange. There have been scanty reports on the evaluation of the economic losses in naira or dollars in Nigeria. Adedeji et al., (2017) attempted to estimate the monetary value of twenty-three (23) Holstein Friesian calves that died during repeated outbreaks of LSD to be N3, 180,000 ($17,377.05), while Limon et al., (2020) estimated the losses in both the backyard herd (12) and the Transhumance herd (4) to be $2,490.04 and $2,302.09, respectively.

Prevention and Control

Control and prevention of LSD is undertaken through vaccination, quarantines, livestock movement controls, vector control, slaughter of infected and exposed animals, and cleaning and disinfection of the premises (OIE, 2012). Vaccination is considered to be the most effective method for controlling LSD in both endemic and non-endemic areas (EFSA, 2019). At present, only live vaccines are commercially available against LSDV, with different vaccines licensed for use in different countries, although the most common LSDV strain used in attenuated vaccines is the Neethling strain. This strain was highly effective in controlling LSD epidemics in the Balkans (Klement et al., 2018). In Nigeria, the LSD vaccine is commercially available and is produced and marketed by the National Veterinary Research Institute, Vom, Plateau State. However, despite vaccines being available, vaccination is usually self-funded by the farmers and is therefore based on the purchasing power of the farmers and their interest in pursuing vaccination, partly due to low mortality in the affected herds.

Another interesting reason why small-scale farmers and pastoralists are not keen on vaccinating their herds against LSD is that hides are a delicacy locally consumed as "gbomo." The consumption rate of this delicacy may probably exceed that which is exported as leather. These factors, therefore, limit the number of animals that are vaccinated, and as such, commercial farmers with large herds vaccinate their herds while small holder farmers, which constitute the vast majority of livestock holders, do not vaccinate against LSD. The Government should make LSD vaccination mandatory and consistent, as well as educate veterinarians and livestock workers on the importance of timely diagnosis of clinical cases, which will help to slow the spread of the disease (Beard, 2016).

Conclusion

Lumpy skin disease falls under category C of the National Livestock Disease Reporting System (NLDRS) in Nigeria. These are diseases of economic importance controlled, individual outbreaks of which should be reported as they occur. However, with the effect of climate changes and the raising inflation in Nigeria, more emphasis should be made towards prevention rather than control. The Government should make LSD vaccination mandatory and consistent, as well as educate veterinarians and livestock workers on the importance of timely diagnosis of clinical cases, which will help to slow the spread of the disease. In addition, the Government needs to subsidize the cost of the vaccine as well as increase surveillance of LSD and by so doing, timely diagnosis and vaccination may reduce the cost of treatment/control of LSD in Nigeria.

References

Abera Z, Degefu, H., Gari, G. and Kidane, M. 2015. Sero-prevalence of lumpy skin disease in selected districts of west Wollega zone. BMC *Veterinary Research*, 1–9.

Abutarbush, S. M., Ababneh, M. M., Al Zoubi, I. G., Al Sheyab, O. M., Al Zoubi, M. G., Alekish, M. O., and Al Gharabat, R. J. 2013. Lumpy skin disease in Jordan: Disease emergence, clinical signs, complications and preliminary-associated economic losses. *Transboundary and Emerging Diseases*, 62: 549– 554.

Adedeji, A. J., Adole, J. A., Dogonyaro, B. B., Kujul, N., Tekki, I. S., Asala, O., Chima, N. C., Dyek, Y. D., Maguda, A. S., Aba-Adulugba, E. P. 2017. Recurrent outbreaks of lumpy skin disease and its economic impact on a dairy farm in Jos, Plateau State, Nigeria. *Nigerian Veterinary Journal,* 38(2): 151-158.

Adedeji, A. J., Akanbi, O. B., Adole, J. A., Chima, N. C. and Baje, M. 2018. Outbreak of lumpy skin disease in a dairy farm in Keffi, Nasara State, Nigeria. *Sokoto Journal of Veterinary Science*, 16(3): 80-86.

Annandale, C. H., Holm, D. E., Ebersohn, K., and Venter, E. H. 2014. Seminal transmission of lumpy skin disease virus in heifers. *Transboundary and Emerging Diseases*, 61: 443– 448.

Atai, R. B., Olaolu, O. S., Adole, J. A., Haruna, I., Ijoma, S. I., Maurice, N. A., Omoniwa, D. O., Dogonyaro, B. B., and Adedeji, A. J. 2021. Epidemiological features of lumpy skin disease outbreaks amongst herds of cattle in Bokkos, north-central Nigeria. *Sokoto Journal of Veterinary Sciences,* 19(2): 81 - 88.

Babiuk, S., Bowden, T. K., Boyle, D. B., Wallace, D. B. and Kitching, R. P. 2008. Capripoxviruses: an emerging worldwide threat to sheep, Goats and Cattle. *Transboundary and Emerging Diseases*, 55(7): 263-272.

Beard, P. M. 2016. Lumpy skin disease: A direct threat to Europe. *Veterinary Record*, 178(22): 557– 558.

Bhanuprakash, V., Indrani, B. K., Hosamani, M., and Singh, R. K. 2006. The current status of sheep pox disease. *Comparative Immunology, Microbiology and Infectious Diseases*, 29: 27– 60.

Bida, S. A., Ali, I. I., Eid F. L. A and Mustapha, H. B. 1976. Lumpy skin disease outbreak in cattle of northern Nigeria. *Journal of Nigeria Veterinary Medical Association*, 5: 21-26.

Blood, D. C. (2000). *Pocket Companion to Veterinary Medicine*, 9th edi. Saunders W. B. Harcourt publishers limited, Pp. 340-342, 511.

Brenner, J., Bellaiche, M., Gross, E., Elad, D., Oved, Z., Haimovitz M., Wasserman, A., Friedgut, O., Stram, Y., Bumbarov V. and Yadin H. 2009. Appearance of skin lesions in cattle population vaccinated against lumpy skin disease: Statutory Challenge. *Vaccine*, 27: 1500-1503.

Buller, R. M., Arif, B. M., Black, D. N., Dumbell, K. R., Esposito, J. J., Lefkowitz, E. J., McFadden, G., Moss, B., Mercer, A. A., Moyer, R. W., Skinner, M. A., and Tripathy, D. N. 2005. Family Poxviridae. In C. M. Fauquet, M. A. Mayo, J. Maniloff, U. Desselberger, and L. A. Ball (Eds.), *Virus Taxonomy: Classification and Nomenclature of Viruses: Eighth Report of the International Committee on Taxonomy of Viruses,* pp. 117– 133.

Carn, V. M. and Kitching, R. P. 1995. An investigation of possible routes of transmission of lumpy skin disease virus (Neethling). *Epidemiology and Infection*, 114(1): 219–26.

Center for Food Security and Public Health, Iowa State University, 2011.

Chihota, C. M, Rennie, L. F., Kitching, R. P., Mellor, P. S. 2001. Mechanical transmission of lumpy skin disease virus by *Aedes aegypti* (Diptera: Culicidae). *Epidemiology and Infection*, 126(2): 317-321.

Danbirni, S., Kaltungo, B. Y., Ememe, M. U., Adeneike, E. A. and Sinkalu, V. O. 2020. Clinical management of a Lumpy skin disease in a Bunaji bull in Tohu village of Zaria LGA, kaduna State. *The proceedings of the 45th Annual conference of the Nigerian Society of Animal Production* (NSAP) in collaboration with Abubakar Tafawa Balewa University, Bauchi and Federal Polytechnic Bauchi. Theme: Animal *Agriculture: Exploring the Goldmine of Nigeria's Agro-Revolution Held on 15th-19th March*, 2020. Pp. 498-502. ISBN: 978-978-978-981-320-9.

Davies, F. G. 1982. Observations on the epidemiology of lumpy skin disease in Kenya. *Journal of Hygiene* (Lond). 88(1): 95–102.

Davies, F. G. 1991. Lumpy skin disease of cattle: a growing problem in Africa and the near east. *World Animal Review*, 68:37–42.

Doughlas, C. B. 2000. *Pocket Companion to Veterinary Medicine*. Harcourt Publishers Limited, 24-28 Oval Road, London NW1 7DX, Pp. 365 – 366.

European Food Safety Authority. *Lumpy skin disease: vaccination is most effective control method* [internet]. [cited 2019, May 7.

Ezenwa, V. O. 2004. Parasite infection rates of impala (Aepyceros melampus) in fenced game reserves in relation to reserve characteristics. *Biological Conservation*, 118(3): 397–401.

Gari, G., Bonnet, P., Roger, F., Ware – Szkuta, A. 2011. Epidemiological aspects and financial impact of lumpy skin disease in Ethiopia. *Preventive Veterinary Medicine*, 102: 274-283.

Gari G., Waret-Szkuta A, Grosbois, V., Jacquiet, P., Roger, F. R. 2010. Risk factors associated with observed clinical lumpy skin disease in Ethiopia. *Epidemiology of Infections,* Pp. 1657–66.

Givens, M. D. 2018. Review: Risks of disease transmission through semen in cattle. *Animal*, 12(1): 165– 171.

Grabels, F. 2018. *IDvet 34790 Screen® Capripox Double Antigen Multi-species* [Internet]. 2018. Available from: https://www.id-vet.com/produit/id-screen-capripox-double-antigen-multi-species/.

Hailu, B., Tolosa, T., Gari, G. 2014. Estimated prevalence and risk factors associated with clinical lumpy skin disease in North-Eastern Ethiopia. *Preventive Veterinary Medicine*, 115(1–2): 64–68.

Idris, A. A. 1989. *Infectious Diseases of Livestock in Nigeria – An Outline*. First edition by Ahmadu Bello University Press, Ltd, Zaria, Nigeria, Pp. 50 – 52.

Klement, E., Broglia, A, Antoniou, S. E., Tsiamadis, V., Plevraki, E., Petrović, T., Vladimir Polaček, V., Debeljak, Z, Miteva, A., Alexandrov, T., Marojevic, D., Pite, L., Kondratenko, V., Atanasov, Z., Gubbins, S., Stegeman, A., Abrahantes, J. C. 2018. Neethling vaccine proved highly effective in controlling lumpy skin disease epidemics in the Balkans. *Preventive Veterinary Medicine*. doi: 10.1016/j.prevetmed.2018.12.001.

Lamien, C. E., Le Goff, C., Silber, R., Wallace, D. B., Gulyaz, V., Tuppurainen, E., Madani, H., Caufour, P., Adam, T., El-Harrak, M., Luckins, A. G., Albina, E. and Diallo, A. 2011. Use of the Capripox virus homologue of vaccinia virus 30kDa RNA polymerase subunit (RPO30) gene as a novel diagnostic and genotyping target: development of a classical PCR method to differentiate goat pox virus from sheep pox virus. *Veterinary Microbiology*, 149(1-2): 30-39.

Limon, G., Gamawa, A. A., Ahmed, A. I., Lyons, N. A. and Beard, P. M. 2020. Epidemiological characteristics and economic impact of lumpy skin disease, sheep pox and goat pox among subsistence farmers in north east Nigeria. *Frontiers in Veterinary Science*, 7(8): doi: 10.3389/fvets.2020.00008.

Lubinga, Jimmy C, J. C., Sarah J Clift, S. J., Tuppurainen, E. S. M., Stoltsz, W. H., Babiuk, S., Coetzer, J. A. W., Venter, E. H. 2019. Demonstration of lumpy skin disease virus infection in Amblyomma hebraeum and Rhipicephalus appendiculatus ticks using immunohistochemistry. *Ticks Tick Borne Diseases*, 5(2): 113–120.

MacDonald RAS. Pseudo-urticaria of cattle, 1930. Northern Rhodesian Department of Animal Health, *Annual Report* 1930, 20–21.

Magori-Cohen, R., Louzoun, Y., Herziger, Y., Oron, E., Arazi, A., Tuppurainen, E., Shpigel, N. Y. and Klement, E. 2012. Mathematical modelling and evaluation of the different routes of transmission of lumpy skin disease virus. *Veterinary Research*; 43(1):1–13.

Molla, W., Frankena, K., Gari, G., Kidane, M., Shegu, D. and Jong, M. C. M. 2018. Seroprevalence and risk factors of lumpy skin disease in Ethiopia. *Preventive Veterinary Medicine,* 160: 99-104.

Nawathe, D. R., Asagba, M. O., Abegunde, A., Ajayi, S. A. and Durkwa, L. 1982. Some observations on the occurrence of lumpy skin disease in Nigeria. *Zenralbl Veterinarmed B.* 29(1): 31-36.

Nawathe, D. R., Gibbs, E. P. J., Asagba, M. O. and Lawmani, M. J. P. 1978. Lumpy skin disease in Nigeria. *Tropical Animal Health and Production*, 10(1): 49-54.

OIE. 2012. Terrestrial Manual. Aetiology Epidemiology Diagnosis Prevention and Control. *Lumpy Skin Disease*: 1-5.

OIE. 2018. Terrestrial Manual, Chapter 3.4.12, *Lumpy Skin Disease* (NB: Version adopted in May 2017).

Radostitis, O. M., Gay, C. C., Hinchcliff, K. W., and Constable, P. D. 2006. *Veterinary Medicine, A Text Book of the Diseases of Cattle, Sheep, Pigs, Goats and Horses* (10th ed), Pp. 940, 1248-1250, 1411.

Radostits, O. M., Gay, C. C., Blood, D. C. and Hinchcliff, K. W. 2003. *Veterinary Medicine, A Text Book of the Diseases of Cattle, Sheep, Pigs, Goats and Horses*. Ninth edition, by Book power formerly ELST, Pp. 999-1004.

Şevik, M. and Doğan, M. 2017. Epidemiological and molecular studies on lumpy skin disease outbreaks in Turkey during 2014–2015. *Transboundary Emergency Diseases,* 64(4):1268–79.

Somasundaram, M. K. 2011. An outbreak of lumpy skin disease in a Holstein dairy herd in Oman: a clinical report. *Asian Journal of Animal and Veterinary Advances*, 6(8): 851-859.

Stubbs, S., Oura, C. A., Henstock, M., Bowden, T. R., King, D. P., and Tuppurainen, E. S. 2012. Validation of a high-throughput real-time polymerase chain reaction assay for the detection of capripoxviral DNA. *Journal of Virological Methods*, 179: 419– 422.

Tageldin, M. H., Wallace, D. B., Gerdes, G. H., Putterill, J. F., Greyling, R. R., Phosiwa, M. N., Al Busaidy, R. M., Al Ismaaily, S. I. 2014. Lumpy skin disease of cattle: an emerging problem in the Sultanate of Oman. *Tropical Animal Health and Production,* 46(1): 241-6.

Tano Lazare. *Technical Responsible, MERIAL with the Collaboration of Albert Douffissa.*

Tasioudi, K. E., Antoniou, S. E., Iliadou, P., Sachpatzidis, A., Plevraki, E., Agianniotaki, E. I., Fouki, C., Mangana-Vougiouka, O., Chondrokouki, E., and Dile, C. 2016. Emergence of lumpy skin disease in Greece, 2015. *Transboundary and Emerging Diseases*, 63: 260– 265.

Tulman, E. R., Afonso, C. L., Lu, Z., Zsak, L., Kutish, G. F. and Rock, D. L. 2001. Genome of lumpy skin disease virus. *Journal of Virology*, 75(15): 7122-7130.

Tuppurainen E. (2017). Diagnostic assays for the detection of lumpy skin disease virus and antibodies.

Tuppurainen E. S. M. and Oura CA. 2012. Review: lumpy skin disease: an emerging threat to Europe, the Middle East and Asia. *Transboundary Emergency Disease,* 59(1): 40-8.

Tuppurainen, E. S. M., Alexandrov, T., and Beltran-Alcrudo, D. 2017. Lumpy skin disease field manual - A manual for veterinarians. *FAO Animal Production and Health Manual*, 20: 1– 60.

Tuppurainen, E. S. M., Venter, E. H. and Coetzer, J. A. W. 2005. The detection of lumpy skin disease virus in of experimentally infected cattle using different diagnostic techniques. *Onderstepoort Journal of Veterinary Research*, 72(2): 153-164.

United States Animal Health Association. 2008. *Foreign Animal Diseases*, seventh edition, Pp. 213 – 218.

Wood, J. A. 1974. A skin condition of cattle. *Veterinary Record*, 10.1136/vr.95.14.326.

Wood, J. A. 1988. Lumpy skin disease – A review. *Tropical Animal Health and Production,* 20(1): 11-17.

Yaounde, Cameroun. *Manual of Main Ruminant Diseases*. Pp. 45-46. www.merial.com.

Yeruham, I., Nir, O., Braverman, Y., Davidson, M., Grinstein, H., Haymovitch, M. and Zamir, O. 1995. Spread of lumpy skin disease in Israeli dairy herds. *Veterinary Record*, 137(4): 91–3.

Chapter 5

Equine Piroplasmosis in Nigeria

Philip Wayuta Mshelia[1,*], DVM, MS, PhD
and Kelly Sears[2], DVM, MS, PhD, DACVIM
[1] Department of Veterinary Medicine, Equine Unit,
Ahmadu Bello University, Zaria, Nigeria
[2] Large Animal Medicine, Carlson College of Veterinary Medicine,
Oregon State University, Corvallis, Oregon, USA

Introduction

Equine piroplasmosis (EP) is an infectious, tick-borne disease caused by the hemoprotozoan parasites *Theileria equi, Babesia caballi,* and a recently reported new species, *T. haneyi* (Scoles and Ueti, 2015; Knowles et al., 2018). EP has a global distribution, but a few countries are reported to be EP-free (Wise et al., 2013; Scoles and Ueti, 2015). According to Scoles and Ueti (2015), certain genera of Ixodid ticks, namely *Rhipicephalus*, Dermacentor, and *Hyalomma*, are known to transmit these protozoa. These protozoan pathogens cause acute and chronic infections with a mortality rate of up to 50% (de Waal, 1992).

Horses infected with *T. equi* remain persistently infected while those affected by *B. caballi* are infected for an extended period before the immune system naturally eliminates the parasite without therapeutic intervention. Conversely, parasitemia may fall below the level of detection (Friedhoff and Soule, 1996). Chronically infected horses are reservoirs for spreading the pathogens via ticks or iatrogenic transmission (Ueti et al., 2008). In endemic areas, poor management practices have been reported to exacerbate the impact of infection (Scoles and Ueti, 2015). Timoney (2000) suggests that the

* Corresponding Author's Email: pwmshelia@abu.edu.ng.

In: Infectious and Parasitic Diseases of Animals in Developing Countries
Editor: Selwyn Arlington Headley
ISBN: 979-8-88697-504-8

international trade in horses and other equids could lead to an increase in the global spread of equine diseases. Expansion of vectors into previously uninhabited regions due to rising temperatures (Harvell et al., 2002). The recent EP outbreaks in the USA and the Netherlands, without visible premonitory signs and reduced detectability during long-term persistence (Short et al., 2012), have made EP a challenging disease. Nigeria as recorded significant economic losses associated with EP, which include the cost of treatment and deaths.

Aetiology

Theileria equi, first called *Piroplasma equi* but later reclassified as *Babesia equi (B. equi)*, was first discovered in South Africa in 1901 (Laveran, 1901 as cited by Mehlhorn and Schein et al., 1998). It was discovered a few years later that two biologically distinct parasites could infect the erythrocyte and co-habit within it in order to cause pathologies associated with EP (Mehlhorn and Schein, 1998). One of the parasites was larger and so named *Piroplasma caballi*, but now called *Babesia caballi*, whereas the second parasite was the earlier reported *B. equi* (Nuttal and Strickland, 1910, as cited by Mehlhorn and Schein, 1998). The taxonomy of *B. equi* was reclassified to *T. equi* in 1998 because of extra-erythrocytic evidence of the parasite within peripheral blood mononuclear cells (PBMC), absence of transovarial transmission which occurs in other *Babesia* species, presence of small erythrocytic stages measuring only 1.5-2.5 μm in length instead of the 3-6 μm long erythrocytic stages of *Babesia* species, and distinction in the formation and shape of sexual stages of *T. equi* in the tick vector from those of typical *Babesia* species, as well as their surface proteins' close identity to those of other *Theileria* species (Mehlhorn and Schein, 1998). Furthermore, phylogenetic and genomic analyses showed that *T. equi* possesses characteristics of both *Babesia* and *Theileria* lineages (Allsopp et al., 1994; Uilenberg, 2006; Allsopp et al., 2007), thus supporting the concept of a new genus for *T. equi* (Kappmeyer et al., 2012).

There was a serendipitous discovery of *Theileria haneyi* in a horse that wandered into Eagle Pass at the border between the United States and Mexico. Like *T. equi*, it has intraerythrocytic merozoite stages, but they are morphologically distinct owing to their smaller asexual (merozoite) stages. The mean length and width of each *T. haneyi* merozoite are 1.15 ± 0.16 mm and 0.70 ± 0.07 mm respectively (Knowles et al., 2018), while those of *T. equi* are 1.88 ± 0.21 mm and 0.91 ± 0.13 mm respectively (Bork et al., 2003). It is important to note that *Theileria haneyi* is a distinct parasite closely related to *Theileria* species isolated from waterbucks (*Kobus defassa*) and South African mountain zebras based on phylogenetic analysis of their 18S rDNA. Based on the unique differences in morphology and 18S rDNA between this parasite and other *Theileria* species, the parasite was named *T. haneyi* in honour of the veterinarian, Dr. D. Haney, who first restrained and clinically examined a stray horse from which the parasite was detected (Knowles et al., 2018). The global prevalence of *T. haneyi* currently remains unclear as it evades the internationally accepted diagnostics that utilize ema-1 as the primary target. This novel organism lacks the well-conserved *ema-1* gene that has been identified in isolates around the world (Knowles et al., 2018).

Epidemiology

There are many uses for horses in Nigeria, including recreation, sports, and transportation. In northern Nigeria, polo ponies, both exotic and indigenous, are among the most abundant, and a number of horse-related events are held annually. It is traditional for northern states to host horse processions (durbar), as well as polo and horse racing. Nigeria, particularly the ancient cities, sees hundreds of horses transiting, mostly from neighbouring countries. This includes horses from the Niger Republic, Burkina Faso, Mali, Sudan, Chad, and a host of other countries. The region hosts a variety of events, including horse processions (durbars), polo matches, and horse races. In consequence, Northern part of Nigeria has become a significant epidemiological niche for the transmission of EP infection, and adaptation of apicomplexans to new hosts. As a result, EP may cause a variety of clinical manifestations that are not yet fully understood (Mshelia et al., 2020).

Markets in Katsina, Jigawa, and Yobe State share a substantial border with the Niger Republic, and they were once part of the centuries-old network of markets when the region played an important role as a trans-Saharan trade hub. These livestock markets are linked to road networks and settlement patterns, which makes it easier to transport animals across Nigeria. (Mshelia et al., 2020). The movement of horses across the northern borders of Nigeria from Burkina Faso, Chad, Sudan, and the Niger Republic for various purposes could have been responsible for the persistence of EP in this region. Piroplasmosis is one of the most important parasitic diseases of horses in Nigeria (Mayaki, 2017). Authors, such as Oduye (1976), and Leeflang and

Ilemobade (1977), were the first to report EP in Nigeria. These early reports were followed by those of Aliu (1983) and Oladosu and Dipeolu (1983). The study by Lawal et al. (1999) reported *T. equi* and *B. caballi* infections in horses and found them to occur with prevalence rates of 33% and 2%, respectively, in Zaria, Northwest Nigeria. Other microscopic and serological studies have been reported with varying prevalence in all the geopolitical zones of Nigeria (Takeet et al., 2009; Garba et al., 2011a; Garba et al., 2011b; Garba et al., 2012; Sanusi et al., 2014; Turaki et al., 2014; Oladipo et al., 2015; Mshelia et al., 2016; Idoko et al., 2020).

Recently, molecular studies have been carried out to characterise the etiologic agents in Nigeria (Idoko et al., 2020; Mshelia et al., 2020; Onyiche et al., 2020; Takeet et al., 2020). Idoko et al., 2020 screened 57 donkeys and 47 horses from Kaduna state, Nigeria. They were horses used for traditional horse procession (durbar) and polo, while the donkeys were typically used as pack animals. Twenty-five (43.8%) donkeys had *T. equi* infection, five (8.8%) donkeys had *B. caballi* infection, and three (5.3%) of these donkeys were co-infected with *B. caballi* and *T. equi* by PCR. An analysis of the 18S rRNA gene sequences of PCR-positive amplicons from 25 infected donkeys revealed four monophyletic clades: seven parasites in clade A, three in clade B, 11 in clade C, and four in clade D.

Mshelia et al., 2020 tested 300 samples, 33.3% (110/300) were positive for 18S rDNA. By using 18S rDNA positive samples, individual nPCRs and sequences were conducted to determine the species of organisms infecting horses. Results for species-specific reactions yielded 13.0% (39/300) *T. equi*, 3.3% (10/300) *Babesia caballi*, and 2.7% (8/300) *T. haneyi*. There was a double infection with *T. equi* and *B. caballi* in 2.7% of horses (8/300), while a triple infection with *T. equi*, *B. caballi*, and *T. haneyi* was detected in 0.6% (2/300) horses. (Table 1). The 18S rDNA sequence of two horses was positive for *B. bovis* and confirmed by specific nPCR. Based on the sequence similarity to the query sequence, the familiar clades for *Theileria* were 28 as clade A, 13 as clade C, and 16 as clade D. Except for clades B and E, all the familiar clades were found in Nigeria.

Onyiche et al., 2020 analyzed 468 blood samples from horses and donkeys and 201 pooled samples of ticks using polymerase chain reaction (PCR). A minimum infection rate (MIR) of 7.6% was observed for *Babesia caballi* amplified in *Rhipicephalus evertsi evertsi* in tick pools while *T. equi* was observed in *R. e. evertsi* (MIR, 61.6%), *H. truncatum* (MIR, 50.0%) and *Hyalomma dromedarii* (MIR, 23.7%). In horses, the prevalence of *T. equi* was

(39.9%; 112/281) and *B. caballi* (41.2%; 77/187). In the donkeys' *T. equi* (1.4%; 4/281) and (1.6%; 3/187) for *B. caballi*.

Molecular detection and sequence analysis carried out by Takeet et al., 2020 in 3 states of the South West revealed that 7 (6.9%) horses out of a total of 102 horses had *T. equi* (Table 2).

Table 1. Result of nPCR targeting species-specific equine piroplasmids in horses from northwestern Nigeria

Area	Total number of samples	Breed	Positive samples		
			T. equi	*B. caballi*	*T. haneyi*
Kaduna					
Igabi	80	Argentine polo ponies	43 (53.8%)	-	-
	8	Thoroughbred	5 (62.5%)	-	-
	3	Criollo	2 (66.7%)	-	-
Zaria	127	West African Barb	7 (5.5%)	4 (3.1%)	5 (3.9%)
	25	West African Barb	3 (12%)	1 (4%)	1 (4%)
Katsina					-
Mai'adua	32	West African Barb	11 (34.4%)	4 (12.5%)	2 (6.25%)
Jigawa					
Maigatari	25	West African Barb	1 (4%)	1 (4%)	-

Mshelia et al., 2020.

Table 2. Prevalence of *Theileria equi* in naturally infected horses from three western states in Nigeria detected by the polymerase chain reaction

	Argentine horses (%)		Local horses (%)		Sudanese horses (%)		
	Infected	Non infected	Infected	Non infected	Infected	Non infected	Total
Abeokuta	0 (0)	3 (13.6)	4 (18.2)	13 (59.1)	0 (0)	2 (9.1)	22
Ibadan	1 (2.1)	17 (36.2)	1 (2.1)	17 (36.2)	0 (0)	11 (23.4)	47
Lagos	1 (3.0)	12 (36.4)	0 (0)	12 (36.4)	0 (0)	8 (24.2)	33
Total	2 (1.9)	32 (31.4)	5 (4.9)	42 (41.2)	0 (0)	21 (20.6)	102

Takeet et al., 2020.

Life Cycle

The life cycle of the aetiologic agents of equine piroplasmosis, *B. caballi*, and *T. equi*, involves three distinct stages; the asexual transmission stage (sporozoite), asexual blood-stage (merozoite), and the sexual blood stage (gametocyte) (Moltmann et al., 1983; Scoles and Ueti, 2015; Knowles et al., 2018) (Figures 1, 2). Variations in tick species can impact the development of the parasites within the tick vector (Wise et al., 2013). Regardless of variations in the infesting tick species, the infectious sporozoites of *B. caballi*, *T. equi*, as well as *T. haneyi* are transmitted through tick-saliva during blood meal intake (Uilenberg, 2006).

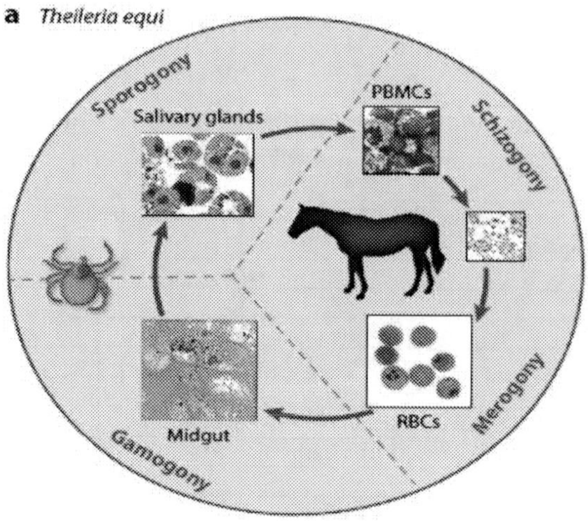

Figure 1. Developmental stages of *T. equi* within the tick vector (sexual stages) and equine host (asexual stages) adapted from Scoles and Ueti (2015).
Keys: PBMCs (peripheral blood mononuclear cells); RBCs (red blood cells).

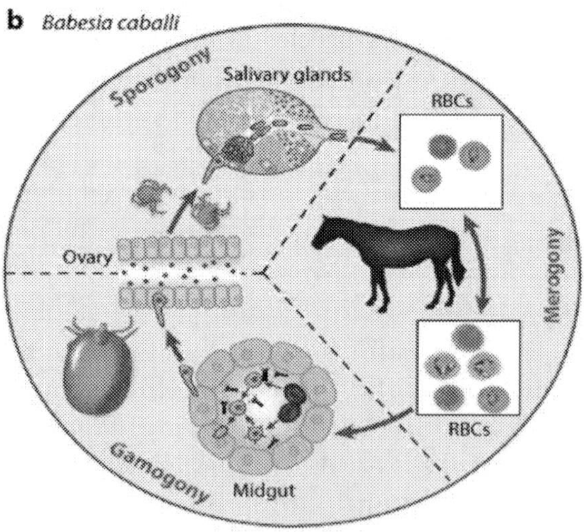

Figure 2. Developmental stages of *B. caballi* within the tick vector (sexual stages) and equine host (asexual stages) adapted from Scoles and Ueti (2015).
Keys: PBMCs (peripheral blood mononuclear cells); RBCs (red blood cells).

The precise duration of the extrinsic acquisition feeding; parasite replication time within the tick vector and transmission feeding (incubation period) is not well defined. Once the *B. caballi* is in the host-parasite, the sporozoites directly invade erythrocytes where they multiply and develop first into trophozoites and later into merozoites. These blood stages (merozoites) are subsequently released and invade the uninfected erythrocytes, leading to erythrocyte rupture. On the other hand, *T. equi* and *T. haneyi* initial invasion is different in that it first enters peripheral blood mononuclear cells (PBMCs) (Mehlhorn and Schein, 1998; Knowles et al., 2018). This particular life cycle event for *T. equi* partly accounted for the taxonomic reclassification as *Theileria* (formerly *Babesia equi*) (Kappmeyer et al., 2012). Once inside the PBMCs, the sporozoites develop into large schizonts and then merozoites about 9 days after invasion. These merozoites are released and invade erythrocytes.

Asexual replication results in an expanding population of merozoites and parasitized erythrocytes. Some of the merozoites develop into gametocyte forms within equine peripheral blood and, upon ingestion of merozoites and/or gametocytes by a competent tick vector; the parasites undergo sexual reproduction, with the gametocytes developing into gametes, which combine to form zygotes within the tick midgut (Mehlhorn and Schein, 1998; Uilenberg, 2006). The zygotes develop differently depending on the tick species and the parasite. *Babesia caballi* zygotes multiply and invade numerous tissues and organs of the ticks, including the ovaries. *Babesia caballi* infection can be passed transovarially to the next tick generation, and development to an infective stage for horses occurs in the salivary glands of immature and adult ticks (Uilenberg, 2006; Rothschild and Knowles, 2007). In contrast, *T. equi* zygotes develop into kinetes, which invade the ticks' hemolymph and salivary gland cells (Mehlhorn and Schein, 1998; Uilenberg, 2006; Rothschild and Knowles, 2007). After 6–24 days, continued development results in the presence of sporozoites within the salivary gland of the tick (Moltmann et al., 1983; Zapf and Schein, 1994; Guimaraes et al., 1998).

The close interaction between the life cycles of ticks and the pathogens they carry determines the mode of transmission of tick-borne pathogens (Scoles and Ueti, 2015). Tick-borne transmission can be biological when the parasites undergo asexual and sexual developmental stages within the equine host and vectors; mechanical, by contaminated mouthparts; or iatrogenically by contaminated needles or blood transfusion. Successful pathogen transmission is dependent on a host of complex interactions between tick population dynamics, host density, and closely associated vector-host behaviors. Intrastadial transmission, in which one life stage of the tick acquires the pathogen and transmits it; interstadial or transtadial transmission, in which one life stage of the tick acquires the pathogen and the subsequent stage transmits it; and transovarial transmission, in which a female tick acquires the pathogen, and her offspring transmits it (Ueti et al., 2008). For example, *B. caballi* are transovarially transmitted by one-host ticks, whereas *T. equi* is intrastadially or transstadially transmitted by only the nymphal or adult ticks (Scoles and Ueti, 2015). Persistently infected horses are also reservoirs for transmission, aside from biological transmission.

Clinical Findings

As EP clinical signs vary from horse to horse and are non-specific (Rothschild and Knowles, 2007), the severity of clinical disease in horses vary based on the region in which the horse resides, the strain of parasite, and the horse's overall health (Wise and Sellon 2015). Wise and Sellon, 2015 noted that comparing disease severity across geographic locations in different parts of the world illustrates how clinical manifestations differ in severity across different regions. Acute infections are often life-threatening in South Africa and Nigeria. While the outbreak in Texas in 2009 had no overt clinical signs Co-infections of *T. equi* and *B. caballi, T. equi* and *T. haneyi,* and a combination of the three parasites has been reported (Mshelia et al., 2020; Idoko et al., 2020), but there has been no report on variations in clinical manifestations in the presence of co-infections, nor on the clinical implication of parasite strains on clinical disease severity.

In response to the discovery of *Theileria haneyi*, there was some uncertainty regarding the possibility of naturally occurring co-infections between *T. equi* and *T. haneyi*. Mshelia et al. (2020) findings show that *T. equi* and *T. haneyi* can co-infect naturally as well as with *B. caballi. T. equi* and *T. haneyi* co-infection experiments have been recorded (Sears et al., 2019).

Babesia caballi, T. equi, and *T. haneyi* infections cannot be distinguished clinically, but differentiation between the three infections using molecular tools may be important for successful treatment and control of the disease (Rothschild and Knowles, 2007; Knowles et al., 2018).

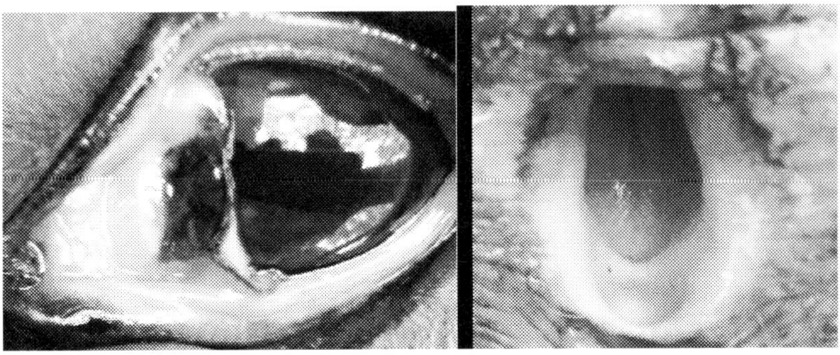

(A) (B)

Figure 3. Jaundice of the mucous membranes of the eye (A) and vulva (B). The mucous membrane of the vulva in the mare gives a clearer picture of the state of the cardiovascular system.

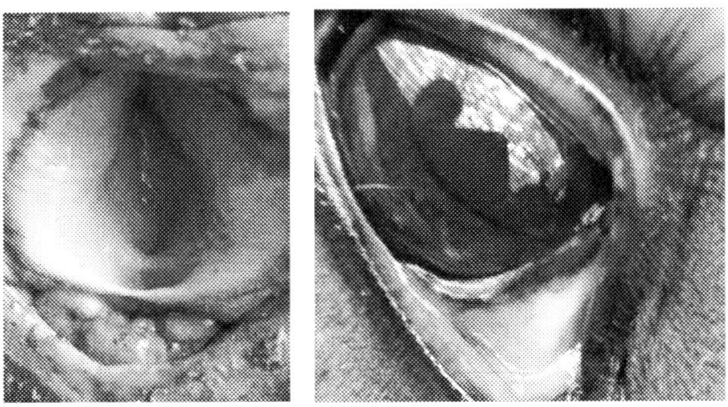

(A) (B)

Figure 4. (A) Mucous membrane of the vulva and eye (B) 3 days after treatment with imidocarb.

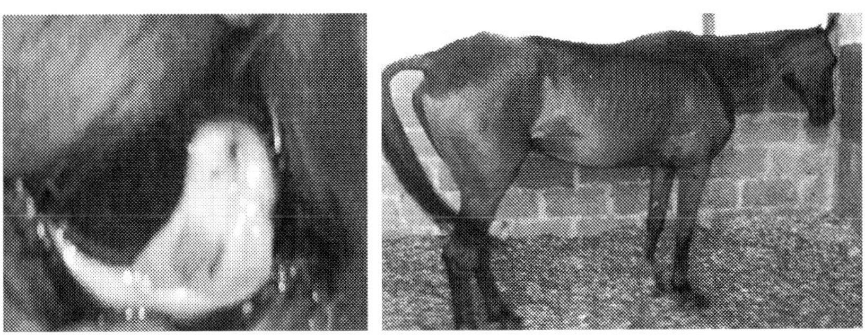

(A) (B)

Figure 5. (A) Petechiae hemorrhage of the ocular mucous membrane and (B) Erect tail, malaise and poor body condition in an Argentine polo pony that arrived Nigeria before onset of clinical signs.

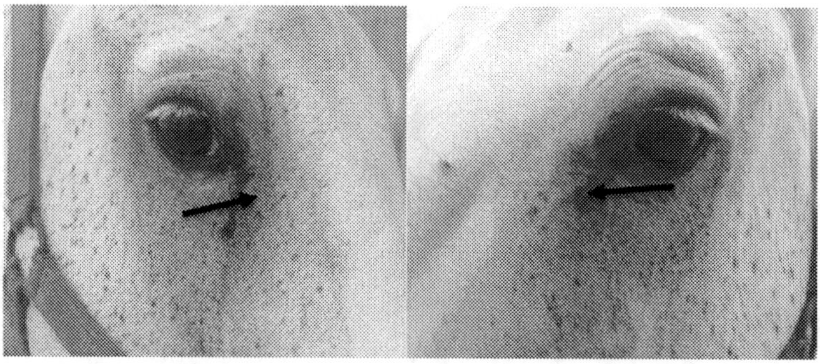

(A) (B)

Figure 6. Bilateral ocular serous discharge (arrow), (A) Left eye and (B) Right eye.

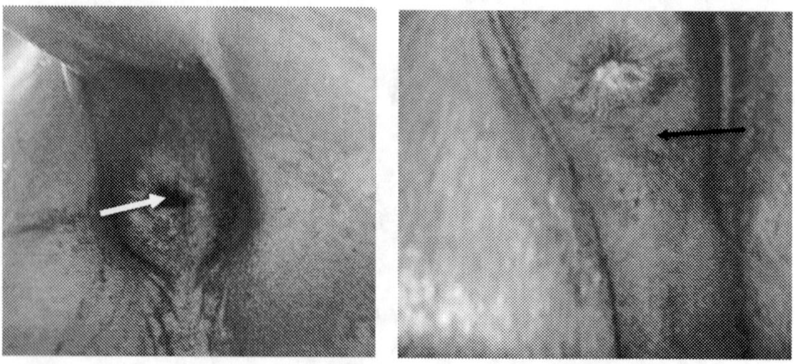

(A) (B)

Figure 7. (A) Relaxation of the anal sphincter (white arrow) and (B) Anal sphincter 24-hours after treatment with Imidocarb (black arrow).

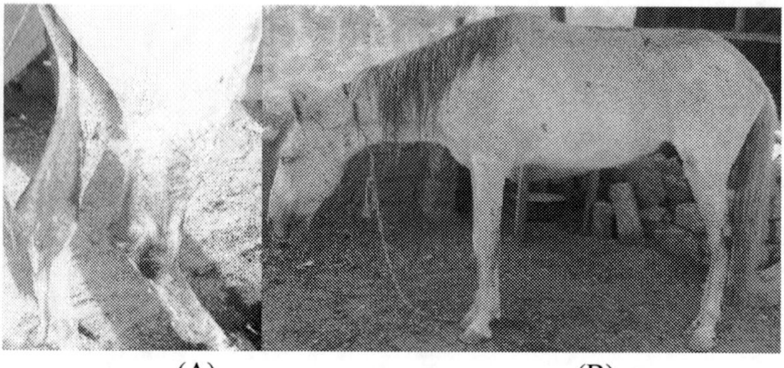

(A) (B)

Figure 8. (A) Evidence of diarrhoea-matted hock, (B) Lethargy, peripheral edema at the ventral part of the neck, weakness, anorexia.

The incubation period, or time from infection to manifestation of clinical signs, ranges from 10 to 30 days for *B. caballi*, 12 to 19 days for *T. equi* (de Waal, 1992), and 14 to 30 days for *T. Haneyi*. Knowles et al. (2018) demonstrated this in splenectomised horses. The course of the disease may be per acute, acute, subacute, or chronic (Rothschild and Knowles, 2007).

At the incipient stage of the infections acute signs are characterized by nonspecific signs (Wise and Sellon, 2015) which include pyrexia (up to 42°C/107.6°F), decreased appetite, lethargy, edema of the dependent parts (Figure 8A), icterus (3A and 3B), anemia, petechiae hemorrhages on mucous membranes including the third eyelids (3A) due to thrombocytopenia, hemoglobinuria (Figure 10A), or bilirubinuria, splenomegaly, digestive or respiratory signs (Figure 9), and occasionally, death (de Waal, 1992; Ambawat et al., 1999; Deger et al., 2009; Laus et al., 2013; Abedi et al., 2014). EP is typically severe in Argentine polo ponies (APP). The majority of clinical findings are severe, including a relaxed anal sphincter (which begins to resolve within 24 hours of imidocarb treatment) (Figure 7A and 7B).

EP typically manifests as bilateral serous ocular discharges (6A and 6B) 1-2 weeks before nonspecific clinical signs such as partial anorexia, malaise, and decreased performance. In the 1980s, the mortality rate for Argentine polo ponies was reported to be high (Lawal et al., 1999). Relaxation of the anal sphincter (Figure 7A) [possibly involving a caudal rectal branch of the pudendal nerve, but not proved] is more prevalent in APP than in West African barbs (WAB). In the absence of piroplasmosis preventative medication, freshly imported APP exhibits EP-like symptoms after 3 to 4 weeks, depending on stable management methods. This EP-like syndrome begins with bilateral serous ocular discharges, then progresses to intermittent pyrexia and inappetance. *Theileria equi* infection was reported in a case by the authors that presented respiratory signs, nervous symptoms, relaxation of the anal sphincter, diarrhoea, liver disease, and multiple organ malfunction. *B. caballi* cases rarely show clinical signs as reported from other parts of the world. In most cases, acute infections are successfully treated when appropriate supportive therapy is applied at the earliest opportunity. Nevertheless, unregulated and indiscriminated imidocarb use could lead to the development of resistance in the future. Some horses found dead without a known cause have been reported to have per acute infections.

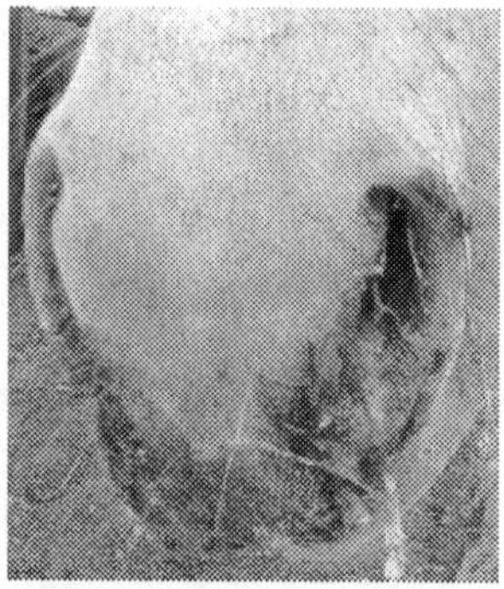

Figure 9. Respiratory involvement.

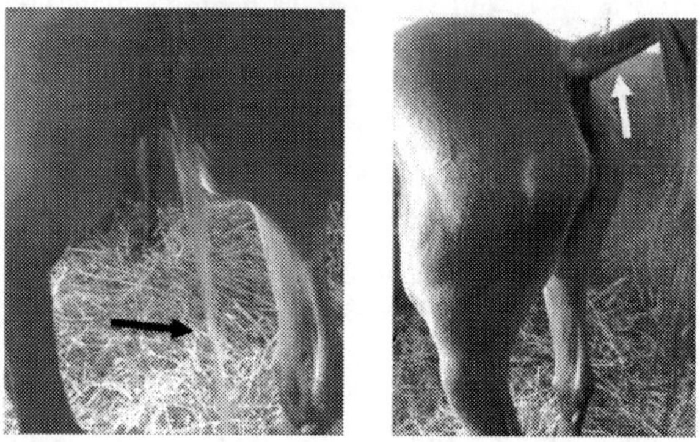

(A) (B)

Figure 10. (A) Colored urine (black arrow), (B) Erect tail in a 12-year-old Argentine polo pony (white arrow).

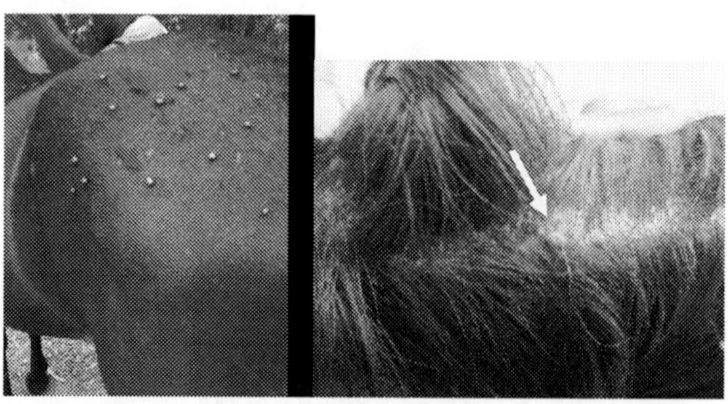

(A) (B)

Figure 11. (A) Ticks infesting hind quarter (orange arrow) of a West African Barb horse, (B) Ticks in the mane (white arrow).

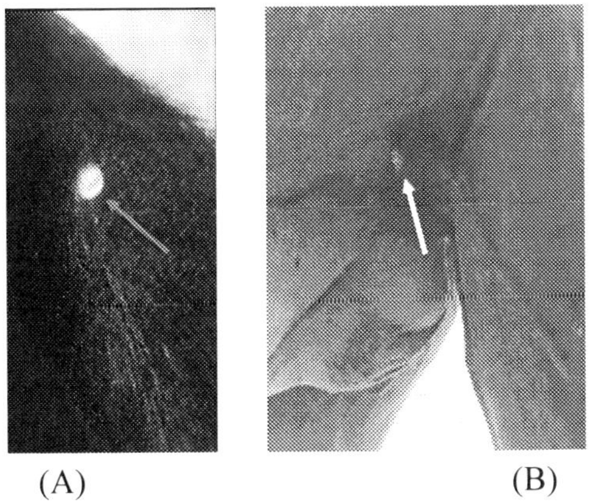

Figure 12. (A) Ticks on the dock of an Argentine polo pony (blue arrow), (B) and in the groin (white arrow).

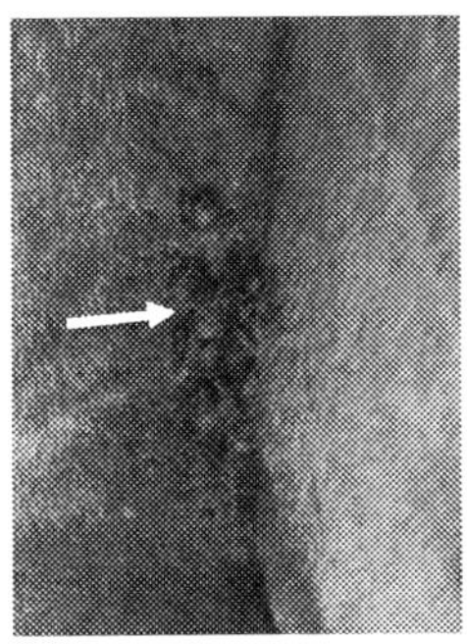

Figure 13. Ticks in the groin (white arrow).

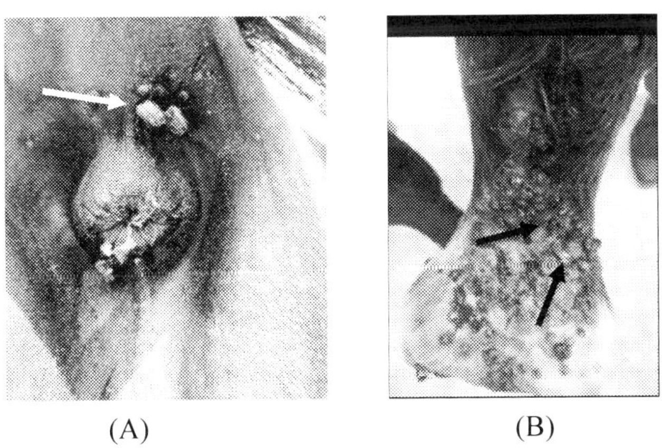

Figure 14. (A) Ticks infesting the base of the tail (white arrow), (B) and caudal part of the pastern (black arrows).

Clinically, chronic piroplasmosis is indistinguishable from other chronic inflammatory diseases and is characterized by nonspecific signs such as inappetance, poor body condition, poor performance, and weight loss (Kappmeyer et al., 2012; Montes-Cortes et al., 2017). There's splenomegaly on rectal palpation. Anemia may be minimal (Wise and Sellon, 2015) or absent in horses with chronic or persistent infection; these animals are termed carriers and are reservoirs for tick and iatrogenic transmission (via blood transfusion, use of contaminated needles or intravenous sets, or an ethno veterinary practice of bloodletting introduced to Nigeria by horse merchants from Chad) (Rothschild and Knowles, 2007; Mshelia et al., 2020).

Pathology

Horse-matured erythrocytes are round, elastic, and biconcave, with a central pallor. The diameter is 5-6μm, there are no nuclei or organelles, and it has a lifespan of 140–165 days (Carter et al., 1974). Equine reticulocytes mature within the bone marrow even in the presence of increased erythropoiesis, explaining the uncommon presence of immature polychromatophilic cells in horse peripheral blood (Latimer and Rakich, 1992; Grondin and Dewitt, 2010). As a result, assessing regenerative responses is dependent on measuring parameters such as red blood cell distribution width (RDW), a coefficient of the degree of anisocytosis of circulating erythrocytes. This parameter's value is significantly altered in microcytic and/or macrocytic anaemias (Kramer, 2000).

An assessment of the alteration of erythrocytes as well as anemia development in EP is necessary in order to understand the mechanism that is critical to successful immune invasion by merozoites and subsequent erythrocyte colonization and multiplication. In addition, pathophysiological mechanisms such as the direct mechanical effect of merozoites on erythrocytes; intra-erythrocyte trophozoite and merozoite binary fission; decreased life span due to sialic acid chelation; alteration of other components of the erythrocyte membrane; and suppression of bone marrow erythropoiesis have been proposed to explain the development of anemia in EP (De waal, 1992; Hailat et al., 1997; Ambawat et al., 1999; AlSaad et al., 2010); the effect of the toxic hemolytic factors produced by the parasites on the erythrocyte membrane (De Gopegui et al., 2007; Zygner et al., 2007); and the immune-mediated mechanism by autoantibodies directed against erythrocyte membrane components both in the infected and uninfected cells (Oladosu and

Olufemi, 1992; Knowles et al., 1994; De Gopegui et al., 2007; Zygner et al., 2007). The consequences of the parasites' toxic metabolites' deleterious effect on erythrocyte membrane components are lipid peroxidation, as evidenced by elevated MDA levels, and oxidative stress (Ambawat et al., 1999; Nazifi et al., 2008; Salem and El-Sherif, 2015). Anemia can cause tissue hypoxia, which can lead to anaerobic metabolism and hyperlactatemia (McMichael et al., 2005; Ayers and Warrington, 2008). Tissue hypoxia is characterized by a decrease in the percent of haemoglobin saturation with oxygen, which can lead to metabolic acidosis.

This anemic condition is characterized by decreases in blood pH, bicarbonate, base access, and oxygen saturation percentage, as well as an increase in the anion gap, which indicates titrational metabolic acidosis (Alsaad, 2014). In addition, anemic hypoxia is associated with panting, which manifests clinically as tachypnoea and tachycardia (Radostitis et al., 2000). Continuous cellular lysis releases endogenous pyrogens, which stimulate the hypothalamic thermoregulatory centres, resulting in pyrexia (Svendson and Carter, 1984). The severity of the pyrexia can be influenced by parasitemia, the clinical stage of the disease, and systemic involvement (Krause, 2002). Furthermore, increased plasma Aspartate aminotransferase (AST) and Alanine aminotransferase (ALT) levels may occur as a result of erythrocyte membrane disruption and ischemia-induced hepatocellular damage. Another consequence of anemia, particularly hemolytic anemia in EP, is a decrease in haptoglobin concentration, an important plasma protein that binds free haemoglobin, sequesters the hem component of haemoglobin, and prevents iron-utilizing pathogens from benefiting from the hemolysis (Tecles et al., 2005; Cary et al., 2009). The clinical significance of the decrease in haptoglobin concentration is the excessive breakdown of haemoglobin into heme and globin components. The globin or protein components are usually recycled, whereas the cytotoxic hem component, in addition to being used by some pathogens, is first converted to a green pigment called biliverdin, and then to an orange pigment called unconjugated or indirect bilirubin in a reaction catalysed by biliverdin reductase (Radostitis et al., 2008; Cary et al., 2009; Salib et al., 2013).

As a result, the emergence of anemia is central to the EP's variable, non-specific clinical signs (Deger et al., 2009; Kappmeyer et al., 2012; Laus et al., 2013; Abedi et al., 2014). Anemia in EP may be microcytic hypochromic (Al-Obaidi et al., 2015), macrocytic normochromic (Takeet et al., 2009), or macrocytic hypochromic (Alsaad and Al-Mola, 2006; Zobba et al., 2008; Ibrahim et al., 2011; Mahmoud et al., 2016; Idoko et al., 2018). Leukocytosis due to lymphocytosis (Sandhu, 1998; Ike et al., 2005; Alsaad and Al-Mola, 2006; Zobba et al., 2008; Ibrahim et al., 2011) is possibly caused by bone marrow stimulation, lymphoid depletion, and disorganisation with massive lymphocytosis (Mohri and Sardari, 2000). In addition, leucocytosis caused by neutrophilia and eosinophilia has been reported in diseases caused by a cellular response to parasite antigens and tick infestations (Ibrahim et al., 2011; Al-Obaidi et al., 2015).

In EP, thrombocytopenia is a common clinical sequela (Radostitis et al., 2008; Al-Obaidi et al., 2015; Osman, 2017), that is frequently accompanied by an increase in the mean platelet volume (MPV), indicating that juvenile platelets are growing larger and more active, suggesting a regenerative response. When platelets are activated, their shapes change from biconcave to spherical discs, resulting in the formation of pseudopods. Clinically, an increase in MPV could indicate a severe infection, systemic inflammatory process (Margetic, 2012), or other chronic disorders where platelet consumption and sequestration in the spleen and/or reticuloendothelial system is evident, or it could be due to small fibrin clots or platelets clumping.

The overall clinical sequelae of EP's haematological changes are systemic inflammatory syndrome, which leads to multi-systemic dysfunction and hyper coagulopathy (Donnellan and Marais, 2009). Liver transferases (ALT and AST) should be considered not only as regular tests that detect hepatocellular damage, but also as contributors to the pathophysiology of anemia development in hemolytic disorders (Sookoian and Pirola, 2012). This is significant because the enzymes, particularly ALT, are entirely responsible for erythrocyte alanine synthesis, and both enzymes contribute to the majority of the cytosolic glutamate needed for erythrocyte glutathione biosynthesis (Ellinger et al., 2011).

Because the erythrocyte membrane is glutamate-impermeable (Young et al., 1987), erythrocytes rely on *de novo* glutamate production to meet their intracytosolic amino acid needs, which are met by transferases (Ellinger et al., 2011). Aside from modifications in erythrocyte membrane transferases, EP shows differences in serum activity of ALT, AST, alkaline phosphatase (ALP), gamma-glutamyl transferase (GGT), lactate dehydrogenase (LDH), and creatine kinase (CK) (Camacho et al., 2005). These changes are caused by centrilobular hepatocelular degeneration and necrosis, as well as hypoxia-induced hepatobiliary system damage caused by anemia and icterus (Camacho et al., 2005).

The same applies to hemolytic anemia, as it may lead to hypoproteinemia or low blood osmolality. Hyperbilirubinemia due to high indirect bilirubin manifests clinically as icterus in *B. caballi* and *T. equi* infected horses (OIE, 2008; Radostitis et al., 2008; Rothschild, 2013) and is also a net result of hemolytic anemia. The continuous formation of unconjugated bilirubin can cause an elevation in hepatic enzymes (ALT, AST, and ALP) (Radostitis et al., 2008).

Transportation, severe exertion during polo, racing, and durbar procession, as well as intraerythrocytic activities of merozoites, all induce a slew of behavioral and physiological changes that affect heart and respiratory rates as well as stress-related hormones (Jagri et al., 2012). These alterations have an effect on haematological, biochemical, and oxidative stress parameters via producing reactive oxygen species (Uchino et al., 2012; Kumar et al., 2013; Wessely-Szponder et al., 2015). Because erythrocyte membranes have a high polyunsaturated fatty acid content, they are extremely vulnerable to oxidative damage manifested by hemolysis, reduced deformability, and impairment of transport via microcirculation. Horse erythrocytes are more susceptible to oxidative damage and have less deformability than human erythrocytes (Baskurt et al., 1997). The process of lipid peroxidation is a common side effect of oxidative stress and is associated with changes in the structure and function of the erythrocyte membrane, as well as increased osmotic fragility and decreased cell fluidity.

Furthermore, lipid peroxidation is associated with changes in plasma sialic acid levels (Iijima et al., 2009). Desialylation of the erythrocyte membrane results in the loss of the critical high molecular weight glycoprotein mucin, a hydroxyl radical scavenger and essential component of sialic acids.

This, in turn, renders underlying structures more vulnerable to oxidative damage and affects the biophysical and biochemical functioning of the cells (Ogasawara et al., 2007; Mehdi et al., 2012). Similarly, infections can use sialic acid removal to circumvent host immune responses via "molecular mimicry" (Vimr et al., 2004). The harmful effects of reactive oxygen species and lipid peroxides are mitigated by a variety of endogenous antioxidant defence mechanisms that operate as free radical scavengers (Kolanjiappana et al., 2002). Changes in the surface membrane molecules of erythrocytes are produced by invading merozoites of apicomplexan parasites other than *T. equi* have been frequently described (Harvey et al., 2014). Apicomplexan parasites, particularly those from the genera Babesia and Theileria, have major antioxidant systems that they use to maintain redox homeostasis and survival against host immune responses (Bosch et al., 2015). Thioredoxin and glutaredoxin systems are examples of antioxidant systems. The close synergistic effect of thiol/disulfide couples in these systems regulates intracellular redox homeostasis.

The antioxidant capacity of the cell is regulated by the major redox pairs glutathione/glutathione disulfide (GSH/GSSG), whereas thioredoxins (Trxred/Trxox) create a complementary redox system that interacts with a separate subset of proteins (Jones and Go, 2010). In addition to the thiol/disulfide pairs, enzymatic antioxidants, which are generically classed as primary and secondary antioxidants, are present.

Secondary antioxidants participate in the regeneration of low molecular weight antioxidant species, whereas primary antioxidants react directly with prooxidants (Bosch et al., 2015). Primary antioxidant enzymes include catalase (CAT) and superoxide dismutase (SOD). The CAT catalyses the reduction of hydrogen peroxide to water and oxygen ($2H_2O_2 \rightarrow 2H_2O + O_2$), thereby decreasing its cellular buildup. SODs, on the other hand, are metallo- (M-) proteins that catalyse superoxide anion dismutation, resulting in the production of molecular oxygen and hydrogen peroxide (Bosch et al., 2015).

Both humoral and cellular immunologic components are engaged in equine piroplasmosis as protective immunological responses to the aetiologic agents (Mealey et al., 2011). When sporozoites are released into the plasma following a tick bite, immunoglobulin G (IgG), especially IgG3 antibodies, inhibits infection by binding and neutralising the sporozoites before they target the peripheral blood mononuclear cells (PBMCs) (Awinda et al., 2013). As the initial line of defence between the time the parasite enters the circulation and the time it invades the target cells, the humoral immune response is crucial (Homer et al., 2000). In immunocompromised horses, this stage may be preceded by intraerythrocytic infection, in which sporozoites override humoral immune responses and change into merozoites, infecting circulating erythrocytes and causing hemolysis. Following lysis, two important processes occur. First, the parasites re-enter the circulation to begin a fresh round of invasion. The recurring cycle of invasion and infection of fresh erythrocytes causes parasitemia to rise and acute disease to occur. On the other hand, haemoglobin (Hb) is released from lysed infected erythrocytes, scavenging nitric oxide, which is a major regulator of smooth muscle relaxation, endothelial adhesion molecule production, platelet activation, and platelet aggregation (Rother et al., 2005). Because free haemoglobin is hydrophobic, it interacts with and disturbs lipid membranes and other lipophilic structures (Balla et al., 1993).

Free Hb, which may act as a secondary modulator of Hp's anti-inflammatory role, can be removed from the circulation via three major mechanisms: high-affinity binding of Hb to haptoglobin (Hp); high-affinity binding of the hem to hemopexin (Hpx); and low-affinity binding of Hb to a cluster of differentiation 163 (CD163). The mechanisms involving Hpx and CD163 appear to function during massive or localized hemolysis, where Hp concentration is overwhelmed or limited (Quaye, 2008). The innate immune system cells are expected to regulate parasite growth and parasitemia.

The inhibition is accomplished by the production of soluble factors such as gamma interferon (IFN-γ), tumor necrosis factor-alpha (TNF-α), nitric oxide (NO), and reactive oxygen species (ROSs) by the natural killer cells (NK cells) and macrophages (Mϕ). The absence of these cellular protective immune responses will result in the development of higher parasitemia and a cascade of systemic effects (Krause et al., 2007).

Protective maternal antibodies can be detected in foals up to 5 (Heerden, 1996) or 6 months of age. These foals are thought to be protected by passively acquired immunity and non-specific factors during the first 6–9 months of age (de Waal and Heerden, 2004). Transmission feeding by competent ticks during this time usually produces only subclinical disease, but with constant superinfections, a stable immunity may develop (Phipps et al., 1996). Cross-immunity in mixed infection of *B. caballi* and *T. equi* is unlikely (Schein et al., 1988; Donnellan et al., 2003), but co-infection with both parasites is common (Donnelly et al., 1980). Maternal immunity is transient, and as it fades, foals become more vulnerable to neonatal EP (Kumar et al., 2008). The specific function or significance of the nine ema gene family members in the *T. equi* life cycle or the host innate response is unknown (Kappmeyer et al., 2012).

High antibody titers against these proteins appear between 2–6 weeks of natural infection (Cunha et al., 2006) and may remain for life or for a long period with or without parasite chemotherapeutic elimination (Cunha et al., 2006; Ueti et al., 2012). The persistence of antibody titres in the absence of current infection is attributed to "memory" B cells' continual release of antibodies, particularly IgG, in the absence of ongoing antigenic stimulation (Slifka and Ahmed, 1998; Bernasconi et al., 2002).

Diagnosis

Diagnosis is accomplished through clinical examination, microscopic examination of Giemsa-stained blood smears, molecular detection via polymerase chain reaction (PCR) (Vial and Gurenflot, 2006; Knowles et al., 2018), serological detection via complement fixation test (CFT), enzyme-linked immunosorbent assay (ELISA), and an indirect fluorescent antibody test (IFAT) (OIE, 2008; Rothschild, 2013), and animal. These methods are useful for accurate diagnosis and epidemiological research (Terkawi et al., 2012).

Clinical Examination

History and physical examination alone are not sufficient to provide a reliable diagnosis of EP. In addition, EP has non-specific clinical signs that can also be observed in diseases like equine ehrlichiosis, African horse sickness, equine infectious anemia, equine viral arteritis, purpura haemorrhagica, immune-mediated hemolytic anemia, and red maple leaf toxicity.(Alward et al., 2006; World Animal Health Information Database, 2012). The diagnosis of this condition requires a thorough history, clinical examination, and laboratory confirmation of the causative microorganisms. (Rothschild and Knowles, 2007; Centre for Food Security and Public Health, 2008).

Microscopic Examination

The parasites within erythrocytes can be identified using Giemsa stain to diagnose clinical cases of *B. caballi, T. equi*, and *T. haneyi* (Donnellan and Marais, 2009; Knowles et al., 2018). Blood smears must be meticulously analyzed because parasitemia levels might be low even in severe instances. A typical *Theileria equi* trophozoite can reach a diameter of 3 µm. Infective merozoites are often four piriform parasites measuring 1.5 µm in length, forming a Maltese cross, amoeboid, or signet-ring shaped with a halo. In clinically sick horses, the percentage of parasitized erythrocytes is generally 1 to 5%, but it can reach 20% (Donnellan and Marais, 2009). *T. equi* parasitemia typically affects 1-7% of erythrocytes, with a high of 95% (Rothschild and Knowles, 2007).

T. equi. and *T. haneyi* are smaller than *Babesia caballi*. *Babesia caballi* trophozoites are oval or elliptical in shape, with pear-shaped basophilic-staining merozoites that occur in pairs and are around 4 µm in length in a single erythrocyte (Retief, 1964). The percentage of detectable erythrocytes in peripheral blood parasitized by *B. caballi* is usually less than 1% and can be as low as 0.1% (Rothschild and Knowles, 2007; Donnellan and Marais, 2009).

Using thick blood smears can improve the sensitivity of identifying parasitized erythrocytes (Rothschild and Knowles, 2007). Additionally, blood samples obtained and kept cold before slide preparation, as well as parasitized cell concentration by centrifugation, are useful processes that maximise parasitemia detection (Theiler, 1902; Sippel et al., 1962).

The PCR method is based on the amplification of DNA from EP pathogens and the identification of specific, unique DNA components.

For detecting *Babesia* and *Theileria* parasites, four types of PCR tests are used: primary or conventional PCR, which uses one set of primers; real-time PCR, which quantifies the parasite level in peripheral blood; nested PCR, which uses two sets of primers to increase sensitivity; and nested PCR with hybridization (probe specific for gene target results in enhanced sensitivity and specificity) (Bashiruddin et al., 1999; Battsetseg et al., 2001). The molecular mass of the band, restriction endonuclease treatment of the band, sequencing of the band, and hybridization with particular probes may all be used to define PCR specificity (Schwint et al., 2009; Bhoora et al., 2010; Wise et al., 2013). A real-time PCR can also detect *B. caballi* and *T. equi* quantitatively (Bhoora, 2010). The quantification of the parasite in the blood would enable research into factors that may influence parasitemia levels. A nested PCR for *T. equi* based on the sequencing of the ema-1 gene found parasitemia comparable to 0.000006 percent (Nicolaiewsky et al., 2001). Nested PCR identifies 3.6 times more infections than microscopy and 2.2 times more infections than conventional PCR (Rampersad et al., 2003). To evaluate the PCR's diagnostic sensitivity and specificity, research should involve testing horses in endemic regions, identifying the transmission risk posed by a seropositive but PCR-negative horse, and defining the animal's status from a transmission and regulatory standpoint (United States Department of Agriculture APHIS National Centre for Risk Analysis, 2011).

Serology

Knowles et al. (1991) created the competitive inhibition ELISA (cELISA), which employs the *T. equi* immunodominant and highly conserved surface antigen, ema-1, as specific monoclonal antibodies for the detection of *T. equi* infection. This was later enhanced by employing recombinant protein instead of culture-derived complete parasites (Knowles et al., 1992). The use of recombinant proteins simplified cELISA standardization and eliminated the necessity for in vitro growth of *T. equi* as well as experimental infection of horses for antigen generation, making this diagnostic tool the best screening test for both *Babesia* and *Theileria* infections (Rothschild and Knowles, 2007). Kappmeyer et al. (1999) created the recombinant *B. caballi* rhoptry-associated protein (rap-1) as a cELISA diagnostic test for diagnosing *B. caballi* infection. Veterinary Medical Research and Development (VMRD) eventually commercialized cELISA into two test kits, one for identifying *T. equi* antibodies and the other for detecting *B. caballi* antibodies (Rothschild and Knowles, 2007).

The cELISA is licenced by the USDA-APHIS-VS Centres for Veterinary Biologics (CVB) and authorised by the World Organization for Animal Health (OIE) as a regulatory test for Equine Piroplasmosis serodiagnosis (OIE, 2005). This test is extremely effective in diagnosing chronic infection in horses that are negative for PCR and the Complement Fixation Test (CFT) (Brüning, 1996). The test can also identify experimental *T. equi* infection as early as 21 days post-infection and five weeks after tick transmission (Knowles et al., 1991).

The complement fixation test is based on the fixation of complement during an antigen-antibody response (Brüning, 1996; Friedhoff and Soulé, 1996). A CFT is deemed positive when a positive response occurs at a 1:5 dilution. It is a fairly specific test for acute infections and can detect antibodies as early as 8 days after infection; however, its sensitivity in chronic and inapparent infections is limited because certain antibodies produced in chronic infections do not fix complement (Friedhoff and Soulé, 1996).Other disadvantages of CFT include the possibility of false-negative findings, the requirement for large amounts of antigens, and the cross-reactivity between antibodies against *T. equi* and *B. caballi* (Donnelly et al., 1982; Brüning, 1996).

Ristic and Sibinovic (1964) developed the indirect fluorescent antibody test (IFAT) to identify antibodies against *B. caballi* in chronically infected horses. The test, which is more sensitive than the CFT, involves attaching parasite antigens to a glass slide and enabling it to react with test sera (Wise et al., 2013). Following the binding of fluorescein-labelled antiequine sera, the bound antibodies are detectable under ultraviolet light (Tenter and Friedhoff, 1986). If the test sera exhibit significant fluorescence of the parasites at a dilution of 1:80 or greater, they are termed "positive" (Mosqueda et al., 2012). Antibody responses with the IFAT were detected in horses experimentally infected with *T. equi* and *B. caballi* as early as 3 to 20 days post-infection, with significant titres even in chronic infection (Weiland, 1986). The downsides of IFAT include time limits, the need for additional antigens, and the difficulty in standardisation due to subjectivity in fluorescence interpretation (Huang et al., 2006).

Giemsa-Stained Blood Smears

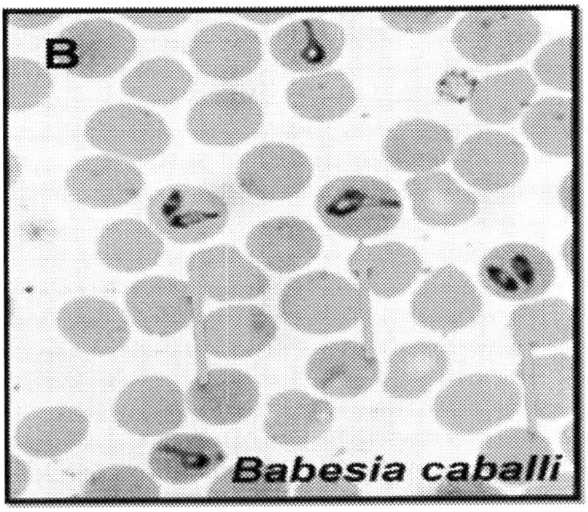

Figure 16. Blood smear showing pyriform merozoites of *Babesia caballi* (B) in erythrocytes as indicated by arrows. Adapted from Kumar et al. (2008).

The presence of diagnostic characteristics, such as enormous paired pyriform intraerythrocytic forms linked at their posterior ends and reaching 2-5 μm in length and 1.3-3.0 μm in diameter, indicates the presence of *B. caballi* merozoite stages (Mehlhorn and Schein, 1998) (Figure 16). Microscopically, the arrangement of four pear-shaped merozoites that form a tetrad known as a 'Maltese cross' indicates *T. equi* (Figure 17) (Yokoyama et al., 2003; OIE, 2014). *T. haneyi's* Maltese cross has a lower mean length (1.15 0 ± 16 mm) and width (0.70 ± 0.07 mm) than *T. equi's* (1.88 0.21 mm) and width (0.91 ± 0.13 mm) (Figure 18) (Knowles et al., 2018). Furthermore, the least and maximal lengths of each Maltese cross mass for *T. equi* are 1.57 mm and 2.32 mm, respectively, whereas those for *T. haneyi* are 0.87 mm and 1.57 mm. Similarly, the least and maximal widths of the Maltese crosses for *T. equi* are 0.72 mm and 1.39 mm, respectively, but for *T. haneyi* n. sp., they are 0.56 mm and 0.9 mm (Knowles et al., 2018).

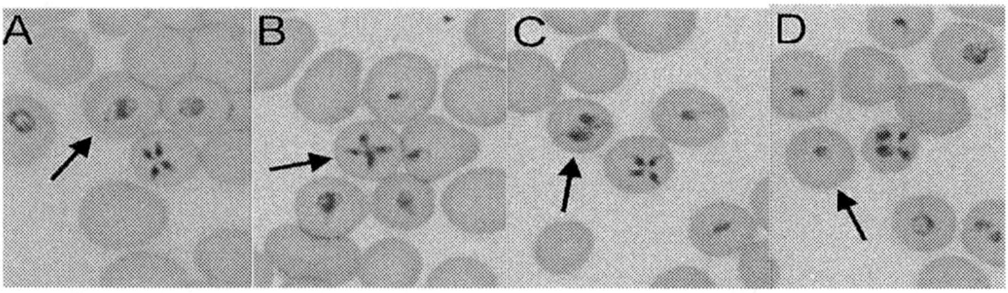

Figure 17. Intra-erythrocytic (merozoite) forms of *Theileria equi* (A-D) in Giemsa-stained blood film. Arrows indicate forms (merozoites and Maltese crosses) within the infected erythrocytes. Merozoites may be spherical or pyriform (pear-shaped) (Mehlhorn and Schein, 1998). Maltese crosses are characterized by an arrangement of four merozoites. Arrows in A-D for *T. equi* indicate different phases of merozoites and Maltese crosses. Adapted from Knowles et al. (2018).

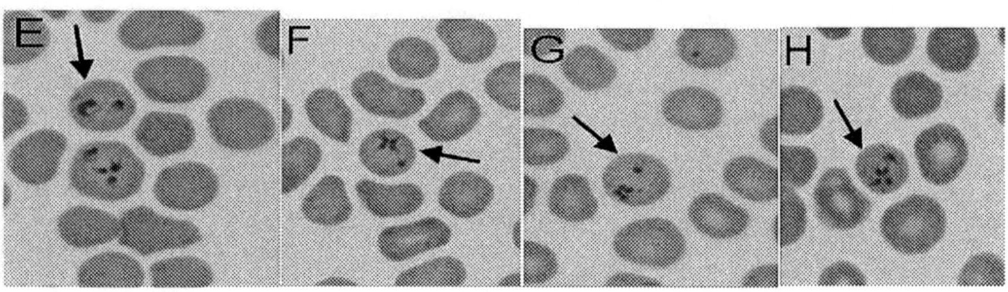

Figure 18. Intraerythrocytic forms of *Theileria haneyi* in Giemsa-stained blood film. Arrows indicate forms (merozoites and Maltese crosses) within the infected erythrocytes. Merozoites may be spherical or pyriform (pear-shaped) (Mehlhorn and Schein, 1998). Maltese crosses are characterized by an arrangement of four merozoites. Arrows in E-F for *T. haneyi* n. sp. indicates different phases of merozoites and Maltese crosses. Width and length measurements of merozoites were performed on individual masses of Maltese crosses. Adapted from Knowles et al. (2018).

Clinical Management of Piroplasmosis

Generally, chemotherapy is designed to minimize the systemic effects of parasitic apicomplexan diseases, however, the persistence of equine piroplasmosis makes effective treatment difficult, particularly in horses infected with *Theileria equi* (Kerber et al., 1999). In endemic countries, it might be advantageous to emphasize symptomatic treatment rather than complete elimination, as this promotes adaptive immunity, however, such treated horses remain chronically infected and continue to harbour parasites that survived previous drug exposure. This is a risk factor for the development of drug resistance and a reservoir for the transmission of disease to naive horses by competent ticks (Ueti et al., 2012).

Antiprotozoal agents such as imidocarb dipropionate have been used for many years (Frerichs et al., 1973; Ueti et al., 2012), diminazene aceturate, atovaquone (Hildebrandt et al., 2013), the combination of N-acetyl-L-cysteine and diminazene aceturate, parvaquone (Kuttler et al., 1987), buparvaquone (Zaugg and Lane, 1992), Miltefosine (AbouLaila et al., 2014), artemisinin derivative and bumped kinase inhibitors 1294 (BKIs 1294) (Hines et al., 2015) have been used for the treatment of equine piroplasmosis with variable challenging success rate. Challenges such as inadequate confirmatory tests for successful parasite clearance, extended time between chemotherapeutic clearance of parasites and development of seronegative status, and the variability of these drugs' susceptibilities among different strains of the causative pathogens are impediments to successful treatment (Bruning, 1996; Schwint et al., 2009; Ueti et al., 2012). Efforts to determine the in vitro efficacy of certain drugs against *T. equi* have been undertaken with minimal success (Bork et al., 2003; Nagai et al., 2003; Munkhjargal et al., 2012; Salama et al., 2013; Wise et al., 2013; Salama et al., 2014) due to a lack of biological relevance or feasibility for use in horses (Hines et al., 2015).

Imidocarb Dipropionate (ID)

Imidocarb dipropionate (ID) is a dicationic diamidine of the carbanilide series [3,3'-bis (2-imidazoline-2- yl)-carbanalidae] of antiprotozoal compounds, commonly used to treat equine piroplasmosis caused by *B. caballi, T. equi* and *T. haneyi* (Knowles et al., 2018). The precise mechanism of action of this drug is unknown but causes chromatin clumping, dissolution of the nuclear membrane, and cytoplasmic vacuolization of intraerythrocytic stages within 48 hours post-administration (Belloli et al., 2002). Other mechanisms, such as interfering with the production and/or utilisation of polyamines, or preventing the entry of inositol into parasitized erythrocytes, have been reported. It is administered as a dihydrochloride or dipropionate salt either subcutaneously or intramuscularly to horses (3.4 mg/kg body weight BW) (Donnellan and Marais, 2009). In endemic countries, four doses of the drug at 4 mg/kg BW 72-hourly are recommended, with a second dose to be repeated after two weeks (Ueti et al., 2012). Despite this established protocol, treatment failures persist (Hines et al., 2015). Imidocarb dipropionate lacks efficacy against

Theileria haneyi and fails to consistently clear *Theileria equi* in Horses co-infected with *T. haneyi* (Sears et al., 2020).

Anticholinesterase effects such as sweating, diarrhea, colic, and signs of agitation are toxicity signs associated with the drug (Adam, 1981) and can be mitigated using intravenous injection of 0.3 mg/kg N-butylscopolammonium bromide (Buscopan®) (Ueti et al., 2012) and atropine sulfate (Heerden, 1996). The abuse of Imidocarb is rapidly spreading among quacks and grooms, encouraged by some veterinarians, especially in the past 3 years. This could lead to an unprecedented development of resistance in the equine population.

Diminazene Aceturate (DA)

This drug is the most available and affordable for treating equine piroplasmosis, but it is associated with several clinical challenges. It is associated with massive swelling of the muscles of the neck, especially when the DA granules are not well dissolved and also relapse is a common feature. It irritates, and some horses tend to show no sign of swelling after 5 days. But overt swelling could be seen even after 3 weeks of the injection.

Supportive Therapy

Supportive therapy is essential when dealing with EP, particularly when severe symptoms are present. The disease is endemic in Nigeria, where treatment aims to alleviate clinical symptoms and improve recovery times. Since chronic infection induces lifelong immunity, eliminating the organism serves a limited purpose. Acute infections require emergency treatment in sub-Saharan Africa.

- Liver protectants and Lipotropics (Thioctic acid): It ameliorates the negative effects of piroplasmosis and improves liver metabolism.
- Ayurveda herbal liver tonic (Yakrivit^R^) with a combination of 20 herbs). In the author's experience, the use of this herb has decreased recovery times, alleviated clinical signs, and reduced mortality rates, especially in acute cases where horses are too weak to tolerate ID and DM treatment.

- Fluid therapy: identification of potential losses and biochemical status of electrolytes in the blood. Normal saline (0.9%) is indicated for hyperkaliemia, hyponatremia, hypochloremia (e.g., renal disturbances in EP), and metabolic alkalosis. If hypoglycemia or hyperkaliemia is present, 5% dextrose can be administered.
- In some cases, the temperature can reach 42 degrees Celsius (107 degrees Fahrenheit).
- Institute therapy that will improve hepatic and renal function.
- Use antioxidant and immune booster.
- Use oral hematinic and maintain the body's electrolyte and glucose level.
- Monitor the animal for anemia, thrombocytopenia, hypoglycemia, and azotemia.

Clinical Points to Consider before or during Therapy

- The use of steroids such as dexamethasone is not recommended as they suppress the immune system and increase parasitemia.
- Non-steroidal anti-inflammatory drugs (NSAIDS) should not be given to horses and foals that are dehydrated.
- When administering imidocarb or any other available medication, it is important to consider the horse's clinical condition.
- The administration of iron dextran to horses should be avoided. At low doses, the drug can cause adverse reactions, while at high doses, it can cause sudden death.

Conclusion

There is evidence of *Theileria equi, Theileria haneyi*, and *Babesia caballi* being present in Nigeria. Horses infected with these pathogens may play a critical role in spreading them through their specific tick vectors. There is, however, no knowledge of which ticks are vector competent in Nigeria. Identifying the various competent tick vectors responsible for parasite transmission warrants further investigation. Hence, surveillance and restrictions on the international movement of equids are necessary to prevent the introduction of infected animals into Nigeria in order to prevent the spread of pathogens. Parasite-free erythrocytes are also removed from the circulation, but the cause of this phenomenon is unknown. In some cases of piroplasmosis, nervous symptoms are observed. However, the mechanism behind these symptoms is unknown. In endemic areas, it is widely accepted that protective immunity is present following an initial parasitic infection, however no studies have been conducted directly addressing this issue. There is considerable evidence that innate immunity plays a central role in controlling some *Babesia* and *Theileria* parasites, although its relevance to EP is unclear. Currently, there is limited information available demonstrating how cellular immunity contributes to EP control.

Additional studies are required to determine the role of Ayurvedic herbal liver tonic in reducing recovery times and alleviating clinical manifestations, especially in acute cases where horses are too weak to tolerate ID and DM treatment.

References

Abedi, V., Razmi, G., Seifi, H. and A, Naghibi. 2014. Molecular and serological detection of Theileria equi and Babe-sia caballi infection in horses and ixodid ticks in Iran. *Ticks and Tick-Borne Diseases,* 5: 239–244.

Aboulaila, M., Batadoj, D., Salama, A., Munkhjargal, T., Ichikawa-Seki, M. A., Terkawi, M., Yokoyama, N. and I, Igarashi. 2014. Evaluation of the inhibitory effects of miltefosine on the growth of *Babesia* and *Theileria* parasites. *Veterinary Parasitology*, 204 (3-4):104-110.

Adams, L. G. 1981. Clinicopathological aspects of imidocarb dipropionate toxicity in horses. *Research in Veterinary Science,* 31: 54–61.

Aliu. Y. O. 1983. Tick-borne diseases of domestic animals in Nigeria: Current treatment procedure. *Veterinary Bulletin*. 53: 233- 251.

Allsopp, M. T., Cavalier-Smith, T. and D. T. De Waal. 1994. Phylogeny and evolution of the piroplasms. *Parasitology*, 108 (Pt 2):147–152.

Allsopp, M. T., Lewis, B. D. and B. L. Penzhorn. 2007. Molecular evidence for transplacental transmission of Theileria equi from carrier mares to their apparently healthy foals. *Veterinary Parasitology*, 148:130–136.

Al-Obaidi, Q. T., Al-Sultan, I. I., Arshad, M. M., Mohd-Azam, K. G. K. and A. M. Mimi. 2015. Clinical case of acute equine piroplasmosis in a Malaysian Mare. *Research Opinion in Animal and Veterinary Science,* 5(6): 270-274.

Alsaad, K. M. 2014. Evaluation of haemogram, acute phase response, acid base balance and blood gas analysis in newborn foals infected with Babesiosis. *Journal of Animal and Plant Science*, 24: 738-742.

Alsaad, K. M., Alsaad, E. A. and H.A Al-Derawie. 2010. Clinical and diagnostic study of equine babesiosis in drought horses in some areas of Basrah Province. *Research Journal of Animal Science,* 4 (1):16-22.

Alward, A., Corriher, C. A. and M. H. Barton. 2006. Red maple (Acer rubrum) leaf toxicosis in horses: A retrospective study of 32 cases. *Journal of Veterinary Internal Medicine*, 20: 1197–1201.

Alsaad, K. M. and G. M. AL-Mola. 2006. Clinical and pathological study of equine babesiosis in drought horses in Mosul. *Iraqi Journal of Veterinary Science*, 20 (1): 89-101.

Ambawat, H. K., Malhotra, D. V. and S. Kumar. 1999. Erythrocyte associated haemato-biochemical changes in *Babesia equi* infection experimentally produced in donkeys. *Veterinary Parasitology*, 85:319–324.

Awinda, P. O., Mealey, R. H., Williams, L. B., Conrad, P. A., Packham, A. E and K. E. Reif. 2013. Serum antibodies from a subset of horses positive for *Babesia caballi* by competitive enzyme-linked immunosorbent assay demonstrate a proteinrecognition pattern that is not consistent with infection. *Clinical Vaccine and Immunology*, 20:1752–1757.

Ayers, P. and L. Warrington. 2008. Diagnosis and treatment of simple acid-base disorders. *Nutrition and Clinical Practice*, 23 (2): 122-127.

Balla, J., Jacob, H. S., Balla, G., Nath, K., Eaton, J. W., and G. M. Vercellotti. 1993. Endothelial-cell heme uptake from heme proteins: Induction of sensitization and desensitization to oxidant damage. *Proceeding of National Academy of Science*, 90: 9285–9289.

Bashiruddin, J. B., Camma, C. and E. Rebelo. 1999. Molecular detection of *Babesia equi* and *Babesia caballi* in horse blood by PCR amplification of part of the 16S rRNA gene. *Veterinary Parasitology*, 84: 75–83.

Baskurt, O. K., Temiz, A. and Meiselman, H. J. 1997. Red blood cell aggregation in experimental sepsis. *Journal of Laboratory and Clinical Medicine,* 130(2): 183-190.

Battsetseg, B., Xuan, X. and H. Ikadai. 2001. Detection of *Babesia caballi* and *Babesia equi* in *Dermacentor nuttalli* adult ticks. *International Journal of Parasitology*, 31: 384–386.

Belloli, C., Crescenzo, G., Lai, O., Carofiglio, V., Marang, O. and P. Ormas. 2002. Pharmacokinetics of imidocarb dipropionate in horses after intramuscular injection. *Equine Veterinary Journal*, 34 (6):625-629.

Bernasconi, N., Traggiai, E. and A. Lanzavecchia, 2002. Maintenance of serological memory by polyclonal activation of human memory B cells. *Science*, 298: 2199–2202.

Bhoora, R., Quan, M., Matjila, P. T., Zweygarth, E., Guthrie, A. J. and N. E. Collins. 2010. Sequence heterogeneity in the equi merozoite antigen gene (*ema-1*) of *Theileria equi* and development of an ema-1-specific TaqMan MGB assay for the detection of *T. equi*. *Veterinary Parasitology,* 172: 33–45.

Bork, S., Yokoyama, N., Matsuo, T., Claveria, F. G., Fujisaki, K. and I. Igarashi. 2003. Growth inhibitory effect of triclosan on equine and bovine Babesia parasites. *American Journal of Tropical Medicine and Hygiene*, 68: 334-340.

Bosch, S. S., Kronenberger, T., Meissner, K. A., Zimbres, F. M., Stegehake, D., Izui, N. M., Schettert, I., Liebau, E. and C. Wrenger. 2015. "Oxidative Stress Control by Apicomplexan Parasites", *Bio Med Research International*, ID 351289: 1-10.

Bruning, A. 1996. Equine piroplasmosis an update on diagnosis, € treatment and prevention. *Brazilian Veterinary Journal*, 152: 139–151.

Camacho, A. T., Guitian, F. J., Pallas, E., Gestal, J. J., Olmeda, A. S., Habela, M. A., Telford, S. R. and Spielman, A. 2005. *Theileria* (*Babesia*) *equi* and *Babesia caballi* infections in horses in Galicia, Spain. *Tropical and Animal Health Production*, 37: 293–302.

Carter, E. I., Valli, V. E., McSherry, B. J., Milne, F. J., Robinson, G. A., and J. H. Lumsden. 1974. The kinetics of hematopoiesis in the light horse I. the lifespan of peripheral blood cells in the normal horse. *Canadian Journal of Comparative Medicine*, 38: 303-313.

Cary, C., Zaias, J. and N. H. Altman. 2009. Acute Phase Response in Animals: A Review. *Comparative Medicine*, 59 (6):517-526.

Cunha, C. W., McGuire, T. C. and Kappmeyer, L. S. 2006. Development of specific immunoglobulin Ga (IgGa) and IgGb antibodies correlates with control of parasitemia in Babesia equi infection. *Clinical Vaccine and Immunology,* 13:297–300.

De Gopegui, R. R., Penalba, B., Goicoa, A., Espada, Y., Fidalgo, L. E. and L. Espino. 2007. Clinicopathological findings and coagulation disorders in 45 cases of canine babesiosis in Spain. *Veterinary Journal*, 174: 129–132.

De Waal, D. T. 1992. Equine piroplasmosis: A review. *Brazilian Veterinary Journal*, 148:6–14.

De Waal, D. T. and Heerden, J. V. 2004. Equine piroplasmosis. In *Infectious Diseases of Livestock, Volume One*, (Ed. 2), 425-434.

Deger, S., Deger, Y. and K. Bicek, 2009. Status of lipid peroxidation, antioxidant and oxidation products of nitric oxide equine babesiosis: status of antioxidant and oxidant in equine babesiosis. *Journal of Equine Veterinary Science*, 29: 743-747.

Donnellan, C., Page, P., Nurton, P., van den Berg, J. S. and A. Guthrie. 2003. Piroplasmosis – current trends. *Conference Proceedings of the Equine Practioners Group of South Africa*, 86-87.

Donnellan, C. M. and H. J. Marais. 2009. Equine Piroplasmosis. *In: Mair TS, Hutchinson RE, editors: Infectious Disease of Horses, UK, EVJ Ltd*, pp 333-340.

Donnelly, J., Joyner, L. P., Graham-Jones, O. and C. P. Ellis. 1980. A Comparison of the complement fixation and immunofluorescent antibody tests in a survey of the prevalence of Babesia equi and Babesia caballi in horses in the Sultanate of Oman. *Tropical Animal Health and Production*, 12 (1): 50-60.

Ellinger, J. J., Lewis, I. A. and J. L. Markley. 2011. Role of aminotransferase in glutamate metabolism of human erythrocytes. *Journal of Biomolecular NMR*, 49: 221-229.

Ememe, M. U., Onyegbula, O., Egwuogu, F. C., Nlebedum, C. U. and C. C. Ogbu. 2018. *Babesia caballi* infection in a 6-month-old colt. *Sokoto Journal of Veterinary Sciences*, 16 (1): 102-106.

Frerichs, W. M., Allen, P. C. and A. A. Holbrook, 1973. Equine piroplasmosis (*Babesia equi*): Therapeutic trials of imidocarb dihydrochloride in horses and donkeys. *Veterinary Records*, 93: 73–75.

Friedhoff, K. T. and Soule, C. 1996. An account on equine babesioses. *Revue Scientifique et Technique,* 15 (3): 1191-1201.

Garba, U. M., Sackey, A. K. B., Agbede, R. I. S., Tekdek, L. B. and M. Bisalla. 2012. Plasma Total Protein, Serum Calcium and Inorganic Phosphate Levels in Nigerian Horses with Natural Piroplasmosis. *Journal of Physiology and Pharmacology Advances,* 2 (2): 117 121.

Garba, U. M., Sackey, A. K. B., Agbede, R. I. S., Tekdek, L. B. and M. Bisalla. 2011a. Serum urea and creatinine levels in Nigerian local horses naturally infected with *Babesia. Pakistan Veterinary Journal*, 31 (2): 163-165.

Garba, U. M., Sackey, A. K. B., Tekdek, L. B., Agbede, R. I. S and M. Bisalla. 2011b. Clinical manifestations and prevalence of piroplasmosis in Nigerian royal horses. *Journal of Veterinary Advances*, 1 (1): 11 – 15.

Grondin, T. M. and S. F. Dewitt. 2010. Normal Hematology of the Horse and Donkey. In *Schalm's Veterinary Hematology, 6th edition.* Weiss DJ, Wardrop KJ, editors. Wiley-Blackwell Publishing Ltd, Ames, Iowa, USA, pp. 821-828.

Guimaraes, A. M., Lima, J. D. and M. F. Ribeiro. 1998. Ultrastructure of sporogony in Babesia equi in salivary glands of adult female Boophilus microplus ticks. *Parasitology Research*, 84: 69–74.

Hailat, N. Q., Lafi, S. Q., Al-Darraji, A. M. and F. K. Al-Ani. 1997. Equine babesiosis associated with strenuous exercise: clinical and pathological studies in Jordan. *Veterinary Parasitology*, 69: 1–8.

Harvell, C. D., Mitchell, C. E., Ward, J. R., Altizer, S., Dobson, A. P., Ostfeld, R. S. and Samuel, M. D. 2002. Climate warming and disease risks for terrestrial and marine biota. *Science*, *296* (5576): 2158-2162.

Harvey, K. L., Yap, A., Gilson, P. R., Cowman, A. F., and B. S. Crabb. 2014. Insights and controversies into the role of the key Apicomplexan invasion ligand, Apical Membrane Antigen 1. *International Journal of Parasitology*, 44(12): 853-857.

Heerden, J. V. 1996. Equine babesiosis in South Africa: a report of two cases. *Equine Veterinary Education*, 8, 3-5.

Hildebrandt, A., Gray, J. S. and Hunfeld, K. P. 2013. Human babesiosis in Europe: what clinicians need to know. *Infection*, 41(6): 1057-1072.

Hines, S., Ramsay, J., Kappmeyer, L., Lau, A., Ojo, K., Van Voorhis, W., Knowles, D. and Mealey, R. 2015. Theileria equi isolates vary in susceptibility to imidocarb dipropionate but demonstrate uniform in vitro susceptibility to a bumped kinase inhibitor. *Parasites and Vectors,* 8: 33.

Homer, M. J., Aguilar-Delfin, I., Telford III, S. R., Krause, P. J. and Persing, D. H. 2000. Babesiosis. *Clinical Microbiology Reviews*, 13(3): 451-469.

Huang, X., Xuan, X., Yokoyama, N., Katayama, Y., Anzai, T., and I. Igarashi. 2006. Evaluation of enzyme-linked immunosorbent assays with recombinant antigens for the serodiagnosis of equine Babesia infections. *Veterinary Parasitology*, 140: 158-161.

Ibrahim, A. K., Gamil, I. S., Abdelbaky, A. A., Hussein, M. M. and A. A. Tohamy. 2011. Comparative molecular and conventional detection methods of *Babesia equi* (*B. equi*) in Egyptian Equine. *Global Veterinaria*, 7:201-210.

Idoko S. I., Abalaka, S. E., Mshelia, P. W., Edeh, R. E., Kolo, H. N. and K. Y. Adeyanju. 2018. Ureamic Syndrome in *Theileria equi*-infected Argentine Polo Pony: A Case Report. *Abuja Journal of Veterinary and Biomedical Sciences*, 1 (1): 74 – 79.

Iijima, H., Patrzyc, H. B., Budzinski, E. E., Freund, H. G., Dawidzik, J. B., Rodabaugh, K. J. and H. C. Box. 2009. A study of pyrimidine base damage in relation to oxidative stress and cancer. *British Journal of Cancer*, 101: 452 – 456.

Jagri, M. S., Nemec Svete, A., Zrimek, P., Kramari, P., Kos, K. V., Vovk, T. and K. Silvestra. 2012. Plasma Malondialdehyde, Biochemical and Haematological Parameters in Standardbred Horses during a selected field Exercise Test. *Acta Veterinaria (Beograd),* 62 (1): 53-65.

Jones, D. P. and Go, Y. M. 2010. Redox compartmentalization and cellular stress. *Diabetes, Obesity and Metabolism*, 12, 116-125.

Kappmeyer, L. S., Thiagarajan, M., Herndon, D. R., Ramsay, J. D., Caler, E., Djikeng, A., Gillespie, J. J., Lau, A. O. T., Roalson, E. H., Silva, J. C., Silva, M. G., Suarez, C. E., Ueti, M. W., Nene, V. M., Mealey, R. H., Knowles, D. P. and K. A. Brayton. 2012. Comparative genomic analysis and phylogenetic position of *Theileria equi*. *BMC Genomics*, 13:603.

Kerber, C. E. Ferreira, F., and M. C. Pereira. 1999. Control of equine piroplasmosis in Brazil. *Onderstepoort Journal of Veterinary Research*, 66:123–127.

Knowles, D. P., Kappmeyer, L. S., Haney, D., Herndon, D. R., Fry, L. M., Munro, J. B., Sears, K., Ueti, M. W., Wise, L. N. and M. Silva. 2018. Discovery of a novel species, *Theileria haneyi* n. sp., infective to equids, highlights exceptional genomic diversity within the genus Theileria: Implications for apicomplexan parasite surveillance. *International Journal of Parasitology,* 48: 679–690.

Knowles Jr., D. P., Kappmeyer, L. S., Stiller, D., Hennager, S. G., L. E. Perryman. 1992. Antibody to a recombinant merozoite protein epitope identifies horses infected with *Babesia equi*. *Journal of Clinical Microbiology*, 30: 3122–3126.

Kolanjiappana, K., Manoharana, S. and M. Kayalvizhi. 2002. Measurement of erythrocyte lipids, lipid peroxidation, antioxidants and osmotic fragility in cervical cancer patients. *Clinica Chimica Acta*, 326: 143–149.

Kramer, J. W. 2000. Normal Hematology of the Horse. In: Feldman BF, Zinkl JG, Jain NC editors. *Schalm's Veterinary Hematology,* 5th edition. Lippincott, Williams and Wilkins, Philadelphia, USA, pp. 1069-1074.

Krause, P. J. 2002. Equine Babesiosis. *Medical Clinics of North America*, 86: 361-373.

Krause, P. J., Daily, J. and S. R. Telford. 2007. Shared features in the pathobiology of babesiosis and malaria. *Trends Parasitology*, 23, 605-610.

Kumar, K. J., Yang, H. L., Tsai, Y. C., Hung, P. C., Chang, S. H., Lo, H. W., Shen, P. C., Chen, S. C., Wang, H. M., Wang, S. Y., Chou, C. W. and Y. C. Hseu. 2013. Lucidone protects human skin keratinocytes against free radical-induced oxidative damage and inflammation through the up-regulation of HO-1/Nrf2 antioxidant genes and down-regulation of NF-κB signaling pathway *Food and Chemical Toxicology*, 59: 55-66.

Kumar, S., Kumar, R., Gupta, A. K. and Dwivedi, S. K. 2008. Passive transfer of *Theileria equi* antibodies to neonate foals of immune tolerant mares. *Veterinary Parasitology*, 151: 80-85.

Kuttler, K. L., Zaugg, J. L. and Gipson, C. A. 1987. Imidocarb and parvaquone in the treatment of piroplasmosis (Babesia equi) in equids. *American Journal of Veterinary Research*, 48(11): 1613-1616.

Latimer, K. S., and P. M. Rakich, 1992. Peripheral Blood Smears. In *Cytology and Hematology of the Horse, 1st edition.* Cowell RL, Tyler RD, editors. American Veterinary Publications, Goleta, California, USA, pp. 191-207.

Laus, F., Veronesi, F., Passamonti, F., Paggi, E., Cerquetella, M., Hyatt, D., Tesei, B., and D. Piergili Fioretti. 2013. Prevalence of tick borne pathogens in horses from Italy. *Journal of Veterinary Medicine and Science,* 75: 715-720.

Laveran, A. 1901. Contribution to the study of *Piroplasma equi. CR Sessions Society of Biology Paris*, 53:2.

Lawal, A. I., Kwanashie, G., Okubanjo, O. O., Natala, A. J. and Idoko, R. 1999. The prevalence of piroplasmosis and microflaria infections in local and exotic horses in Zaria. *Zaria Veterineriya*, 6: 16-22.

Leeflang, P., and A. A. Ilemobade. 1977. Tick-borne diseases of domestic animals in northern Nigeria. *Tropical Animal Health and Production*, 9 (4): 211-218.

Mahmoud, M. S., El-Ezz, N. T., Abdel-Shafy, S., Nassar, S. A., El Namaky, A. H., Khalil, W. K., Knowles, D., Kappmeyer, L., Silva, M. G. and C. E. Suarez. 2016. Assessment of Theileria equi and Babesia caballi infections in equine populations in Egypt by molecular, serological and haematological approaches. *Parasites and Vectors*, 9 (1): 260.

Margetic, S. 2012. Inflammation and haemostasis. *Biochemia Medica (Zagreb)*, 22: 49–62.

Mayaki, A. M. 2017. Retrospective study of equine cases at the Veterinary Teaching Hospital, Usmanu Danfodiyo University, Sokoto, Nigeria (2001-2015). *Nigerian Veterinary Journal*, *38*(3): 208-214.

McMichael, M. A., Lees, G. E., Hennessey, J., Sanders, M. and M. Boggess. 2005. Serial plasma lactate concentrations in 68 puppies aged 4 to 80 days. *Journal of Veterinary Emergency and Critical Care*, 15 (1): 17–21.

Mealey, R. H., Kappmeyer, L. S., Ueti, M. W., Wagner, B., and D. P. Knowles. 2011. Protective Effects of Passively Transferred Merozoite-Specific Antibodies against *Theileria equi* in Horses with Severe Combined Immunodeficiency. *Clinical and Vaccine Immunology*, 100 –104.

Mehdi, M. M., Singh, P. and S. I. Rizvi. 2012. Erythrocyte sialic acid content during aging in humans: Correlation with markers of oxidative stress. *Disease Markers*, 32: 179–186.

Mehlhorn, H. and E. Schein. 1998. Redescription of Babesia equi Laveran, 1901 as *Theileria equi* Mehlhorn, Schein. *Parasitology Research*, 84: 467–475.

Mohri, M. and K. Sardari. 2000. Clinical and laboratory findings in equine piroplasmosis. *Journal of Equine Veterinary Science*, 20: 857-859.

Moltmann, U. G., Mehlhorn, H. and E. Schein, 1983. Fine structure of Babesia equi Laveran, 1901 within lymphocytes and erythrocytes of horses: An in vivo and in vitro study. *Journal of Parasitology*, 111–120.

Montes-Cortés, M. G., Fernández-García, J. L., and M. A. H. Martínez-Estéllez, 2017. Seroprevalence of *Theileria equi* and *Babesia caballi* in horses in Spain. *Parasite*, 24 (14): 1-11.

Mosqueda, J., Olvera-Ramírez, A., Aguilar-Tipacamú, G. and G. J. Cantó, 2012. Current Advances in Detection and Treatment of Babesiosis. *Current Medicinal Chemistry,* 19: 1504-1518.

Mshelia, P. W., Kappmeyer, L., Johnson, W. C., Kudi, C. A., Oluyinka, O. O., Balogun, E. O., Richard, E. E., Onoja, E., Sears, K. P. and M. W. Ueti, 2020. Molecular detection of *Theileria species* and *Babesia caballi* from horses in Nigeria. *Parasitology Research*, 119: 2955–2963.

Mshelia, W. P., Sambo, W. K., Adamu, S. Edeh, E. R. and I. Onoja. 2016. Persistence of equine piroplasmosis in horses in Nigeria. *Journal of Equine Veterinary Science*, 39: S104-S105.

Munkhjargal, T., Aboulaila, M., Terkawi, M. A., Sivakumar, T., Ichikawa, M. and B. Davaasuren, 2012. Inhibitory effects of pepstatin A and mefloquine on the growth of Babesia parasites. *American Journal of Tropical Medicine and Hygiene*, 87:681–688.

Nagai, A., Yokoyama, N., Matsuo, T., Bork, S., Hirata, H. and X. Xuan. 2003. Growth-inhibitory effects of artesunate, pyrimethamine, and pamaquine against Babesia equi and Babesia caballi in in vitro cultures. *Antimicrobial Agents and Chemotherapy,* 47:800–803.

Nazifi, S., Razavi, S. M., Mansourian, M., Nikahval, B. and M. Moghaddam. 2008. Studies on correlation among parasitaemia and some hemolytic indices in two tropical diseases (Theileriosis and Anaplasmosis) in Fars province of Iran. *Tropical Animal Health and Production*, 40: 47-53.

Nicolaiewsky, T. B., Richter, M. F. and V. R. Lunge. 2001. Detection of *Babesia equi* (Laveran, 1901) by nested polymerase chain reaction. *Veterinary Parasitology*, 101: 9–21.

Nuttal, G. H. and C. Strickland 1910. Die parasiten der pferdepiroplasmose response der biliary fever [*The parasites of the equine piroplasmosis response of biliary fever*]. *Zentralbl Bakteriol*, 1: 2.

Oduye, O. O. 1976. Survey of blood parasites of horses in Ibadan, Western Nigeria. *Wiad Parazytology*, 22: 155-159.

Ogasawara, Y., Namai, T., Yoshino, F., Lee, M. C. and K. Ishii. 2007. Sialic acid is an essentialmoiety ofmucin as a hydroxyl radical scavenger. *FEBS Letters,* 581: 2473–2477.

Oladipo, T. A., Adekunle, O. F., Okuneye, O. J., Adebayo, M. D., Adeoye, A. T. and O. J. Banjoko. 2015. Pre and Post Polo Competition Prevalence of Equine Babesiosis in Stable Horses in Ibadan, Oyo state, Nigeria. *International Journal of Research in Agriculture and Forestry*, 2 (8): 6-9.

Oladosa, L. A. and Olufemi, B. E. (1992). Hematology of experimental babesiosis and enrlichiosis in steroid immuno-suppresscal horse. *Journal of Veterinary Medicine*, 39: 345-352.

Oladosu, L. A. and O. O. Dipeolu, 1983. The clinico-pathological features and control strategies of equine Babesiosis in Nigeria. *Proceedings of National Symposium on control of ticks and tick-borne diseases in Nigeria.*

Onyiche, T. E., Taioe, M. O., Ogo, N. I., Sivakumar, T., Biu, A. A., Mbaya, A. W., Xuan, X., Yokoyama, N. and Thekisoe, O. 2020. Molecular evidence of *Babesia caballi* and

Theileria equi in equines and ticks in Nigeria: Prevalence and risk factors analysis. *Parasitology*, 147 (11): 1238-1248.

Osman, S. A. 2017. Clinical, haematological and therapeutic studies on babesiosis in Arabian horses in the Qassim region, central of Saudi Arabia. *Journal of Applied Animal Research*, 45 (1): 118-121.

Phipps, L.P. and A. Otter. 2004. Transplacental transmission of *Theileria equi* in two foals born and reared in the United Kingdom. *Veterinary Records*, 154: 406-408.

Quaye, I. K. 2008. Haptoglobin, inflammation and disease. *Transactions of the Royal Society of Tropical Medicine and Hygiene*, 102(8): 735-742.

Radostitis, O. M., Gay, C. C., Blood, D. C., and K. W. Hinchliff. 2000. *Veterinary Medicine: A Text Book of the Diseases of Cattle, Sheep, Goats and Horses.* 9 Ed. WB Saunders Co. London, New York, Philadelephia, pp: 1289-1296.

Rother, R. P., Bell, L., Hillmen, P. and Gladwin, M. T. 2005. The clinical sequelae of intravascular hemolysis and extracellular plasma hemoglobin: a novel mechanism of human disease. *Jama*, 293(13): 1653-1662.

Rothschild, C. and D. Knowles. 2007. Equine piroplasmosis. In: Sellon, D. C. and Long, M. T. (eds.) *Equine Infectious Diseases*. Elsevier, St. Louis, MO, p.465-473.

Salama, A. A., Aboulaila, M., Moussa, A. A., Nayel, M. A., El-Sify, A. and M. A. Terkawi. 2013. Evaluation of in vitro and in vivo inhibitory effects of fusidic acid on Babesia and Theileria parasites. *Veterinary Parasitology*, 191:1–10.

Salama, A. A., Aboulaila, M., Terkawi, M. A., Mousa, A., El-Sify, A. and M. Allaam. 2014. Inhibitory effect of allicin on the growth of Babesia and *Theileria equi* parasites. *Parasitology Research*, 113:275–283.

Salem, N. Y. and M. A. El-Sherif. 2015. Malondialdehyde status, trace minerals and hematologic results of anemic - *T. equi* infected Egyptian horses. *International Journal of Veterinary Science*, 4 (3): 118-122.

Salib, F. A., Youssef, R. R., Rizk, L. G. and S. F. Said. 2013. Epidemiology, diagnosis and therapy of *Theileria equi* infection in Giza, Egypt. *Veterinary World*, 6 (2): 76-82.

Sandhu, G. S. 1998. *Histopathological, biochemical and hematological studies in cross-bred calves and hematological studies in cross bred calves*, M.V.Sc. Thesis, Punjab Agricultural University, Ludhiana.

Sanusi, M., Ahmed, I. A., Tahir, I., Mai, H. M., Kalla, D. J. U. and I. Shuaibu. 2014. Survey of equine piroplasmosis in savanna areas, Bauchi State, North-east Nigeria. *Ippologia-Cremona*, 25 (1): 3-8.

Schein, E., Rehbein, G. and W. P. Voigt, 1981. Babesia equi (Laveran 1901) 1. Development in horses and in lymphocyte culture. *Tropical Entomology and Medical Parasitology*, 32:223–227.

Schwint, O. N., Ueti, M. W. and G. H. Palmer. 2009. Imidocarb dipropionate clears persistent *Babesia caballi* infection with elimination of transmission potential. *Antimicrobial Agents and Chemotherapeutics*, 53: 4327–4332.

Scoles, G. A. and Ueti, M. W. 2015. Vector ecology of equine piroplasmosis. *Annual Review of Entomology*, 60: 561–580.

Sears, K. P., Kappmeyer, L. S., Wise, L. N., Silva, M., Ueti, M. W., White, S., Reif, K. E. and Knowles, D. P. 2019. Infection dynamics of *Theileria equi* and *Theileria haneyi*, a newly discovered apicomplexan of the horse. *Veterinary Parasitology*, 271: 68-75.

Sears, K., Knowles, D., Dinkel, K., Mshelia P. W., Onzere. C., Silva, M., Fry, L. 2020. Imidocarb Dipropionate Lacks Efficacy against Theileria haneyi and Fails to Consistently Clear Theileria equi in Horses Co-Infected with T. haneyi. *Pathogens,* 9(12): 1035.

Sellon, DC, Long, MT. 2014. 56/ Piroplasmosis. In: Wise LN, Knowles DP, Rothschild CM, *Equine Infectious Diseases*. 2 ed., Saunders Elsevier, China, p. 650.

Short, M. A., Clark, C. K., Harvey, J. W., Wenzlow, N., Hawkins, I. K., Allred, D. R., Knowles, D. P., Corn, J. L., Grause, J. F., Hennager, S. G. and Kitchen, D. L. 2012. Outbreak of equine piroplasmosis in Florida. *Journal of the American Veterinary Medical Association,* 240(5): 588-595.

Slifka, M. and R. Ahmed.1998. Long-lived plasma cells: a mechanism for maintaining persistent antibody production. *Current Opinion in Immunology*, 10: 252–258.

Sookoian, S. and C. J. Pirola. 2012. Alanine and aspartate aminotransferase and glutamine-cycling pathway: Their roles in pathogenesis of metabolic syndrome. *World Journal of Gastroenterology*, 18 (29): 3775-3781.

Sunday Idoko, Idoko, Tirosh-Levy, Sharon, Leszkowicz Mazuz, Monica, Adam, Babagana Mohammed, Garba, S., Nafarnda, D. W. and Steinman, A. 2020. Genetic Characterization of Piroplasms in Donkeys and Horses from Nigeria. *Animal*, 10 (324): 1-9.

Svendson, P., and A. M. Carter, 1984. *An Introduction to Animal Physiology.* 2nd Edn, MTP Press, Boston, USA, pp: 156-159.

Takeet, M. A, Ademola., I. O., Adejinmi, J. O., Mosaku, E. I., Abakpae, S. A. V. and Peters, S. O. 2020. Molecular Detection and Genetic Analysis of *Theileria equi* Detected in Apparently Healthy Horses in Nigeria. *Folia Veterinaria*, 64: 9 – 16.

Takeet, M., Adeleye, A., Adebayo, O. and F. Akande. 2009. Haematology and serum biochemical alteration in stress induced equine theileriosis. A case report. *Science World Journal,* 4: 19–21.

Tecles, F., Spiranelli, E., Bonfanti, U., Ceron, J. J. and S. Paltrileiri. 2005. Preliminary studies phase protein concentrations in hematologic and neoplastic diseases in dogs. *Journal of Veterinary Internal Medicine,* 19: 865–870.

Tenter, A. M., and K. T. Friedhoff. 1986. Serodiagnosis of experimental and natural *Babesia equi* and *B. caballi* infections. *Veterinary Parasitology*, 20: 49–61.

Terkawi, M. A., Alhasan, H., Huyen, N. X., Sabagh, A., Awier, K., Cao, S., Goo, Y. K., Aboge, G., Yokoyama, N., Nishikawa, Y., Kalb-Allouz, A. K., Tabbaa, D., Igarashi, I., and X. Xuan. 2012 Molecular and serological prevalence of *Babesia bovis* and *Babesia bigemina* in cattle from central region of Syria. *Veterinary Parasitology*, 187: 307-311.

Timoney, P. J. 2000. The increasing significance of international trade in equids and its influence on the spread of infectious diseases. *Annals of the New York Academy of Sciences*, *916*(1): 55-60.

Turaki, U. A., Kumsha, H. A., Biu, A. A. and Bokko, P. B. 2014. Prevalence of Piroplasmosis amongst local horses in Northeastern Nigeria. *IOSR Journal of Agriculture and Veterinary Science (IOSR-JAVS),* 7 (12; 4): 04-07.

Uchino, Y., Kawakita, T., Miyazawa, M., Ishii, T., Onouchi, H., Yasuda, K., Ogawa, Y., Shimmura, S., Ishii, N. and Tsubota, K. (2012). Oxidative stress induced inflammation initiates functional decline of tear production. *PLoS One*, 7.

Ueti, M. W., Mealey, R. H., Kappmeyer, L. S., White, S. N., Kumpula-McWhirter, N. and Pelzel, A. M. 2012. Re-emergence of the apicomplexan *Theileria equi* in the United States: elimination of persistent infection and transmission risk. *PLoS One,* 7:e44713.

Ueti, M. W., Palmer, G. H., Kappmeyer, L. S., Statdfield, M., Scoles, G. A.and Knowles, D. P. 2005. Ability of the vector tick Boophilus microplus to acquire and transmit Babesia equi following feeding on chronically infected horses with low-level parasitemia. *Journal of Clinical Microbiology*, 43: 3755–3759.

Ueti, M. W., Palmer, G. H., Scoles, G. A., Kappmeyer, L. S. and Knowles, D. P. 2008. Persistently infected horses are reservoirs for intrastadial tick-borne transmission of the apicomplexan parasite *Babesia equi*. *Infection and Immunity*,76 (8): 3525–3529.

Uilenberg, G. 2006. Babesia-A historical overview. *Veterinary Parasitology*, 138:3–10.

Vial, H. J. and A. Gurenflot. 2006. Chemotherapy against babesiosis. *Veterinary Parasitology*. 138:147-160.

Vimr, E. R., Kalivoda, K. A., Deszo, E. L. and S. M. Steenbergen. 2004. Diversity of microbial sialic acid metabolism, *Microbiology and Molecular Biology Reviews,* 68: 132–153.

Wessely-Szponder, J., Bełkot, Z., Bobowiec, R., Kosior-Korzecka, U. and M. Wójcik. 2015. Transport induced inflammatory responses in horses. *Polish Journal of Veterinary Sciences,* 18 (2): 407–413.

Wise, L. N., Kappmeyer, L. S., Mealey, R. H., and D. P. Knowles. 2013. Review of equine piroplasmosis. *Journal of Veterinary Internal Medicine,* 27: 1334–1346.

World Organisation for Animal Health (OIE). 2005. *Laboratory Criteria: OIE Manual of Standards for Diagnostic Tests and Vaccines for Terrestrial Animals 2008,* Chapter 2.5.8 (OIE, 2005).

World Organisation for Animal Health (OIE). 2008. *Equine Piroplasmosis (Equine Babesiosis, Equine Theileriosis, Biliary Fever).* August 29, 2008. Pp: 1-5.

World Organisation for Animal Health (OIE). 2014. *World Animal Health Information Database (WAHID).* www.oie.int/wahis_2/public/wahid.php.

World Organization for Animal Health (OIE). 2018. *OIE-Listed Diseases, Infections and Infestations In Force in 2018.*

Young, J. D., Wolowyk, M. W., Fincham, D. A., Cheeseman, C. I., Rabenstein, D. L. and J. C. Ellory. 1987 Conflicting evidence regarding the transport of alpha-glutamyl-dipeptides by human erythrocytes. *Biochemistry Journal*, 242:309–311.

Zapf, F., and E. Schein. 1994. The development of *Babesia (Theileria) equi* (Laveran, 1901) in the gut and the haemolymph of the vector ticks. *Hyalomma species. Parasitology Research*, 80: 297–302.

Zaugg, J. L. and Lane, V. M. 1992. Efficacy of buparvaquone as a therapeutic and clearing agent of Babesia equi of European origin in horses. *American Journal of Veterinary Research*, 53 (8):1396-1399.

Zobba, R., Ardu, M., Niccolini, S., Chessa, B., Manna, L., Cocco, R. and M. L. Pinna Parpaglia. 2008. Clinical and laboratory findings in equine piroplasmosis. *Journal of Equine Veterinary Science,* 28: 301–308.

Zygner, W., Gojska, O., Rapacka, G., Jaros, D. and H. Wędrychowicz, 2007. "Hematological changes during the course of canine babesiosis caused by large Babesia in domestic dogs in Warsaw (Poland)," *Veterinary Parasitology*, 145 (1-2):146–151.

Chapter 6

Parasitic Infections in Cattle in the Northeastern Part of the Province of Corrientes (Argentina)

Sergio Ivan Jorge Lobayan[1,*]
and Javier Hernán Schapiro[2,3]

[1] School of Veterinary Medicine,
Faculty of Agricultural and Veterinary Sciences,
University of Salvador (USAL), Corrientes, Argentina
[2] Institute of Pathobiology-IPVET, CICVyA,
National Institute of Agricultural Technology (INTA)
Castelar, Buenos Aires, Argentina
[3] School of Veterinary Medicine,
Faculty of Agricultural and Veterinary Sciences,
University of Salvador (USAL), Buenos Aires, Argentina

Introduction

The Argentine Republic has a total surface area of 4025695 km^2 (2795695 km^2 without the Argentine Antarctic), with a latitudinal range that goes from approximately 21°50' S to the pole and altitudes that vary from sea level to more than 7000 meters, which means that it has a wide range of climates and microclimates (Cabrera 1971).

This amplitude allows the existence of different eco-regions described by Cabrera (1971) and Burkart (1999), among which is the "*district of the fields*" comprising the northeast of the province of Corrientes, where plains

---

* Corresponding Author's Email: sergio.lobayan@usal.edu.ar.

In: Infectious and Parasitic Diseases of Animals in Developing Countries
Editor: Selwyn Arlington Headley
ISBN: 979-8-88697-504-8

grasslands predominate alternating with wooded areas, in an undulating relief in the north and flat in the south.

The climate in this region is humid subtropical with annual rainfall of around 1500 mm, uniform throughout the year, and the soils are lateritic, red, acidic, formed by fine particles (Cabrera 1971).

Natural grasslands and implanted pastures predominate in this region of the country, being most of the species that compose it of summer growth, with a very seasonal pattern of 7 months with strong regrowth from October to April and 5 months of little growth (Pizzio 2018).

Cattle ranching is mostly extensive in nature, with most production systems on pastoral systems.

The cattle stock of the Argentine Republic as of December 2020 was 54460799 heads, and that of the province of Corrientes was 4569387, corresponding to 8.3% of the national total (MAGyP 2020; SENASA 2021).

The province of Corrientes is the second most important cattle raising area in the country and the most important of the areas considered marginal.

Cattle raising activity is carried out on 686000000 hectares, which represents 75% of the provincial surface. The main activity is cattle breeding, even so, in the last years the activities of rebreeding and wintering of steers have been incorporated, especially in the fields of the south of the province.

The type of cattle in this region is predominantly zebu crossbred in different proportions, with a predominance of the synthetic breeds Braford and Brangus.

One of the factors that negatively affect cattle production is verminous gastroenteritis, caused by gastrointestinal nematodes. These are the most frequent parasites of grazing ruminants worldwide generating important economic losses in livestock production (Soulsby 1987, 241; Cordero del Campillo 1999, 237; Bowman 2011, 158; Caracostantogolo 2012, 135).

The importance of this is reflected by Steffan (2011) in the chapter: "*History and evolution of the main research and teaching groups in Veterinary Parasitology in Southern Latin America*" where he refers to the fact that in Argentina gastrointestinal parasitosis of ruminants constitute 18% of the thematic areas involved in research work.

Definition

Bovine verminous gastroenteritis is a parasitic disease produced by several species of nematodes located in the abomasum, small and large intestines. It can have an acute, subacute or chronic course, with low mortality and generally occurs in endemic processes. It affects mainly young animals, and is characterized by progressive emaciation, digestive disturbances, anemia and trophic disorders of the skin, producing serious economic damage to the livestock farm (Cordero del Campillo 1999, 237; Caracostantogolo 2012, 135).

Etiology

The most important genera and species of gastrointestinal nematodes in terms of their epidemiological involvement belong to the Class Nematoda and the Superfamily Trichostrongyloidea.

The most important species of each genus are: *Trichostrongylus colubriformis*, *T. axei*, *Ostertagia ostertagi*, *Haemonchus placei*, *Cooperia curticei*, *C. punctata*, *C. pectinata*, *C. oncophora*, *Nematodirus spathiger*, *N. fillicolis*, *N. helvetianus* and *Oesophagostomum radiatum* (Soulsby 1987, 140-211; Bowman 2011, 158-178; Caracostantogolo 2012, 32-41; Fiel 2013, 35-36).

Biological Cycle

The general life cycle of the Class Nematoda includes the stages of: egg, larva 1 (L_1), larva 2 (L_2), larva 3 (L_3), larva 4 (L_4), larva 5 (L_5) preadults that evolve into adult stages of separate sexes (Bowman 2011, 153; Caracostantogolo 2012, 31).

Regarding the characteristics of trichostrongylids, in the digestive tract the males fertilize the females and these eliminate blastomorphic eggs that go out into the environment with the fecal stool. There, an embryonation process takes place and after 24-48 hours the eggs hatch and the L_1 emerge, which then molt to L_2 and finally to L_3, keeping molt 2 as a protective sheath. The latter L_3 is the infective stage that emerges from the fecal stool by its own means, or by taking advantage of the dispersion caused by rainfall or trampling of animals, to go to the pastures in the vicinity of the depositions. Hosts ingest them and larval development continues in mucosa and gastrointestinal glands, where they molt to L_4, then emerge into the lumen of the digestive tract as L_5, adult male and female worms (Soulsby 1987, 185-238; Cordero del Campillo

1999, 238-252; Bowman 2011, 158-178; Caracostantogolo 2012, 32-41; Fiel 2013, 35-36).

Table 1. Anatomical location and biotic potential of gastrointestinal nematodes

Genus	Localization	Biotic potential
Haemonchus sp.	Abomasum	5000 to 15000
Ostertagia sp.	Abomasum	100 to 200
Trichostrongylus sp.	Abomasum and small intestine	100 to 200
Cooperia sp.	Small intestine	1000 to 3000
Nematodirus sp.	Small intestine	50 to 100
Oesophagostomum sp.	Small intestine	5000 to 10000

Adapted from: Soulsby (1987, 168 - 232) and Hansen (1994, 19).

The number of eggs produced by an adult female can be influenced by several factors: the number of adult parasites lodged in the organs, the male-female ratio, the level of immunity, age, the physiological state of the host, and the consistency of the faeces (Soulsby 1987, 241).

According to Armour (1980), "each female may expel several thousand eggs over her lifetime, which may vary from about four weeks to twelve months, establishing differences in the biotic potential of each genus of parasite due to differences in oviposition" (Cited in Fiel 2013, 35).

The anatomical location of trichostrongylid adult specimens in the digestive tract of hosts and the daily egg laying by adult and sexually mature females are observed in Table 1.

Epidemiology

Gastrointestinal nematodes are widely distributed where pastures constitute the food base of ruminants (Soca 2005), and are characterized by their close relationship with the environment and hosts, so this interdependence causes both generic and species diversity, or the density of populations to vary according to climate and farm management (Fiel 2013, 61).

Generally, gastrointestinal parasitic infections are mixed, involving two or more genera and several species, which explains the general denomination of "*verminous gastroenteritis*" (Cordero del Campillo 1999).

Climatic conditions determine the predominance of certain species in different areas of the country. In general terms, it can be established that

Ostertagia sp. and *Nematodirus* sp. are well adapted to cold climatic conditions, *Cooperia* sp. and *Trichostrongylus* sp. in temperate climates, while *Haemonchus* sp. and *Oesophagostomum* sp. develop favorably in warm climates (Fiel 2013, p. 36).

In the northeastern region of the province of Corrientes with a subtropical climate, cattle breeding activity predominates on permanent pastures, being these the favorable environmental conditions for the development of gastrointestinal nematodes throughout the year (Fiel 2005).

Most of the epidemiological studies carried out in this region were based on fecal egg counts and quantification and identification of L_3 from stool cultures.

Regarding parasitic genera in the northeastern region of Argentina, in chapter 4 of Fiel (2013, 93), Romero reviews studies based on coprology, where he observed a predominance of the genera *Haemonchus* sp. and *Cooperia* sp. over *Ostertagia* sp., *Oesophagostomum* sp. and *Trichostrongylus* sp.

Meanwhile, in a research work carried out in Mercedes (Corrientes) on calves from 4 to 6 months of age (Rosa 1973), the predominant parasitic genera, in decreasing order and through the coprocultures, were: *Cooperia* sp., *Oesophagostomum* sp., *Haemonchus* sp., *Ostertagia* sp. and *Trichostrongylus* sp.

In the survey conducted by Lobayan et al. (2016) on gastrointestinal nematodes in cattle in open pastoral systems in southern Misiones and northeastern Corrientes, the genera they were able to identify were: *Haemonchus* sp. (30%), *Trichostrongylus* sp. (26%), *Cooperia* sp. (24%) and *Oesophagostomum* sp. (20%).

In another study, conducted by Schapiro et al. (2018) in the province of Misiones in reference to the distribution of gastrointestinal nematode genera in both open grazing systems and under tree cover, they were able to identify the genera *Haemonchus* and *Cooperia* as the most prevalent, with values of 60% and 30% respectively, and in lower percentage *Oesophagostomum* with 10%.

Invariably, throughout the subtropical region, stool cultures establish *Haemonchus* sp. and *Cooperia* sp. as the predominant genera (Nari 1994).

Parasite load in hosts has a large individual variation, and sampling in general evidences a positive binomial positive curve, where few animals have high counts, while most have moderate, low or very low loads (Fiel 2013).

Rosa (1973) in his research study indicated that the average egg counts were 310, which was maintained in January, decreased at the end of February (average of 55), registered an increase in April (average of 156), and then fluctuated in values close to 100 eggs per gram of fecal matter.

In the egg counts on the total samples of the three years of study conducted by Lobayan et al. (2016), 70% were between 1 and 206 eggs per gram of fecal stool, 13% between 207 and 41, 3% with counts between 414 and 2090, and with 14% of animals with no egg shedding.

According to Suárez (1997) in cattle, the loads considered low would oscillate in egg counts lower than 245 and 146, moderate loads would not exceed 700 and 363 and high loads would exceed these figures respectively in cattle younger than one year and older than 18 months of age.

Based on the aforementioned studies, it could be considered that the parasite loads recorded are moderate in the extensive pastoral systems of northeastern Corrientes, even the egg counts in feces on some occasions could be overestimated, taking into account that the predominant genus was *Haemonchus* sp., which has a high biotic potential (Bowman 2011, 166).

Pathogenesis

Gastrointestinal nematodes cause pathophysiological alterations that lead to losses in productive parameters, especially in young animals (Rosa 2012).

Under natural conditions, several species of gastrointestinal nematodes coexist in the same host with different mechanisms of pathogenic action and localization in different sections of the gastrointestinal tract. The total pathogenic action, whose severity depends on the age of the animals and the intensity of the infection, is the sum of the pathogenic action of each of the species involved (Cordero del Campillo 1999, 245-246).

The genus *Haemonchus* sp. is located in the abomasum and, being hematophagous, can cause anemia (Vignau 2005, 104).

The genus *Trichostrongylus* sp. has species that parasitize the abomasum and small intestine, generally located deep in the epithelium and altering its functionality (Vignau 2005, 104).

The genus *Cooperia* sp. is found in the small intestine, they are not very pathogenic species that produce superficial lesions in the crypts of Lieberkühn, they feed on secretions and desquamated cells of the epithelium hindering the absorption of nutrients (Vignau 2005, 104).

In the genus *Oesophagostomum* sp. the adult stages produce a deep lesion in the mucosa of the large intestine when feeding on material of the lamina propria, the lesion in this stage is characterized by local inflammation with thickening of the mucosa and anemia due to hemorrhages (Vignau 2005, 105).

Immunity

There are somatic antigens, present in the body structures of gastrointestinal nematodes, and functional antigens, substances produced by the parasites during their parasitic life. Agglutination reactions with the formation of immune complexes in the mouth, vulva, cloaca and anus of nematodes hinder their penetration into tissues, feeding or reproduction, and alter the ability to copulate or posture in adult females (Vignau 2005, 112-113).

The immune response in young cattle manifests itself to a lesser degree, but they acquire a good immune response capacity (with assured nutrition and health) from 18 months of age (Fiel 2005).

Losses

Weaning calves are susceptible to gastrointestinal nematodes due to their lack of immunity, but due to management issues they are often exposed to pastures with high contamination and infectivity, resulting in the most damaged category of the herd (Meana Irigoyen 2000).

If pasture infection is very high, the animals develop clinical manifestations of parasitic gastroenteritis with severe weight losses (40-60 kg/animal), and in the most severe cases, even mortality. However, the usual presentation of the disease is subclinical - without symptoms - causing variable losses that can reach up to 20-40 kg/animal (Fiel 2005).

Currently, clinical parasitosis with death of animals has become sporadic, as a consequence of experience and a higher annual deworming regime. For this reason, bovine cattle production systems are affected by lower levels of parasitism, but which are expressed subclinically on weight gain and lower development of growing animals (Fiel 2014).

Bulman (2012, 108-110) describes the substantial economic losses caused by gastrointestinal nematodoses in cattle due to lack of or incorrect control, and in addition to the phenomenon of resistance to antiparasitics.

Diagnosis

Diagnosis is made on the basis of clinical data, epidemiological history and laboratory analysis (Cordero del Campillo 1999, 248).

Epidemiological studies of bovine gastrointestinal nematodosis can be based on quantitative coprology, stool cultures, pasture washings and parasitic necropsies (Ueno 1988; Cordero del Campillo 1999, 158-177; Bowman 2011, 295-371; Fiel 2011; Rosa 2012, 291-305).

To perform quantitative coprology, individual samples of 40 to 60 g of fecal stool are taken with polyethylene bags or gloves of the same material, introducing two fingers and rubbing the rectal ampulla using circular movements to stimulate defecation through the anal reflex (Ueno 1988; Hansen 1994; Gibbons 2011; Fiel 2011, 16-28; Rosa 2012, 291-305).

Each sample is given a gastrointestinal nematode egg count, which is expressed in eggs per gram of fecal matter using the modified McMaster technique (Roberts 1949; Ueno 1988; Hansen 1994; Gibbons 2011; Fiel 2011; Rosa 2012).

Coprocultures are performed to obtain L_3 using the technique of Corticelli and Lai (1963) or Henriksen and Korsholm (1983), and then identified and counted using the keys of Niec (1968) (Ueno 1988; Gibbons 2011; Fiel 2011, 30-49; Rosa 2012, 291-305).

Grass washing is used for L_3 recovery, quantification, and identification (Hansen 1994; Fiel 2011, 56-64).

Parasitic necropsy is used for counting and identification of adult nematode populations present in the gastrointestinal tract (Lukovich 1981; Ueno 1988; Hansen 1994; Fiel 2011; 66-88).

Data obtained from studies based on periodic slaughter of animals for parasitic necropsy are considered much more accurate, but due to the high cost of such studies, most information is obtained by fecal egg counts and stool cultures (Fiel 2005; Fiel 2013, 33).

Control

The control of verminous gastroenteritis can be carried out with chemical methods involving the administration of antiparasitic treatments, or with non-chemical methods such as grazing manipulation and proper management of grazing animals, or with integrated systems that include these two facets

(Soulsby 1987, 251; Caracostantógolo 2012, 141), in what is known as integrated management of parasitosis (Smith 1966).

The drugs currently used in cattle belong to the following groups: benzimidazoles and probenzimidazoles, imidazothiazoles, macrocyclic lactones, organophosphates, and salicylanides (Cordero del Campillo 1999, 249; Soulsby 1987, 248-249).

For many years the use of antiparasitics was the main tool used for the control of gastrointestinal nematodes, but the long-term sustainability of their use was affected by the emergence of anthelmintic resistance, toxicity and residuality of these chemicals (Waller 2003).

During the Technical Cooperation Project of the Food and Agriculture Organization of the United Nations (FAO) (PCT/RLA/2364) on anthelmintic resistance, developed in 1994-1995, 43% of the farms sampled in Argentina had gastrointestinal nematodes resistant to antiparasitic drugs. The results showed that in cattle, resistance was present in 60% of the herds studied and most of them (55%) were resistant to the ivermectin group (Caracostantogolo 2005).

This problem, far from diminishing, continued to advance, and so it is that in the study of prevalence of anthelmintic resistance carried out in the northeast of the province of Corrientes by Lobayan et al. (2017) it was found that resistance to ivermectin was 100%, and to benzimidazoles was 25% of the establishments surveyed. The resistant parasitic genera were *Haemonchus* sp. and *Cooperia* sp.

Total dependence on a single control method based on the use of anthelmintics in real production systems has proven to be unsustainable and inefficient in the medium and long term, mainly due to the appearance of antiparasitic resistance, so integrated parasite control is an adequate control tool to control parasite populations without affecting production levels (Rossanigo 2005).

The control tools used to date are insufficient, and this situation has stimulated the development of alternative or complementary control methods. Some of them are oriented towards the control of the parasites inside the animal and others, attacking the non-parasitic phases that develop in the environment (Saumell 2009).

Eradication of the disease from a field is impossible so far, so the key to control is to live with the disease without affecting the productivity of the animals. The key to efficient control of gastrointestinal worms is based on the use of antiparasitic treatments combined with adequate animal and pasture management (Fiel 2005).

It should be taken into account that epidemiological knowledge provides guidance on the trend of the evolution of verminous gastroenteritis in both animals and pastures in a given agroecological area. However, the establishment of common control programs for certain areas or regions does not seem to be an appropriate measure, since there may be nearby livestock farms with similar production plans, but with different parasitic problems (Steffan 2005).

It should also be taken into account that there are some observations that suggest that climate change is modifying the traditional patterns of presentation of gastrointestinal nematode infections, or at least is contributing, together with other factors, to the observed changes (Uriarte 2013).

Márquez Lara (2013) also lists a wide menu of control alternatives, some implemented and others under development so far, based on the epidemiology and population dynamics of these parasites, among which the following stand out: rational management of anthelmintics, pasture management, selection of resistant animals, biological control, use of pastures with concentrated tannins, etc.

In general, the use of anthelmintic treatments to avoid losses due to subclinical parasitosis is very frequent and is not subject to professional control, nor is a diagnosis made prior to treatment, and the choice of the antiparasitic obeys commercial reasons rather than the veterinarian's indication (Caracostantogolo 2005).

The role of the veterinarian is fundamental to preserve the useful life of the antiparasitic drugs in use, for which the methods of parasite control must necessarily take into account the local epidemiological characteristics together with the correct diagnosis of the parasitic situation of the herd in particular (Fiel 2013 b).

Silvopastoral Systems

Corrientes is the Argentine province with the largest area of implanted forests, about 450 thousand hectares (Ministry of Finance 2018) which can be taken as a competition for livestock or as a profit and diversification strategy, developing both productions combined in silvopastoral systems (Esquivel 2004).

Silvopastoral systems are a natural combination or a deliberate association of one or several woody components (shrubs and/or trees) within a pasture of grass and herbaceous legume species, native or cultivated, and their use with grazing animals (Combe 1979).

Implanted forestations contribute to mitigate the process of climate change, so that coexistence with livestock activity results in beneficial effects, among which we can highlight the natural control of gastrointestinal nematodoses (Soca 2000; Mendonca 2014; Schapiro 2018).

Conclusion

In 2011, Daniel Rearte wrote an article in the Latin American Association of Animal Production on the "current and prospective situation of Argentine livestock farming", in which he pointed out that the area devoted to livestock farming was considerably reduced (more than 15 million hectares) due to the growth of soybean crops. This scenario is repeated in other countries such as Uruguay, where cattle raising has ceded more than 900000 hectares per year to soybean cultivation, while only Brazil and Paraguay can show an increase in production from an increase in stock due to the possibility of expanding their cattle frontiers, but resorting to the clearing of forest areas.

This reduction in surface area is no longer temporary but permanent, since the area gained by agriculture is never returned to livestock farming.

In another article published by the Institute for the Promotion of Argentine Beef in 2021 under the title "*Livestock farming is not part of the problem, but part of the solution*", the challenge of sustainable meat production is raised, based above all on natural processes in harmony with nature, which is a strength and an opportunity because it requires little economic investment due to the fact that it is more associated with process technologies than with inputs.

In this context, the vast majority of Argentine livestock production has a low dependence on external inputs, since extensive breeding systems based on natural pastures require little or no input and use of agrochemicals and fertilizers, and feed that is not produced on the farm. For this reason, several of the management technologies to improve or sustain Argentine livestock production in these environments converge in the same direction.

In the socioeconomic study on the "*Causes that affect the adoption of technology in beef cattle farming in the province of Corrientes*" (Giancola 2013), it emerges that there is agreement on the importance of general sanitation and deworming, however, the diagnosis of the degree of parasitization through the use of egg counts in fecal matter and the rotation of deworming drugs do not seem to be prioritized among producers. Deworming is carried out systematically and periodically, at their discretion, and exceptionally it is implemented according to technical recommendations.

There are few producers who are informed about the technique of counting eggs in feces but do not do it due to logistic problems, and there is a concern about the lack of laboratories available in the area to perform this technique.

Therefore, the challenge for official research and extension institutions, university educational institutions and veterinarians working with livestock producers in this region is to bring these process technologies for the efficient management of bovine verminous gastroenteritis, and in this way, cattle ranching in Corrientes on pastoral systems will maintain a differential status in terms of environmental sustainability.

References

Armour, J. (1980). The epidemiology of helminth disease in farm animals. *Vet. Parasitol.*, 6, 7-46. https://doi.org/10.1016/0304-4017(80)90037-0.

Bowman, D. D. (2011). Georgis. *Parasitología para Veterinarios. Novena edición* [*Parasitology for Veterinarians*. Ninth edition]. Elsevier España S.L. 453 p. ISBN: 978-84-8086-705-4.

Bulman, M. G. (2012). Pérdidas económicas directas e indirectas por parásitos internos y externos de los animales domésticos en Argentina [*Direct and indirect economic losses due to internal and external parasites of domestic animals in Argentina*]. The Original Work was presented in a Special Session of the National Academy of Agronomy and Veterinary Medicine (Buenos Aires, Argentina), on May 29, 2012, and published in *ANALES, Volume LXVI*, 66, 76-176, 2012. http://sedici.unlp.edu.ar/bitstream/handle/10915/32935/Documento_completo.pdf?sequence=1.

Burkart, R., Bárbaro, N. O., Sánchez, R. O., and Gómez, D. A. (1999). *Eco-regiones de la Argentina* [*Eco-regions of Argentina*]. Environmental Education Component, Secretariat of Natural Resources and Sustainable Development. Presidency of the Nation. Compendium of the work on eco-regions prepared by the Secretariat of Natural Resources and Sustainable Development through the Environmental Institutional Program (PRODIA) and the National Parks Administration. ttps://sib.gob.ar/archivos/Eco_regiones_de_la_Argentina_1999.pdf.

Cabrera, A. L. (1971). *Fitogeografía de la República Argentina* [*Phytogeography of the Argentine Republic*]. Volúmen XIV, Noviembre 1971. N° 1-2. *Boletín de la Sociedad Argentina de Botánica.* 1-42. http://naturalis.fcnym.unlp.edu.ar/repositorio/_documentos/sipcyt/bfa003895.pdf.

Caracostantogolo, J., Castaño, R., Cutullé, C., Cetrá, B., Lamberti, R., Olaechea, F., Plorutti, F., Ruiz, M., Schapiro, J., Martínez, M., Balbiani, G., Castro, M., Morici, G., and y Eddi, C. (2005). Evaluación de la resistencia a los antihelmínticos en rumiantes en Argentina [*Evaluation of anthelmintic resistance in ruminants in Argentina*]. 7-34. In: *Resistencia a los antiparasitarios internos en Argentina*. FAO Animal Production and Health Study, Food and Agriculture Organization of the United Nations, Rome.

Caracostantogolo, J., Schapiro, J., Morici, G., Castaño Zubieta, R., and Martínez, M. (2012). Rumiantes. Gastroenteritis verminosa [*Ruminants. Verminous gastro-enteritis*]. In: Rosa A., Ribicich M. 2012. *Parasitología y enfermedades parasitarias en veterinaria*. Editorial Hemisferio Sur. 325 p. ISBN 978-950-504-618-8.

Combe, J., and G. Budowski G. (1979). Classification of agroforestry techniques: a literature review. In: G. de las Salas (ed.). *Workshop Agrofor. Systems Latin Amer. Turrialba, Costa Rica*. UNU/CATIE: pp 17-47. https://www.cabdirect.org/cabdirect/abstract/19806734178.

Cordero del Campillo, M., and Rojo, F. (1999). *Parasitología Veterinaria* [*Veterinary Parasitology*]. Editorial Mc Graw- Hill. España. 967 p. ISBN: 84-486-0236-6.

Corticelli, B., and Lai, M. (1963). Studies on the technique of culture of infective larvae of gastrointestinal strongyles of cattle. *Acta Med. Vet. Napoli*, 9, 347-357.

Esquivel, J., Fassola, H. E., Lacorte, S. M., Colcombet, L., Pachas, N., and Keller, A. (2004). Sistemas Silvopastoriles – Una sólida alternativa de sustentabilidad ambiental, económica y social [*Silvopastoral systems - A solid alternative for environmental, economic and social sustainability*]. 11as. *Jornadas Técnicas Forestales Y Ambientales*.7 – 9/ Octubre. UNaM FCF, INTA Montecarlo. Eldorado, Misiones, Argentina. https://aulavirtual.agro.unlp.edu.ar/pluginfile.php/80061/mod_resource/content/0/Clase_14_Sistemas_agroforestales/C7_Lacorte_Esquivel_Lectura.pdf.

Fiel, C. (2013b). *Parasitosis gastrointestinal de los bovinos: Epidemiología Control y Resistencia a Antihelmínticos* [*Gastrointestinal parasitosis of cattle: Epidemiology, Control and Anthelmintic Resistanc*]. Argentine Animal Production Site. https://www.produccion-animal.com.ar/sanidad_intoxicaciones_metabolicos/parasitarias/parasitarias_bovinos/53-Parasitosis_gastrointestinal.pdf.

Fiel, C. A. (2014). De norte a sur del país. Hay mucho por hacer [*From north to south of the country. There is much to do*]. In: *Ganadería y compromiso*. N° 75. Instituto de promoción de la carne vacuna argentina (IPCVA). http://www.ipcva.com.ar/files/gyc/75.pdf.

Fiel, C. A., and Nari, A. (2013a). *Enfermedades Parasitarias de importancia clínica y productiva en rumiantes. Fundamentos epidemiológicos para su prevención y control* [*Parasitic diseases of clinical and productive importance in ruminants. Epidemiological basis for their prevention and control*]. Editorial Agropecuaria Hemisferio Sur. 745 p. ISBN: 978-9974-674-35-6.

Fiel, C. A., Steffan, P., and Ferreyra, D. (2011). *Diagnóstico de las parasitosis más frecuentes en rumiantes: Técnicas de laboratorio e interpretación de resultados* [*Diagnosis of the most frequent parasitosis in ruminants: Laboratory techniques and interpretation of results*]. Ed: Área de Parasitología FCV-UNCPBA y Pfizer Sanidad animal. 131 p. ISBN 978-987-33-1502-2.

Fiel, C. A., Universidad del Centro de la Provincia de Buenos Aires. (2005). Parasitosis gastrointestinales de los bovinos: epidemiologia y control [*Gastrointestinal parasitosis of bovines: epidemiology and control*]. *XXXIII Uruguayan Conference on*

Buiatrics, Paysandú, Uruguay, 143-155. https://bibliotecadigital.fvet.edu.uy/bitstream/handle/ 123456789/321/JB2005_143-155.pdf?sequence=1&isAllowed=y.

Giancola, S., Calvo, S., Sampedro, D., Marastoni, A., Ponce, V., Di Giano, S., and Storti, M. (2013). Causas que afectan la adopción de tecnología en la ganadería bovina para carne de la provincia de Corrientes. Enfoque cualitativo [*Causes affecting technology adoption in beef cattle raising in the province of Corrientes. Qualitative approach*]. Ediciones INTA. *Socioeconomic Studies of Technology Adoption Series, (2).* ISSN: 2314-1727. ISBN: 978-987-679-212-7.

Gibbons, L. M., Jacobs, D. E., Fox, M. T., and Hansen, J. (2011). *La Guía RVC/FAO para el diagnóstico parasitológico veterinario. Examen fecal para determinación de helmintos parásitos* [*The RVC/FAO Guide for Veterinary Parasitological Diagnosis. Fecal examination for helminth parasite*]. https://www.rvc.ac.uk/Review/Parasitology_ Spanish/Index/Index.htm.

Hansen, J., and Perry, B. (1994). *The epidemiology, diagnosis and control of helminth parasites of ruminants. A handbook.* https://hdl.handle.net/10568/49809.

Henriksen, S. A., and Korsholm, H. (1983). A method for culture and recovery of gastrointestinal strongyle larvae. *Nordisk Veterinærmedicin,* 35(11), 429-430.

Instituto de promoción de la carne vacuna argentina (IPCVA). (2021). *Carne argentina, carne sustentable: La ganadería no es parte del problema, sino parte de la solución* [*Argentine beef, sustainable beef: Livestock farming is not part of the problem, but part of the solution*]. http://www.ipcva.com.ar/documentos/2402_1631020822_sustentabilidad.pdf.

Lobayan, S. I., Schapiro, J. H., Fiel, C. A., Zabalo, M. M. y Roselli, J. G. (2017). *Resistencia a los antihelmínticos en bovinos del nordeste de Corrientes (Argentina)* [*Anthelmintic resistance in cattle from northeastern Corrientes, Argentina*]. *Revista veterinaria*, 28(2), 138-140. https://revistas.unne.edu.ar/index.php/vet/article/view/2540.

Lobayan, S. I., Tuzinkievicz, T. M., Fiel, C. A., Nápoli, J. N., and Dalzotto, A. P. (2016). Relevamiento de nematodes gastrointestinales en bovinos del sur de Misiones y nordeste de Corrientes (Argentina) [*Identification of gastrointestinal nematodes in cattle in southern Misiones and northeastern Corrientes, Argentina*]. *Revista veterinaria*, 27(2), 137-140. https://revistas.unne.edu.ar/ index.php/ vet/issue/view/142/showToc.

Lukovich, A. (1981). *Identificación de las formas adultas de los nematodos gastrointestinales y pulmonares de los rumiantes en la República Argentina* [*Identification of adult forms of gastrointestinal and pulmonary nematodes of ruminants in Argentina*]. INTA-Castelar. 24 p.

Márquez Lara, D. A., and Pallares, J. (2003). *Epidemiología y control del parasitismo gastrointestinal en bovinos* [*Epidemiology and control of gastrointestinal parasitism in cattle*]. Colombian Agricultural Research Corporation – AGROSAVIA PNDA. http://hdl.handle.net/20.500.12324/1615.

Meana Irigoyen, G. R., Lützelschwab, C., and Fiel, C. A. (2000). La epidemiología como base para el control de los nemátodes gastrointestinales del bovino [*Epidemiology as a basis for the control of gastrointestinal nematodes in cattle*]. In: *Sitio Argentino de*

Producción Animal. https://www.produccion-animal.com.ar/sanidad_intoxicaciones_metabolicos/parasitarias/parasitarias_bovinos/18-epidemiologia_como_base.pdf

Mendonca, R. M. A., Leite, R. C., Lana, A. M. Q., Costa, J. O., and Toth, G. (2014). Parasitic helminth infection in young cattle raised on silvopasture and open-pasture in Southeastern Brazil. *Agroforestry Systems*, 88(1), 53-62. https://link.springer.com/article/10.1007/s10457-013-9655-4.

Ministerio de Agricultura, Ganadería y Pesca (MAGyP). República Argentina. 2020. *Informe Serie Stock Bovina a Diciembre 2020* [*Bovine Stock Series Report to December 2020*]. https://www.magyp.gob.ar/sitio/areas/bovinos/informacion_interes/informes/.

Ministerio de Hacienda. Presidencia de la Nación. República Argentina. (2018). *Informes productivos provinciales: Corrientes* [*Provincial production reports: Corrientes*]. Secretariat for Economic Policy Undersecretary for Microeconomic Programming (SSPMicro). https://www.argentina.gob.ar/sites/default/files/sspmicro_informes_ productivos_provinciales_corrientes.pdf.

Nari, A., and Fiel, C. A. (1994). *Enfermedades Parasitarias de Importancia Económica en Bovinos. Bases epidemiológicas para su prevención y control en Argentina y Uruguay* [*Parasitic Diseases of Economic Importance in Cattle. Epidemiological basis for their prevention and control in Argentina and Uruguay*]. Editorial Hemisferio Sur Uruguay. 519 p. ISBN: 9974-556-89-9.

Niec, R. (1968). Cultivo e identificación de larvas infectantes de nematodes gastrointestinales del bovino y ovino [*Culture and identification of infective larvae of gastrointestinal nematodes of cattle and sheep*]. *Manual técnico No° 3*. INTA-Argentina. 1-37.

Pizzio, R. M., Bendersky, D., Barbera, P., and Maidana, C. E. (2018). *Caracterización y manejo de los pastizales correntinos* [*Characterization and management of correntine grasslands*]. Ediciones INTA. https://inta.gob.ar/sites/default/files/inta_caracterizacion_y_manejo_de_los_pastizales_correntinos.pdf.

Rearte, D. (2011). Situación actual y prospectiva de la ganadería argentina, un enfoque regional [*Current and prospective situation of Argentine livestock farming, a regional focus*]. ISSN 1022-1301. 2011. *Latin American Association of Animal Production.* Vol 19, número 3-4, 46-49. https://produccion-animal.com.ar/informacion_tecnica/origenes_evolucion_y_estadisticas_de_la_ganaderia/121-rearte.pdf.

Roberts, F. H. S., and O'Sullivan, P. J. (1949). Methods for Egg Counts and Larvae Cultures for Strongyles Infesting the Gastro-Intestinal Tract of Cattle. *Aust J Agr Res*, 1, 99-102. https://doi.org/10.1071/AR9500099.

Romero, J., Anziani, O., Cetrá, B., and Fiel, C. A. Capítulo 4: Epidemiología e impacto productivo dc ncmatodos en la región del NEA [*Epidemiology and productive impact of nematodes in the NEA region*]. 89-112. 2013. In: Fiel C. A., Nari A. 2013. *Enfermedades Parasitarias de importancia clínica y productiva en rumiantes. Fundamentos epidemiológicos para su prevención y control.* Editorial Agropecuaria Hemisferio Sur. 745 p. ISBN: 978-9974-674-35-6.

Rosa, A., and Ribicich, M. (2012). *Parasitología y enfermedades parasitarias en veterinaria* [*Parasitology and parasitic diseases in veterinary medicine*]. Editorial Hemisferio Sur. 325 p. ISBN 978-950-504-618-8.

Rosa, W., Niec, R., Lukovich, R., Dindart, J., and Barberan, R. (1973). *Etiología y variación estacional del parasitismo gastrointestinal de los ovinos y bovinos en la zona de Mercedes (Provincia de Corrientes)* [*Etiology and seasonal variation of gastrointestinal parasitism in sheep and cattle in the area of Mercedes, (Province of Corrientes)*]. *Revista de Investigaciones Agropecuarias* (RIA), 10 (1), 25- 40.

Rossanigo, C. (2005). Control integrado de parásitos como herramienta para prevenir la resistencia antiparasitaria: evaluación de un sistema de bajo riesgo en invernada [*Integrated pest control as a tool to prevent pest resistance: evaluation of a low-risk system in winter grazing*]. *FAO Magazine Animal Production and Health. Study. Resistance to internal antiparasitics in Argentina*, 74, 79-87.

Saumell, C., Fusé, L., Iglesias, L., Steffan, P., and Fiel, C. (2009). Alternativas adicionales al control químico de nematodes gastrointestinales en animales domésticos [*Additional alternatives to chemical control of gastrointestinal nematodes in domestic animal*]. *Vet Arg*, 21, 80-84.

Schapiro, J., and Pantiu, A. (2018). Capítulo 2: Manejo sostenible del parasitismo gastrointestinal en bovinos en sistemas silvopastoriles [*Sustainable management of gastrointestinal parasitism in cattle in silvopastoral systems*]. 67-85. In: *El suelo como reactor de los procesos de regulación funcional de los agroecosistemas*. Editors: Jorge Ullé and Beatrice M. Diaz. Special issue for the *VII Latin American Congress of Agroecology*. October 2 to 5, Guayaquil, Ecuador. INTA Editions. Collection: Research, Development and Innovation. https://inta.gob.ar/sites/default/files/intasp_ulle_diaz_ed_el_suelo_como_reactor_socla_2018_v5.pdf

Servicio Nacional de Sanidad Animal, República Argentina (SENASA). 2021. *Estadísticas bovinas* [*Bovine statistics*]. http://www.senasa.gob.ar/cadena-animal/bovinos-y-bubalinos/informacion/informes-y-estadisticas.

Smith, R. F., and Reynolds, H. T. (1966). Principles, definitions and scope of integrated pest control. In: *Proc. FAO Symp. Integrated Pest Control*. Roma, Italia, FAO-UN, p. 11-17.

Soca, M., Roque, E., and Soca, M. (2005). Epizootiología de los nematodos gastrointestinales de los bovinos jóvenes [*Epizootiology of gastrointestinal nematodes in young cattle*]. *Pastos y Forrajes* [online]. 2005, 28 (3), 175-185 [Sept. 6, 2021]. ISSN: 0864-0394.

Soca, M., Simón, L., and Francisco, A. G. (2000). Comportamiento de las nematodosis gastrointestinales de bovinos jovenes en un sistema silvopastoril [*Behavior of gastrointestinal nematodes in young cattle in a silvopastoral system*]. *Pastos y Forrajes*, 23(4).

Soulsby, E. J. L. (1987). *Parasitología y enfermedades parasitarias en los animales domésticos* [*Parasitology and parasitic diseases in domestic animals*]. 7a ed. México: Interamericana. 823 p. ISBN 968-25-7371-5.

Steffan, P. E., Fiel, C. A., and Entrocasso, C. M. (Eds). (2011). Historia y Evolución de los Principales Grupos de Investigación y Enseñanza en Parasitología Veterinaria del Sur de América Latina, 23rd [*History and Evolution of the Main Research and Teaching Groups in Veterinary Parasitology in the South of Latin America, 23rd International Conference on Veterinary Parasitology, 23rd International Conference on Veterinary Parasitology, 23rd International Conference on Veterinary Parasitology*]. In:

International Conference of the World Association for the Advancement of Veterinary Parasitology, Towards good management practices in parasite control, Buenos Aires, Argentina, 21-25 August 2011, AAPAVET, Editorial: Tandil: Grupo Tandilia, 166 p. ISBN 978-987-27154-0-3.

Steffan, P. E., Fiel, C. A., Saumell, C., Fusé, C., and Iglesias, L. (2005). El uso de antihelmínticos en los programas de control y el riesgo potencial de resistencia [*The use of anthelmintics in control programs and the potential risk of resistance*]. *FAO, Resistencia a los antiparasitarios internos en Argentina*, 85-94.

Suárez, V. H. (1997). Diagnóstico de las parasitosis internas de los rumiantes en la región de invernada, interpretación y técnicas [*Diagnosis of internal parasitosis in ruminants in the wintering region, interpretation and techniques*]. *Boletín de divulgación técnica (INTA)*. P. 56.

Ueno, H., and Gonçalves, P. C. (1988). *Manual para diagnóstico das helmintoses de ruminantes* [*Manual for the diagnosis of ruminant helminths*]. Vol. 166. 4° Ed. Japan International Cooperation Agency, Tokyo. https://www1.ibb.unesp.br/Home/ Departamentos/Parasitologia/eventos3779/helmintologia/manual_helmintoses_ueno.pdf.

Uriarte Abad, J. y Calvete Margolles, C. (2012). *El cambio climático modifica la epidemiología de los nematodos gastrointestinales* [*Climate change modifies gastrointestinal nematode epidemiology*]. Unidad de Sanidad Animal. Centro de Investigación y tecnología Agroalimentaria de Aragón, Zaragoza. https://citarea.cita-aragon.es/citarea/bitstream/10532/2064/1/2012_262.pdf.

Vignau, M. L., Venturini, L. M., Romero, J. R., Eiras, D. F., and Basso, W. U. (2005). *Parasitología práctica y modelos de enfermedades parasitarias en los animales domésticos* [*Practical parasitology and models of parasitic diseases in domestic animals*]. 1° Edición, Facultad de Ciencias Veterinarias, Universidad Nacional de La Plata. 195 p. ISBN: 987-43-9225-8 http://meran.fcv.unlp.edu.ar/meran/opac-detail.pl?id1=1632#.YYJqXtLMLIU

Waller, P. J. (2003). Global perspectives on nematode parasite control in ruminant livestock: the need to adopt alternatives to chemotherapy, with emphasis on biological control. Final Proceedings of FAO Technical Cooperation Project in Malaysia TCP/MAL/0065 (T) 2002. *Animal Health Research Reviews*., 4 (1), 35-44.

Chapter 7

Neosporosis in Livestock Ruminants from South America

Luiz Daniel de Barros*
Fernando de Souza Rodrigues
and João Luis Garcia
Department of Preventive Veterinary Medicine,
Laboratory of Animal Protozoology,
State University of Londrina, Londrina, PR, Brazil

Introduction

Neosporosis is an infectious disease caused by *Neospora caninum*, a protozoan parasite with worldwide distribution (Dubey et al. 2017). Canids, including domestic dogs (*Canis familiaris*), Australian dingoes (*Canis lupus dingo*), coyotes (*Canis latrans*), and gray wolves (*Canis lupus*), are the only definitive hosts for *N. caninum* so far (Dubey et al. 2011; Gondim et al. 2004; King et al. 2010; McAllister et al. 1998). However, the parasite is able to infect different animals, including ruminants and avian species (de Barros et al. 2018; 2020; Dubey and Schares 2011). In humans, many studies have shown seropositivity against *N. caninum* (Duarte et al. 2020; Abo-Shehada et al. 2021). However, the DNA of the parasite was recently detected in the umbilical cord blood, indicating the zoonotic potential (Duarte, Oshiro, et al. 2020). Still, parasite isolation from human tissues is necessary to confirm *N. caninum* as a zoonotic parasite.

---

* Corresponding Author's Email: ldbarros@uel.br.

In: Infectious and Parasitic Diseases of Animals in Developing Countries
Editor: Selwyn Arlington Headley
ISBN: 979-8-88697-504-8

The disease can be critical in dogs and livestock, leading mainly to neuromuscular and reproductive disorders respectively (Silva and Machado 2016; Dubey et al. 2017). In cattle, neosporosis is responsible for an estimated loss of over USD $1 billion annually, with two-thirds related to the dairy industry (Reichel et al. 2013). The infection can also cause reproductive failure in sheep and goats; however, the economic impact is still unknown (González-Warleta et al. 2014; Campero et al. 2018; Hecker et al. 2019). Buffaloes are susceptible to *N. caninum* infection since serological response and isolation of the parasite have already been described, but the importance of *N. caninum* as an abortive agent remains uncertain (Reichel et al. 2015; de Barros et al. 2020). Based on these, this chapter aims to overview the current knowledge of neosporosis in livestock ruminants.

Life Cycle and Epidemiology

Neospora caninum has three different biological forms: tachyzoites, bradyzoites, and sporozoites, and all of them are infective to the intermediate and definitive hosts (Dubey et al. 2017). Tachyzoites and bradyzoites are intracellular parasites found in tissues from the intermediate hosts. Tachyzoites are around 6 × 2 μm, with an oval or round shape, and multiply quickly inside nucleated cells, causing cellular death and dissemination of the infection. In contrast, bradyzoites are approximately 7 × 2 μm in size, involved by a rounded thick-walled cyst up to 107 μm in diameter, and multiply slowly, being present in the chronic infection. These tissue cysts are found mainly in the central nervous system and muscles (Dubey et al. 2004; Dubey, Schares, and Ortega-Mora 2007).

Sporozoites are elongated at approximately 7.5 × 2.5 μm and present in the sporulated oocysts. The oocysts, shed in the environment by the definitive host as unsporulated oocysts, become infective after 24 to 72 h of sporulation (Dubey, Schares, and Ortega-Mora 2007). Sporulated oocysts comprise eight sporozoites in two sporocysts each, are spherical, measuring 10-12 μm in diameter, and are resistant in the environment in temperatures up to 60°C (McAllister et al. 1998; Silva and Machado 2016; Lindsay and Dubey 2020; Alves Neto et al. 2011).

Neospora caninum has a heteroxenous life cycle, with canids acting as definitive hosts and mammals and birds as intermediate hosts (Dubey et al. 2017). Figure 1 shows the life cycle of *N. caninum*. The parasite is transmitted horizontally or vertically. While the first occurs postnatally by ingestion of food/water contaminated with sporulated oocysts or raw/undercooked meat contaminated with tissue cysts. The second occurs by the transplacental transmission of tachyzoites to a fetus during pregnancy (Dubey, Schares, and Ortega-Mora 2007). Nowadays, there are two widely accepted concepts of vertical transmission: exogenous and endogenous transplacental transmission. Exogenous transmission is characterized by infection of the offspring after the first infection of the dam by sporulated oocysts. Otherwise, endogenous transmission occurs when a chronically infected dam has a recrudescence of infection (Williams et al. 2009; Trees and Williams 2005).

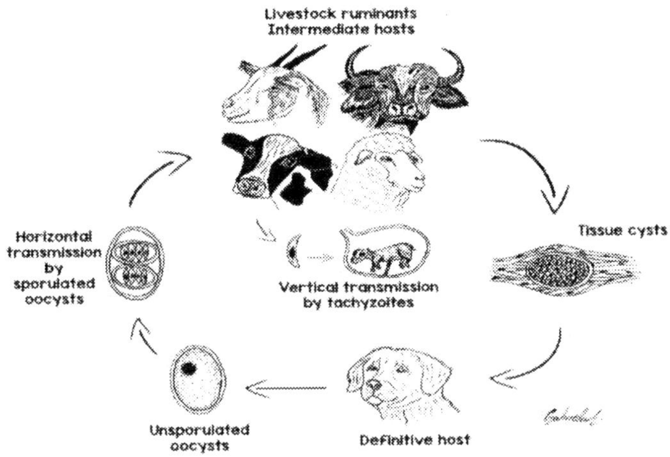

Source: G.A.F. Silva.

Figure 1. Life cycle of *Nespora caninum*.

Vertical transmission is the main route of infection in cattle, with the efficiency estimated at more than 95% (Davison, Otter, and Trees 1999). However, although transplacental is very efficient in cattle, a mathematical modeling study showed that horizontal transmission is necessary for the parasite to persist in the herd (French et al. 1999). Recently, transplacental transmission of *N. caninum* in successive pregnancies of sheep was described, showing that recrudescence of the infection in these species can also occur (Pereira et al. 2021; González-Warleta et al. 2018). Detection of *N. caninum* in semen from bulls has already been described (Ortega-Mora et al. 2003; Ferre et al. 2005); however, venereal transmission is unlikely since an experimental study showed that intrauterine infection occurs using contaminated semen with a high dose of tachyzoites, which is not found from naturally infected bulls (Serrano-Martínez et al. 2007; Ferre et al. 2005). Similarly, calves can be infected by milk, but this route has no epidemiological importance in neosporosis (Davison et al. 2001).

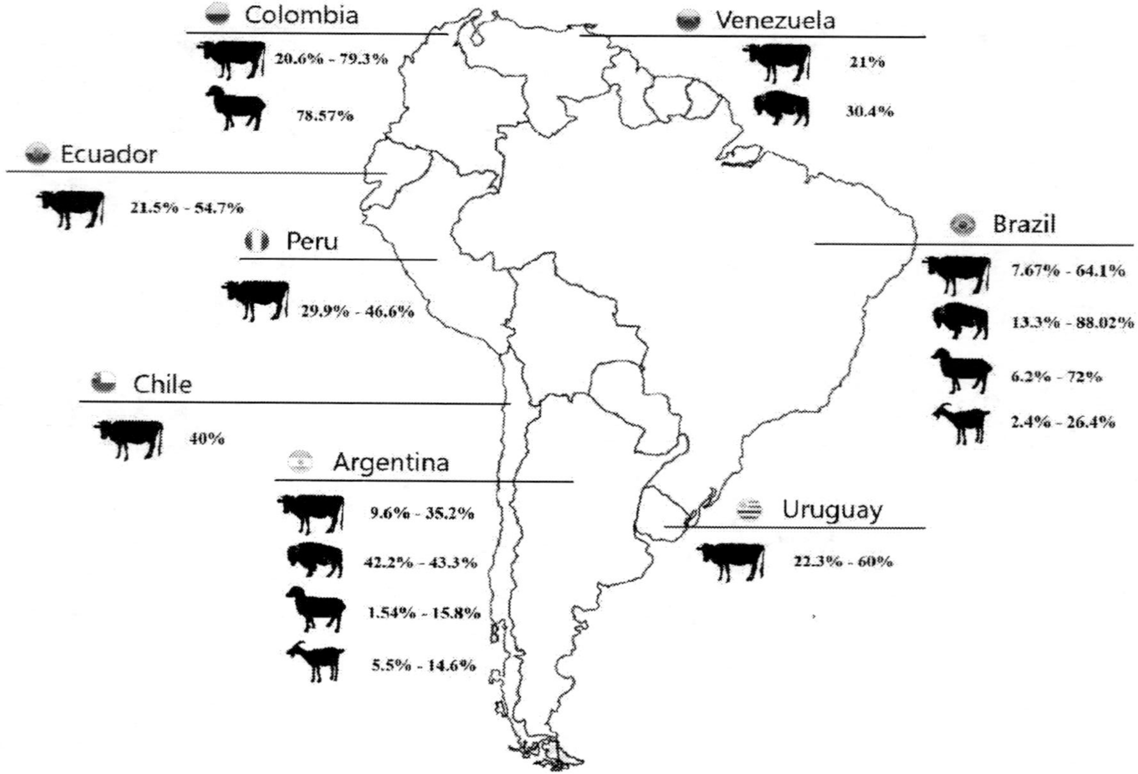

Figure 2. Seroprevalence rates of *Neospora caninum* in livestock ruminants from developing countries in South America.

Table 1. Seroprevalence studies of *Neospora caninum* in cattle from South America

Country	Region	Animals	Number of animals tested	Positive animals (%)	Test	Cut-off	Reference
Argentina	La Pampa	Beef and dairy cattle	4,334	417 (9.6%)	ELISA[a]	n.a.[c]	Fort et al. 2015
Brazil	Amazonas	Beef and dairy cattle	1,073	324 (30,2%)	IFAT[b]	200	Filho et al. 2021
	Mato Grosso	Beef and dairy cattle	2,452	624 (25.44%)	IFAT	100	Schmidt et al. 2018
	Pará	Dairy and beef cows	3,428	503 (14.7%)	IFAT	100	Chiebao et al. 2015
	Paraná	Dairy cows	600	142 (23.67%)	IFAT	100	Snak et al. 2018
	Rio Grande do Sul	Dairy cows	1273	305 (24%)	IFAT	100	Pessoa et al. 2016
	Rondônia	Dairy cattle	416	197 47.36%	IFAT	200	Venturoso et al. 2021
	Santa Catarina	Dairy cows	1518	466 (30.69%)	IFAT	100	Fávero et al. 2017
Chile	O 'Higgins	Dairy cows	45	18 (40%)	ELISA	n.a.	Hervé-Claude et al. 2017
Colombia	Antioquia	Dairy cattle	1,038	294 (28.3%)	ELISA	n.a.	Llano et al. 2018
Ecuador	Sierra	Dairy cows	841	197 (23.4%)	ELISA	n.a.	Maldonado Rivera et al. 2020
Peru	Lima	Dairy cattle	3,407	1,018(29.9%)/ 1,023(31%)	IFAT/ ELISA	200/n.a.	Serrano-Martínez et al. 2018
Uruguay	Salto, Paysandú, Río Negro, Soriano, Colonia, San José, Flores, Durazno, Florida, and Canelones	Dairy cows	4,223 cows	942 (22.3%)	ELISA	n.a.	Macchi et al. 2020
Venezuela	Guárico	Beef and dairy cattle	890	187 (21%)	ELISA	n.a.	Pinilla León and Da Silva Borges 2018

[a] Enzyme-linked immunosorbent assay.
[b] Indirect fluorescent antibody test.
[c] not applied.

Many studies have been published describing the seroprevalence of *N. caninum* in livestock worldwide in the last years. The average worldwide seroprevalence of neosporosis is estimated at 20% for cattle and 5.99% for goats, with the highest prevalence in the American continent (Ribeiro et al. 2019; Rodrigues et al. 2020). In buffaloes, the seroprevalence ranges from 0% to 88.3% (reviewed by de Barros et al. 2020), and in sheep, from 0% to 64% (reviewed by Dubey et al. 2017). Once serologic techniques, cut-off, antigens, and sample size can be different in each study, it is difficult to compare these results (Cerqueira-Cézar et al. 2017; Dubey et al. 2017).

Table 2. Seroprevalence studies of *Neospora caninum* in buffalo from South America

Country	Region	Number of animals tested	Positive animals (%)	Test	Cut-off	References
Argentina	North East	1,350	584 (43.3%)	IFAT[a]	100	Moore et al. 2014
Brazil	Maranhão	338	93 (27.5%)	IFAT	100	Rodrigues et al. 2022
	Pernambuco	345	122 (35.4%)	IFAT	100	Oliveira et al. 2018
Venezuela	Zulia	174	53 (30.4%)	ELISA[b]	n.a.[c]	Valbuena-Carson et al. 2013

[a]Indirect fluorescent antibody test.
[b]Enzyme-linked immunosorbent assay.
[c]not applied.

Table 3. Seroprevalence studies of *Neospora caninum* in sheep from South America

Country	Region	Number of animals tested	Positive animals (%)	Test	Cut-off	References
Argentina	Santa Fe and Entre Ríos	385	55 (14.3%)/ 61 (15.8%)	IFAT[a]/ ELISA[b]	50/ n.a.[c]	Novoa et al. 2020
Brazil	Minas Gerais	488	64 (13.1%)	IFAT	50	da Silva Andrade et al. 2012
	Paraná	1,607	283 (17.6%)	ELISA	n.a.	Romanelli et al. 2021
	Rio de Janeiro	388	24 (6.2%)	ELISA	n.a.	Cosendey et al. 2018
	Rio Grande do Sul	1,800	332 (18.44%)	IFAT	50	Romanelli et al. 2020
	Rondônia	616	373 (60.6%)	IFAT	50	Maia et al. 2021
Colombia	Córdoba	22	28 (78.57%)	ELISA	n.a.	Patarroyo et al. 2013

[a]Indirect fluorescent antibody test.
[b]Enzyme-linked immunosorbent assay.
[c]not applied.

In countries in South America, the disease is responsible for a huge economic impact. In Argentina, the economic loss is estimated at US $87.4

million per annum, while in Brazil, it is estimated at US $513 million per annum (Reichel et al. 2013). Tables 1-4 show all the seroprevalence studies of *N. caninum* in livestock from developing countries in South America in the last years, while Figure 2 shows the seroprevalence ranges.

Table 4. Seroprevalence studies of *Neospora caninum* in goats from South America

Country	Region	Number of animals tested	Positive animals (%)	Test	Cut-off	References
Argentina	Santa Fe and Entre Ríos	1,449	187 (12.9%)/ 212 (14.6%)	IFAT[a]/ ELISA[b]	50 /n.a.[c]	Novoa et al. 2020
Brazil	Maranhão	382	101 (26.4%)	IFAT	100	Rodrigues et al. 2021
	Minas Gerais	667	71 (10.7%)	IFAT	50	Andrade et al. 2013
	Paraná	629	39 (6.2%)	ELISA	n.a.	Romanelli et al. 2020
	Santa Catarina	654	30 (4.58%)	IFAT	50	Topazio et al. 2014

[a]Indirect fluorescent antibody test.
[b]Enzyme-linked immunosorbent assay.
[d] not applied.

Risk factors for *Neospora* infection in livestock have been extensively studied over the years. In general, the seroprevalence in adults is more elevated than in young animals, probably due to higher exposure time (de Souza et al. 2022; Selim, Khater, and Almohammed 2021). The presence of farm dogs was classified as a risk factor for neosporosis in livestock in many studies (Fávero et al. 2017; Ribeiro et al. 2019; Rodrigues et al. 2020). It is an expected finding since canids are the definitive hosts and may shed oocysts that will contaminate the environment; however, other studies have not found an association between the presence of dogs and infection in cattle, which reinforces the importance of endogenous transmission (de Souza et al. 2022). Other risk factors described are feeding dogs with placental, dogs with access to feed shed, contact with fomites, the low hygienic status of the farm, low altitude, season (spring and autumn), low milk production, and extensive breeding (Romanelli et al. 2021; de Souza et al. 2022; Arlan Araujo Rodrigues et al. 2022; Snak et al. 2018; Wei et al. 2022).

Regarding the reproductive parameters, most studies have detected an association between abortion and *N. caninum* infection in cattle. A meta-analysis study showed that seropositive cows were 1.6 times more likely to abort than seronegative (Ribeiro et al. 2019). Cows with many calvings also have a higher risk of infection (Wei et al. 2022). De Souza et al. (2022) evaluated reproductive factors such as placenta retention, abortion, and the birth of weak calves, although only abortion was statistically associated with *N. caninum* seropositivity. However, metritis and stillbirth were associated with seropositivity in dairy cows from Iran (Gharekhani and Yakhchali 2019)

Other studies showed that the number of inseminations to cows become pregnant and the birth interval is higher in seropositive cows (Villa et al. 2022; Lefkaditis et al. 2020). Even in a closed herd, neosporosis affects the reproductive performance of dairy cows (de Barros et al. 2021). The importance of *N. caninum* infection in other livestock remains uncertain; however, recent studies demonstrated an association between seropositivity and history of abortion in sheep and goats (Arlan Araujo Rodrigues et al. 2022; 2020). Although reproductive disorders appear to be less common in buffaloes than in cattle, previous studies described a higher seroprevalence of *N. caninum* in buffalo with a history of abortion and retained fetal membranes (de Barros et al. 2020; Ciuca et al. 2020).

Pathogeny and Clinical Signs

After horizontal infection, the sporozoites are excysted in the gastrointestinal tract and are disseminated to different organs through lymph and blood. Multiplication of tachyzoites in infected organs can cause necrosis and inflammation. Then, with the development of immune response, the parasite differentiates into bradyzoites and forms tissue cysts, mainly in neural and muscular tissues (Dubey et al. 2017).

The main concern about *Neospora* infection is related to pregnant animals since tachyzoites can cross the placental barrier and cause the fetus's infection (called congenital infection), which could lead to reproductive disorders (Dubey, Schares, and Ortega-Mora 2007). The congenital infection occurs by exogenous or endogenous transmission, as mentioned above. The first one usually leads to epidemic abortions, a term employed when the abortion outbreak is short, and at least 15% of dam abort within four weeks. The second one leads to endemic abortions and is related to the reactivation of the infection (Dubey et al. 2017; McAllister et al. 1996).

During pregnancy, pro-inflammatory cytokines, such as IL-2 and IFN-γ, are in low concentrations in the maternal-fetal interface, which helps to maintain the gestation. However, it contributes to parasite proliferation, leading to the recrudescence of infection and transplacental transmission (Innes et al. 2002). Consequently, *N. caninum* causes necrosis in maternal and fetal tissues, leading to an inflammatory response and the clinical signs of infection (Buxton, McAllister, and Dubey 2002).

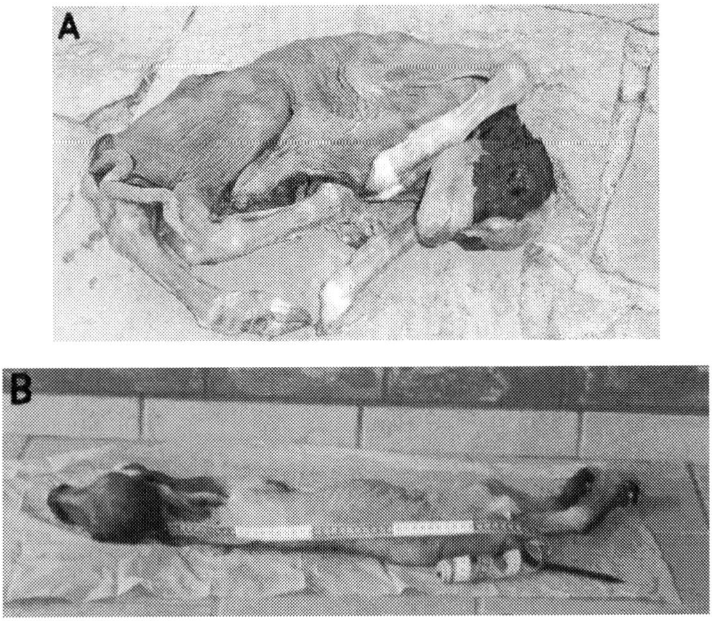

Source: C.A.B. de Macedo and J.L. Garcia.

Figure 3. Reproductive disorders of *Neospora caninum* in livestock ruminants. (A. Mummified fetus; B. Aborted fetus).

Infections in cattle are usually asymptomatic, while reproductive disorders are the main clinical manifestation in pregnant cows (Figure 3). Abortion, usually between 5-8 months of gestation, is the main sign of infection. Other reproductive disorders include fetal reabsorption, impaired calves with neuromuscular alterations such as limb flexion and hyperextension, ataxia, and decreased patellar reflexes (McAllister 2016; Dubey et al. 2017; Dubey and Schares 2011).

Diagnosis

Indirect or direct techniques are employed for the laboratory diagnosis of neosporosis in livestock. The main techniques include serology, histology, immunohistochemistry (IHC), molecular detection, and bioassay.

The serological diagnostic is applied to detect specific antibodies against *N. caninum,* mainly the IgG class, which is at higher levels after six months of infection (Goodswen, Kennedy, and Ellis 2013). There are many techniques available nowadays; however, indirect fluorescent antibody test (IFAT) and enzyme-linked immunosorbent assay (ELISA) are the main methods used worldwide (Francine Alves Sinnott et al. 2017).

IFAT, considered the gold standard among the serological tests, uses the whole tachyzoites maintained in cell culture as antigens (Dubey et al. 2017). This technique may lead to cross-reaction, especially with the apical region of the parasite, with other Apicomplexan parasites, which share the same antigens in the apical organelles. Thus, complete peripheral fluorescence of the parasite and higher dilution cut-offs should be considered to avoid cross-reaction (Gondim, Mineo, and Schares 2017).

The most common ELISA technique for diagnosis is the indirect ELISA; however, other variants have been used, such as competitive, capture, and blocking ELISA (Novoa et al. 2020; Francine A. Sinnott et al. 2014). Many recombinant antigens, including NcGRA6, NcGRA7, NcGRA14, NcCyP, and NcSAG1, were developed for ELISA-based diagnosis of livestock (Hamidinejat et al. 2015; Pinheiro et al. 2015). Comparative analysis of antigens showed that NcSAG1 and NcGRA7 have better performance for diagnosing *N. caninum* infection in aborted cattle (Abdelbaky et al. 2020). Recently, a time resolved-fluorescence immunoassay based on the GRA7 antigen (GRA7-TRFIA) was developed to detect antibodies against *N. caninum* in full-cream milk from sheep. This technique employs a non-invasive, no stressful, and easy-to-perform sample collection and can be applied for monitoring the parasite in sheep flocks with high sensitivity (Huertas-López et al. 2022).

Different organs can be collected for histopathological analysis, including the lung, liver, heart, kidney, spleen (Figure 4A), and brain (Figure 4B). Histological analysis from aborted fetuses usually shows mononuclear inflammatory infiltrate and degenerative lesions in the heart, brain, and placenta (Cabral et al. 2009; Dubey and Schares 2006). Tissue sections stained with hematoxylin-eosin are also examined to detect thick-walled cysts or tachyzoites; however, the latter is very similar to *T. gondii*, leading to a misdiagnosis (Dubey et al. 2017). For this, IHC or PCR should be performed to confirm *N caninum* as the abortive agent. However, monoclonal antibodies targeting the NcSRS2 or NcGRA7 of *N. caninum* are recommended to avoid cross-reaction with *T. gondii* (Uzêda et al. 2013).

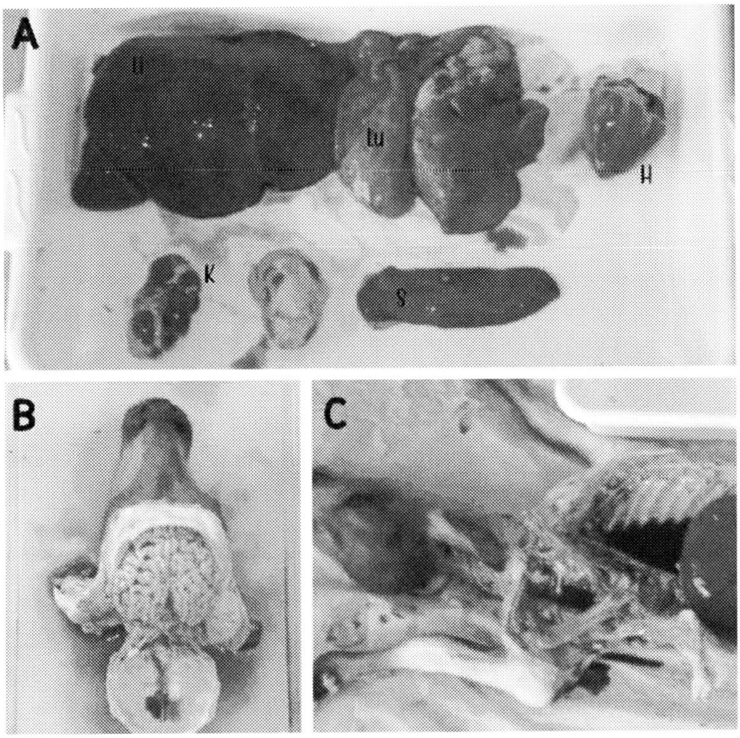

Figure 4. Biological samples collected for histopathological and molecular diagnosis. (A. Tissue samples (Li-liver, Lu-lung, H-Heart, K-Kidney, S-Spleen); B. brain; C. thoracic fluid).

Molecular diagnosis can be performed with many biological samples, such as tissues (Figure 4A-B) and thoracic fluid (Figure 4C). Molecular detection of the parasite is performed by polymerase chain reaction (PCR), a technique with higher sensitivity and specificity that can be used with different biological samples. Nowadays, besides the conventional PCR, other variants of the technique, such as multiplex, nested, and real-time PCR, have been applied for the diagnosis of *N. caninum* in livestock (Qian et al. 2020; Al-Shaeli, Ethaeb, and Gharban 2020; Barry et al. 2019). The genomic sequences of DNA coding for ribosomal RNA (rDNA), such as 18S rDNA and the pNc5 gene, are the main targets used for molecular diagnosis due to their repetitive character (Dubey and Schares 2006). Microsatellites (MS) markers are short tandem nucleotide repeats with mutating rates between 10^3 and 10^6 per cell generation (Vieira et al. 2016). For this, MS analysis has been employed for genetic studies, and previous studies have found that genetic traits could be related to the virulence of the strain (Villa et al. 2021; Dorsch et al. 2020; Campero et al. 2018).

Prevention

Management strategies are the leading measures for preventing and controlling neosporosis in livestock. Avoiding contact between domestic dogs and cattle is mandatory since dogs play an essential role in parasite distribution. Preventing dogs from accessing feedstuffs and water from livestock is also recommended to avoid contamination with oocysts (McAllister 2016). Serological screening followed by removing the seropositive cows is effective but economic evaluation should be performed before implementing this management (Liu, Reichel, and Lo 2020). Replacement heifers and cows must be evaluated serologically before introducing the herd (Dubey et al. 2017).

Reproductive management, such as embryo transfer, is recommended in infected cows with high genetic value. The recipient cow must be seronegative to avoid the recrudescence of infection and, consequently, reproductive disorders (Oliveira et al. 2010). Artificial insemination in dairy cows using beef bull semen is also recommended once a previous study showed that this procedure reduced the risk of abortion in seropositive cows (Lopez-Gatius et al. 2005).

Currently, there is no commercially available vaccine against *N. caninum* infection in livestock. In the past, Bovilis Neoguard®, a killed tachyzoite vaccine based on, was the only licensed vaccine available for cattle; however, this vaccine was withdrawn probably due to its moderate efficacy and possible adverse effects (Romero, Pérez, and Frankena 2004; Weston, Heuer, and Williamson 2012).

Vaccine studies using live and attenuated parasites have shown promising results, with induction of an antibody response and protection against experimental infection (Rojo-Montejo et al. 2013; Weber et al. 2013; Williams et al. 2007; Mazuz et al. 2021). Subunit vaccines based on antigens such as NcSAG1, NcHSP20, and NcGRA7 also induced antibody responses in cattle; however, no protection against transplacental infection was observed (Hecker et al. 2014). Recently, a vaccine based on recombinant *N. caninum*-cyclophilin and -profilin induced a strong immune response and partial protection against abortion and vertical transmission of *N. caninum* in sheep (Tuo et al. 2021).

Conclusion

Livestock farming in South America has made the region one of the main exporters of beef in the world, and the control of neosporosis in these animals is mandatory to reduce the economic impact on the cattle industry. Serological studies show that the parasite is circulating in livestock ruminants from different countrics in South America. Since no commercial vaccine is available, management strategies are the leading measures for preventing and controlling neosporosis in these countries.

References

Abdelbaky, Hanan H., Maki Nishimura, Naomi Shimoda, Jun Hiasa, Ragab M. Fereig, Hiromi Tokimitsu, Hisashi Inokuma, and Yoshifumi Nishikawa. 2020. "Evaluation of Neospora Caninum Serodiagnostic Antigens for Bovine Neosporosis." *Parasitology International*. https://doi.org/10.1016/j.parint.2019.102045.

Abo-Shehada, Mahmoud N., Raida Khalil, Marwan Abu-Halaweh, Kanar Sweis, Zuhair Amr, and Lena Billeh. 2021. "Seroprevalences of Toxoplasma Gondii and Neospora Caninum Infections in Jordanian Women Who Had a Recent Spontaneous Abortion." *Revista Brasileira de Parasitologia Veterinaria*. https://doi.org/10.1590/S1984-29612021076.

Al-Shaeli, Sattar J. J., Ali M. Ethaeb, and Hasanain A. J. Gharban. 2020. "Molecular and Histopathological Identification of Ovine Neosporosis (Neospora Caninum) in Aborted Ewes in Iraq." *Veterinary World*. https://doi.org/10.14202/vetworld.2020.597-603.

Alves Neto, Aldo F., Luciana A. Bandini, Sandra M. Nishi, Rodrigo M. Soares, David Driemeier, Nadia A. B. Antoniassi, Gereon Schares, and Solange M. Gennari. 2011. "Viability of Sporulated Oocysts of Neospora Caninum after Exposure to Different Physical and Chemical Treatments." *Journal of Parasitology*. https://doi.org/10.1645/GE-2571.1.

Andrade, Gislaine da Silva, Fábio Raphael Pascoti Bruhn, Christiane Maria Barcellos Magalhães Rocha, Alessandro de Sá Guimarães, Aurora Maria Guimarães Gouveia, and Antônio Marcos Guimarães. 2013. "Seroprevalence for Neospora Caninum in Goats of Minas Gerais State, Brazil." *Research in Veterinary Science*. https://doi.org/10.1016/j.rvsc.2012.09.026.

Barros, Luiz Daniel de, Alexey Leon Gomel Bogado, Daniella Furlan, Andressa de Melo Jardim, Werner Okano, Luiz César da Silva, Célio Eduardo Sargentin Pereira, Dalton Evert Bronkhorst, Sérgio Tosi Cardim, and João Luis Garcia. 2021. "Effects of Neospora Caninum on Reproductive Parameters in Dairy Cows from a Closed Herd in Brazil." *Veterinary Parasitology: Regional Studies and Reports* 23 (January): 100524. https://doi.org/10.1016/j.vprsr.2020.100524.

Barros, Luiz Daniel de, Ana Carolina Miura, Ana Flávia Minutti, Odilon Vidotto, and João Luis Garcia. 2018. "Neospora Caninum in Birds: A Review." *Parasitology International* 67 (4): 397–402. https://doi.org/10.1016/j.parint.2018.03.009.

Barros, Luiz Daniel de, João Luis Garcia, Katia Denise Saraiva Bresciani, Sérgio Tosi Cardim, Victor Sesnik Storte, and Selwyn Arlington Headley. 2020. "A Review of Toxoplasmosis and Neosporosis in Water Buffalo (Bubalus Bubalis)." *Frontiers in Veterinary Science* 7 (August). https://doi.org/10.3389/fvets.2020.00455.

Barry, Rhiannon, Ruth H. Nissly, Willard Feria, Nagaraja Thirumalapura, Deepanker Tewari, Bhushan M. Jayarao, and Suresh V. Kuchipudi. 2019. "A Probe-Based Real-Time PCR Assay for the Detection of Neospora Caninum in Clinical Samples from Cattle." *Veterinary Parasitology*. https://doi.org/10.1016/j.vetpar.2019.04.002.

Buxton, David, Milton M. McAllister, and J. P. Dubey. 2002. "The Comparative Pathogenesis of Neosporosis." *Trends in Parasitology*. https://doi.org/10.1016/S1471-4922(02)02414-5.

Cabral, Aline Diniz, Clarice Neves Camargo, Nara Thiers Cacciatori Galleti, Liria Hiromi Okuda, Edviges Maristela Pituco, and Claudia del Fava. 2009. "Diagnosis of Neospora Caninum in Bovine Fetuses by Histology, Immunohistochemistry, and Nested-PCR." *Revista Brasileira de Parasitologia Veterinaria*. https://doi.org/10.4322/rbpv.01804003.

Campero, Lucía María, María Laura Gos, Dadin Prando Moore, Javier Regidor-Cerrillo, Juan Manuel Unzaga, Gastón Moré, Luis Miguel Ortega-Mora, and María Cecilia Venturini. 2018. "Microsatellite Pattern Analysis of Neospora Caninum from a Naturally Infected Goat Fetus." *Veterinary Parasitology*. https://doi.org/10.1016/j.vetpar.2018.03.024.

Cerqueira-Cézar, Camila Koutsodontis, Rafael Calero-Bernal, Jitender Prakash Dubey, and Solange Maria Gennari. 2017. "All about Neosporosis in Brazil." *Revista Brasileira de Parasitologia Veterinária* 26 (3): 253–79. https://doi.org/10.1590/s1984-29612017045.

Chiebao, D. P., S. Y. O. B. Valadas, A. H. H. Minervino, V. Castro, A. H. C. N. Romaldini, A. S. Calhau, R. A. B. De Souza, S. M. Gennari, L. B. Keid, and R. M. Soares. 2015. "Variables Associated with Infections of Cattle by Brucella Abortus., Leptospira Spp. and Neospora Spp. in Amazon Region in Brazil." *Transboundary and Emerging Diseases*. https://doi.org/10.1111/tbed.12201.

Ciuca, Lavinia, Giuliano Borriello, Antonio Bosco, Luigi D'andrea, Giuseppe Cringoli, Paolo Ciaramella, Maria Paola Maurelli, Antonio Di Loria, Laura Rinaldi, and Jacopo Guccione. 2020. "Seroprevalence and Clinical Outcomes of Neospora Caninum, Toxoplasma Gondii and Besnoitia Besnoiti Infections in Water Buffaloes (Bubalus Bubalis)." *Animals*. https://doi.org/10.3390/ani10030532.

Cosendey, R. I. J., F. C. R. de Oliveira, E. Frazão-Teixeira, G. N. de Souza, F. Z. Brandão, A. M. R. Ferreira, and W. Lilenbaum. 2018. "Seroprevalence of Anti-Neospora Caninum Antibodies in Sheep from the Rapidly Expanding Flock of Rio de Janeiro, Brazil." *Veterinary Parasitology: Regional Studies and Reports*. https://doi.org/10.1016/j.vprsr.2018.09.001.

Davison, H.C, A. Otter, and A.J Trees. 1999. "Estimation of Vertical and Horizontal Transmission Parameters of Neospora Caninum Infections in Dairy Cattle."

International Journal for Parasitology 29 (10): 1683–89. https://doi.org/10.1016/S0020-7519(99)00129-0.

Davison, H. C., C. S. Guy, J. W. McGarry, F. Guy, D. J. L. Williams, D. F. Kelly, and A. J. Trees. 2001. "Experimental Studies on the Transmission of Neospora Caninum between Cattle." *Research in Veterinary Science* 70 (2): 163–68. https://doi.org/10.1053/rvsc.2001.0457.

Dorsch, Matias A., Javier Regidor-Cerrillo, Luis M. Ortega-Mora, María V. Scioli, Eleonora L. Morrell, Germán J. Cantón, Dadín P. Moore, and Yanina P. Hecker. 2020. "Microsatellite Genotyping Reveals Extensive Genetic Diversity in Bovine Neospora Caninum from the Humid Pampa Region in Argentina." *Parasitology Research*. https://doi.org/10.1007/s00436-020-06922-x.

Duarte, Pâmella Oliveira, Bárbara Guimarães Csordas, Leandra Marla Oshiro, Leandro de Oliveira Souza Higa, Namor Pinheiro Zimmermann, Kauê Rodriguez Martins, Jacqueline Cavalcante Barros, and Renato Andreotti. 2020. "Serological Evaluation of Neospora Caninum in Pregnant Women Treated at Referral Center for Prenatal Screening in Mato Grosso Do Sul, Brazil." *Revista Brasileira de Parasitologia Veterinária* 29 (4). https://doi.org/10.1590/s1984-29612020097.

Dubey, J. P., A. Hemphill, R. Calero-Bernal, and G. Schares. 2017. *Neosporosis in Animals. Neosporosis in Animals*. Boca Raton : Taylor & Francis, 2017.: CRC Press. https://doi.org/10.1201/9781315152561.

Dubey, J. P., C. Sreekumar, E. Knickman, K. B. Miska, M. C. B. Vianna, O. C. H. Kwok, D. E. Hill, M. C. Jenkins, D. S. Lindsay, and C. E. Greene. 2004. "Biologic, Morphologic, and Molecular Characterisation of Neospora Caninum Isolates from Littermate Dogs." *International Journal for Parasitology*. https://doi.org/10.1016/j.ijpara.2004.07.005.

Dubey, J. P., and G. Schares. 2006. "Diagnosis of Bovine Neosporosis." *Veterinary Parasitology* 140 (1–2): 1–34. https://doi.org/10.1016/j.vetpar.2006.03.035.

Dubey, J. P., and G. Schares. . 2011. "Neosporosis in Animals—The Last Five Years." *Veterinary Parasitology* 180 (1–2): 90–108. https://doi.org/10.1016/j.vetpar.2011.05.031.

Dubey, J. P., G. Schares, and L. M. Ortega-Mora. 2007. "Epidemiology and Control of Neosporosis and Neospora Caninum." *Clinical Microbiology Reviews* 20 (2): 323–67. https://doi.org/10.1128/CMR.00031-06.

Dubey, J. P., M. C. Jenkins, C. Rajendran, K. Miska, L. R. Ferreira, J. Martins, O. C. H. Kwok, and S. Choudhary. 2011. "Gray Wolf (Canis Lupus) Is a Natural Definitive Host for Neospora Caninum." *Veterinary Parasitology* 181 (2–4): 382–87. https://doi.org/10.1016/j.vetpar.2011.05.018.

Fávero, Juscivete F., Aleksandro S. Da Silva, Gabriela Campigotto, Gustavo Machado, Luiz Daniel de Barros, João Luis Garcia, Fernanda F. Vogel, Ricardo E. Mendes, and Lenita M. Stefani. 2017. "Risk Factors for Neospora Caninum Infection in Dairy Cattle and Their Possible Cause-Effect Relation for Disease." *Microbial Pathogenesis* 110 (September): 202–7. https://doi.org/10.1016/j.micpath.2017.06.042.

Ferre, Ignacio, Gorka Aduriz, Itziar Del-Pozo, Javier Regidor-Cerrillo, Raquel Atxaerandio, Esther Collantes-Fernández, Ana Hurtado, Carlos Ugarte-Garagalza, and Luis Miguel Ortega-Mora. 2005. "Detection of Neospora Caninum in the Semen and Blood of Naturally Infected Bulls." *Theriogenology* 63 (5): 1504–18. https://doi.org/10.1016/j.theriogenology.2004.07.002.

Filho, Paulo Cesar Gonçalves de Azevedo, Müller Ribeiro-Andrade, Jomel Francisco Dos Santos, Arthêmio Coelho Dos Reis, José Wilton Pinheiro Júnior, Sandra Regina Fonseca de Araújo Valença, Erika Fernanda Torres Samico-Fernandes, and Rinaldo Aparecido Mota. 2021. "Neospora Caninum Infection in Cattle in the State of Amazonas, Brazil: Seroprevalence, Spatial Distribution and Risk Factors." *Revista Brasileira de Parasitologia Veterinaria*. https://doi.org/10.1590/s1984-296120201083.

Fort, Marcelo, Martyn Edelsten, Stephen Maley, and Elisabeth Innes. 2015. "Seroepidemiological Study of Neospora Caninum in Beef and Dairy Cattle in La Pampa, Argentina." *Acta Parasitologica*. https://doi.org/10.1515/ap-2015-0039.

French, N.P, D. Clancy, H.C Davison, and A.J Trees. 1999. "Mathematical Models of Neospora Caninum Infection in Dairy Cattle: Transmission and Options for Control." *International Journal for Parasitology* 29 (10): 1691–1704. https://doi.org/10.1016/S0020-7519(99)00131-9.

Gharekhani, Jamal, and Mohammad Yakhchali. 2019. "Neospora Caninum Infection in Dairy Farms with History of Abortion in West of Iran." *Veterinary and Animal Science*. https://doi.org/10.1016/j.vas.2019.100071.

Gondim, Luís F. P., José R. Mineo, and Gereon Schares. 2017. "Importance of Serological Cross-Reactivity among Toxoplasma Gondii, Hammondia Spp., Neospora Spp., Sarcocystis Spp. and Besnoitia Besnoiti." *Parasitology* 144 (7): 851–68. https://doi.org/10.1017/S0031182017000063.

Gondim, Luis F. P., Milton M. McAllister, William C. Pitt, and Doris E. Zemlicka. 2004. "Coyotes (Canis Latrans) Are Definitive Hosts of Neospora Caninum." *International Journal for Parasitology* 34 (2): 159–61. https://doi.org/10.1016/j.ijpara.2004.01.001.

González-Warleta, Marta, José Antonio Castro-Hermida, Carmen Calvo, Valentín Pérez, Daniel Gutiérrez-Expósito, Javier Regidor-Cerrillo, Luis Miguel Ortega-Mora, and Mercedes Mezo. 2018. "Endogenous Transplacental Transmission of Neospora Caninum during Successive Pregnancies across Three Generations of Naturally Infected Sheep." *Veterinary Research* 49 (1): 106. https://doi.org/10.1186/s13567-018-0601-3.

González-Warleta, Marta, José Antonio Castro-Hermida, Javier Regidor-Cerrillo, Julio Benavides, Gema Álvarez-García, Miguel Fuertes, Luis Miguel Ortega-Mora, and Mercedes Mezo. 2014. "Neospora Caninum Infection as a Cause of Reproductive Failure in a Sheep Flock." *Veterinary Research*. https://doi.org/10.1186/s13567-014-0088-5.

Goodswen, Stephen J., Paul J. Kennedy, and John T. Ellis. 2013. "A Review of the Infection, Genetics, and Evolution of Neospora Caninum: From the Past to the Present." *Infection, Genetics and Evolution* 13 (1): 133–50. https://doi.org/10.1016/j.meegid.2012.08.012.

Hamidinejat, Hossein, Massoud Reza Seifi Abad Shapouri, Mohammad Mehdi Namavari, Parviz Shayan, and Marzieh Kefayat. 2015. "Development of an Indirect ELISA Using Different Fragments of Recombinant Ncgra7 for Detection of Neospora

Caninum Infection in Cattle and Water Buffalo." *Iranian Journal of Parasitology* 10 (1): 69–77. http://www.ncbi.nlm.nih.gov/pubmed/25904948.

Hecker, Yanina P., Eleonora L. Morrell, María A. Fiorentino, Ignacio Gual, Emilia Rivera, Franco Fiorani, Matías A. Dorsch, et al. 2019. "Ovine Abortion by Neospora Caninum: First Case Reported in Argentina." *Acta Parasitologica*. https://doi.org/10.2478/s11686-019-00106-z.

Hecker, Yanina P., Verónica Cóceres, Silvina E. Wilkowsky, José M. Jaramillo Ortiz, Eleonora L. Morrell, Andrea E. Verna, Agustina Ganuza, et al. 2014. "A Neospora Caninum Vaccine Using Recombinant Proteins Fails to Prevent Foetal Infection in Pregnant Cattle after Experimental Intravenous Challenge." *Veterinary Immunology and Immunopathology*. https://doi.org/10.1016/j.vetimm.2014.11.001.

Hervé-Claude, Luis, Alan A. Lavado, Dacil O. Rivera, María Navarrete-Talloni, and Christopher M. Hamilton-West. 2017. "Seroprevalence and Risk Factors for Neospora Caninum in Small Dairy Farms in Central Chile." *Rev.MVZ Córdoba*. https://doi.org/10.21897/rmvz.926.

Huertas-López, Ana, Roberto Sánchez-Sánchez, Carlos Diezma-Díaz, Gema Álvarez-García, Carlos Martínez-Carrasco, Silvia Martínez-Subiela, and José Joaquín Cerón. 2022. "Detection of Anti-Neospora Caninum Antibodies in Sheep's Full-Cream Milk by a Time-Resolved Fluorescence Immunoassay." *Veterinary Parasitology*. https://doi.org/10.1016/j.vetpar.2021.109641.

Innes, Elisabeth A., Aurélie G. Andrianarivo, Camilla Björkman, Diana J. L. Williams, and Patricia A. Conrad. 2002. "Immune Responses to Neospora Caninum and Prospects for Vaccination." *Trends in Parasitology* 18 (11): 497–504. https://doi.org/10.1016/S1471-4922(02)02372-3.

King, Jessica S., Jan Šlapeta, David J. Jenkins, Sarwat E. Al-Qassab, John T. Ellis, and Peter A. Windsor. 2010. "Australian Dingoes Are Definitive Hosts of Neospora Caninum." *International Journal for Parasitology* 40 (8): 945–50. https://doi.org/10.1016/j.ijpara.2010.01.008.

Lefkaditis, M., R. Mpairamoglou, A. Sossidou, K. Spanoudis, and M. Tsakiroglou. 2020. "Neospora Caninum, A Potential Cause of Reproductive Failure in Dairy Cows from Northern Greece." *Veterinary Parasitology: Regional Studies and Reports* 19. https://doi.org/10.1016/j.vprsr.2019.100365.

Lindsay, David S., and J. P. Dubey. 2020. "Neosporosis, Toxoplasmosis, and Sarcocystosis in Ruminants." *Veterinary Clinics of North America: Food Animal Practice* 36 (1): 205–22. https://doi.org/10.1016/j.cvfa.2019.11.004.

Liu, Yue, Michael P. Reichel, and Wing Cheong Lo. 2020. "Combined Control Evaluation for Neospora Caninum Infection in Dairy: Economic Point of View Coupled with Population Dynamics." *Veterinary Parasitology*. https://doi.org/10.1016/j.vetpar.2019.108967.

Llano, Horwald Alexander Bedoya, Marcelo Sales Guimarães, Rodrigo Martins Soares, Gina Polo, and Andréa Caetano da Silva. 2018. "Seroprevalence and Risk Factors for Neospora Caninum Infection in Cattle from the Eastern Antioquia, Colombia." *Veterinary and Animal Science*. https://doi.org/10.1016/j.vas.2018.03.001.

Lopez-Gatius, F., P. Santolaria, J. L. Yaniz, J. M. Garbayo, and S. Almeria. 2005. "The Use of Beef Bull Semen Reduced the Risk of Abortion in Neospora-Seropositive

Dairy Cows." *Journal of Veterinary Medicine Series B* 52 (2): 88–92. https://doi.org/10.1111/j.1439-0450.2004.00818.x.

Macchi, María V., Alejandra Suanes, Ximena Salaberry, Federico Fernandez, José Piaggio, and Andrés D. Gil. 2020. "Epidemiological Study of Neosporosis in Uruguayan Dairy Herds." *Preventive Veterinary Medicine*. https://doi.org/10.1016/j.prevetmed.2020.105022.

Maia, Maerle Oliveira, Maiara Oliveira Maia, Alexandre Redson Soares da Silva, Ana Amélia Domingues Gomes, Daniel Moura de Aguiar, Richard de Campos Pacheco, Alvimar José da Costa, and Thaís Rabelo dos Santos-Doni. 2021. "Seroprevalence of Toxoplasma Gondii and Neospora Caninum in Sheep Intended for Human Consumption in the Rondônia State, Western Brazilian Amazon." *Comparative Immunology, Microbiology and Infectious Diseases*. https://doi.org/10.1016/j.cimid.2020.101599.

Maldonado Rivera, J. E., A. J. Vallecillo, C. L. Pérez, K. M. Cirone, M. A. Dorsch, E. L. Morrell, V. Scioli, et al. 2020. "Bovine Neosporosis in Dairy Cattle from the Southern Highlands of Ecuador." *Veterinary Parasitology: Regional Studies and Reports*. https://doi.org/10.1016/j.vprsr.2020.100377.

Mazuz, Monica L., Benjamin Leibovitz, Igor Savitsky, Elena Blinder, Daniel Yasur-Landau, Yaniv Lavon, Binyamin Sharir, and Sharon Tirosh-Levy. 2021. "The Effect of Vaccination with Neospora Caninum Live-Frozen Tachyzoites on Abortion Rates of Naturally Infected Pregnant Cows." *Vaccines*. https://doi.org/10.3390/vaccines9040401.

McAllister, Milton M. 2016. "Diagnosis and Control of Bovine Neosporosis." *Veterinary Clinics of North America - Food Animal Practice*. https://doi.org/10.1016/j.cvfa.2016.01.012.

McAllister, Milton M., E. M. Huffman, Sharon K. Hietala, Patricia A. Conrad, Mark L. Anderson, and Mo D. Salman. 1996. "Evidence Suggesting a Point Source Exposure in an Outbreak of Bovine Abortion Due to Neosporosis." *Journal of Veterinary Diagnostic Investigation*. https://doi.org/10.1177/104063879600800313.

McAllister, Milton M., J. P. Dubey, David S. Lindsay, William R. Jolley, Rebecca A. Wills, and Angela M. McGuire. 1998. "Rapid Communication." *International Journal for Parasitology* 28 (9): 1473–79. https://doi.org/10.1016/S0020-7519(98)00138-6.

Moore, D. P., J. L. Konrad, S. San Martino, M. P. Reichel, D. B. Cano, S. Méndez, E. J. L. Späth, A. C. Odeón, G. Crudeli, and C. M. Campero. 2014. "Neospora Caninum Serostatus Is Affected by Age and Species Variables in Cohabiting Water Buffaloes and Beef Cattle." *Veterinary Parasitology*. https://doi.org/10.1016/j.vetpar.2014.04.011.

Novoa, María Belén, Nerina Patricia Aguirre, Nadia Ormaechea, Sebastián Palmero, Lisandro Rouzic, Beatriz Susana Valentini, Macarena Sarli, et al. 2020. "Validation and Field Evaluation of a Competitive Inhibition ELISA Based on the Recombinant Protein TSAG1 to Detect Anti-Neospora Caninum Antibodies in Sheep and Goats." *Veterinary Parasitology* 284 (August): 109201. https://doi.org/10.1016/j.vetpar.2020.109201.

Oliveira, Pollyanne Raysa Fernandes de, Larice Bruna Ferreira Soares, Jonas de Melo Borges, Rinaldo Aparecido Mota, and José Wilton Pinheiro Junior. 2018. "Prevalence and Associated Factors with Neospora Caninum Infection in Female Water Buffaloes (Bubalus Bubalis) from Pernambuco, Brazil." *Revista Brasileira de Parasitologia Veterinaria*. https://doi.org/10.1590/s1984-296120180063.

Oliveira, Vanessa Silvestre Ferreira de, Gema Álvarez-Garcia, Luis Miguel Ortega-Mora, Lígia Miranda Ferreira Borges, and Andréa Caetano da Silva. 2010. "Abortions in Bovines and Neospora Caninum Transmission in an Embryo Transfer Center." *Veterinary Parasitology*. https://doi.org/10.1016/j.vetpar.2010.06.028.

Ortega-Mora, Luis Miguel, Ignacio Ferre, Itziar Del-Pozo, Andrea Caetano-Da-Silva, Esther Collantes-Fernández, Javier Regidor-Cerrillo, Carlos Ugarte-Garagalza, and Gorka Aduriz. 2003. "Detection of Neospora Caninum in Semen of Bulls." *Veterinary Parasitology*. https://doi.org/10.1016/j.vetpar.2003.09.015.

Patarroyo S, Joaquin, Marlene Vargas V, José Cardona Á, Rafael Blanco M, and Victor Gomez L. 2013. "Frecuencia de Anticuerpos Anti-Neospora Caninum En Ovinos Del Departamento de Córdoba, Colombia [*Frequency of Anti-Neospora Caninum Antibodies in Sheep from the Department of Córdoba, Colombia*]." *Revista MVZ Córdoba*. https://doi.org/10.218 97/rmvz.161.

Pereira, Kamila Alcalá Gonçalves, Renato Silva de Sousa, Mary Suzan Varaschin, Ana Paula Brenner Busch Becker, Alda Lúcia Gomes Monteiro, Marília de Oliveira Koch, Rafael Carneiro Costa, et al. 2021. "Transplacental Transmission of Neospora Caninum to Lambs in Successive Pregnancies of Naturally Infected Sheep in Southern Brazil." *Veterinary Parasitology: Regional Studies and Reports*. https://doi.org/10.1016/j.vprsr.2021.100537.

Pessoa, Gilson Antonio, Ana Paula Martini, Janislene Mach Trentin, Vanessa Calderaro Dalcin, Carlos Eduardo Porciuncula Leonardi, Fernanda Silveira Flôres Vogel, Manoel Francisco de Sá Filho, Mara Iolanda Batistella Rubin, and Carlos Antonio Mondino Silva. 2016. "Impact of Spontaneous Neospora Caninum Infection on Pregnancy Loss and Subsequent Pregnancy in Grazing Lactating Dairy Cows." *Theriogenology* 85 (3): 519–27. https://doi.org/10.1016/j.theriogenology.2015.09.034.

Pinheiro, Amanda Fernandes, Sibele Borsuk, Maria Elisabeth Aires Berne, Luciano Silva Da Pinto, Renato Andreotti, Talita Roos, Barbara Couto Roloff, and Fábio Pereira Leivas Leite. 2015. "Use of ELISA Based on NCSRS2 of Neospora Caninum Expressed in Pichia Pastoris for Diagnosing Neosporosis in Sheep and Dogs." *Revista Brasileira de Parasitologia Veterinaria*. https://doi.org/10.1590/S1984-29612015015.

Pinilla León, Juan Carlos, and Natalia Da Silva Borges. 2018. "Frecuencia de Neospora Caninum En Bovinos Doble Propósito En Fincas Del Estado Guárico, Venezuela [*Frequency of Neospora Caninum in Dual Purpose Cattle on Farms in Guárico State, Venezuela*]." *Revista Mexicana de Ciencias Pecuarias* 9 (4): 834–44. https://doi.org/10.22319/rmcp.v9i4.4546.

Qian, Weifeng, Wenchao Yan, Chaochao Lv, Rongzhen Bai, Tianqi Wang, Zhiguo Wei, and Min Zhang. 2020. "Molecular Detection and Genotyping of Toxoplasma Gondii and Neospora Caninum in Slaughtered Goats in Central China." *Foodborne Pathogens and Disease*. https://doi.org/10.1089/fpd.2019.2726.

Reichel, Michael P., M. Alejandra Ayanegui-Alcérreca, Luís F. P. Gondim, and John T. Ellis. 2013. "What Is the Global Economic Impact of Neospora Caninum in Cattle – The Billion Dollar Question." *International Journal for Parasitology* 43 (2): 133–42. https://doi.org/10.1016/j.ijpara.2012.10.022.

Reichel, Michael P., Milton M. McAllister, Amar Nasir, and Dadin P. Moore. 2015. "A Review of Neospora Caninum in Water Buffalo (Bubalus Bubalis)." *Veterinary Parasitology* 212 (3–4): 75–79. https://doi.org/10.1016/j.vetpar.2015.08.008.

Ribeiro, Claudia Mello, Isabela Ribeiro Soares, Rodrigo Guerrero Mendes, Paula Andrea de Santis Bastos, Satie Katagiri, Renato Bacarin Zavilenski, Hudson Felipe Porto de Abreu, and Vera Afreixo. 2019. "Meta-Analysis of the Prevalence and Risk Factors Associated with Bovine Neosporosis." *Tropical Animal Health and Production*. https://doi.org/10.1007/s11250-019-01929-8.

Rodrigues, Arlan Araujo, Danilo Rodrigues Barros Brito, Isabelli Sayuri Kono, Sara Silva Reis, Beatriz de Souza Lima Nino, Thiago Vinícius Costa Nascimento, Luiz Daniel de Barros, João Luis Garcia, and Ivo Alexandre Leme da Cunha. 2022. "Seroprevalence of Neospora Caninum and Risk Factors Associated with Infection in Water Buffaloes (Bubalus Bubalis) from Maranhão State, Brazil." *Veterinary Parasitology: Regional Studies and Reports*. https://doi.org/10.1016/j.vprsr.2021.100661.

Rodrigues, Arlan Araújo, Sara Silva Reis, Elinalva da Silva Moraes, José Gracione do Nascimento Souza Filho, Maria Helena dos Santos Reis, Thais Agostinho Martins, Juliana Correa Bernardes, et al. 2021. "Seroprevalence and Risk Factors for Neospora Caninum and Toxoplasma Gondii in Goats of Maranhão State, Brazil." *Veterinary Parasitology: Regional Studies and Reports*. https://doi.org/10.1016/j.vprsr.2021.100634.

Rodrigues, Arlan Araujo, Sara Silva Reis, Milenne Lima de Sousa, Elinalva da Silva Moraes, João Luis Garcia, Thiago Vinicius Costa Nascimento, and Ivo Alexandre Leme da Cunha. 2020. "A Systematic Literature Review and Meta-Analysis of Risk Factors for Neospora Caninum Seroprevalence in Goats." *Preventive Veterinary Medicine* 185 (December): 105176. https://doi.org/10.1016/j.prevetmed.2020.105176.

Rojo-Montejo, Silvia, Esther Collantes-Fernández, Francisco Pérez-Zaballos, Sonia Rodríguez-Marcos, Javier Blanco-Murcia, Antonio Rodríguez-Bertos, Antoni Prenafeta, and Luis Miguel Ortega-Mora. 2013. "Effect of Vaccination of Cattle with the Low Virulence Nc-Spain 1H Isolate of Neospora Caninum against a Heterologous Challenge in Early and Mid-Gestation." *Veterinary Research*. https://doi.org/10.1186/1297-9716-44-106.

Romanelli, Paulo Roberto, Andressa Maria Rorato Nascimento de Matos, Fernanda Pinto-Ferreira, Eloiza Teles Caldart, João Lucas Moura Do Carmo, Nathalia Gomes Dos Santos, Natalia Ribeiro da Silva, et al. 2021. "Anti-Toxoplasma Gondii and Anti-Neospora Caninum Antibodies in Sheep from Paraná State, South Brazil: Prevalence and Associated Factors." *Revista Brasileira de Parasitologia Veterinaria*. https://doi.org/10.1590/S1984-29612021021.

Romanelli, Paulo Roberto, Andressa Maria Rorato Nascimento de Matos, Fernanda Pinto-Ferreira, Eloiza Teles Caldart, Marcelle Mareze, Ricardo Luis Nascimento Matos,

Roberta Lemos Freire, et al. 2020. "Seroepidemiology of Ovine Toxoplasmosis and Neosporosis in Breeding Rams from Rio Grande Do Sul, Brazil." *Transboundary and Emerging Diseases*. https://doi.org/10.1111/tbed.13593.

Romanelli, Paulo Roberto, Andressa Maria Rorato Nascimento de Matos, Fernanda Pinto-Ferreira, Eloiza Teles Caldart, Juliana Silva de Oliveira, Gabriela Anteveli, Brenda Caroline Dos Santos Jeanfelice, et al. 2020. "Toxoplasma Gondii and Neospora Caninum Infections and Factors Associated in Goats in the Parana State, Southern Brazil." *Revista Brasileira de Parasitologia Veterinaria*. https://doi.org/10.1590/s1984-29612020076.

Romero, J. J., E. Pérez, and K. Frankena. 2004. "Effect of a Killed Whole Neospora Caninum Tachyzoite Vaccine on the Crude Abortion Rate of Costa Rican Dairy Cows under Field Conditions." *Veterinary Parasitology*. https://doi.org/10.1016/j.vetpar.2004.06.016.

Schmidt, Ana Carolina, Thábata dos Anjos Pacheco, Janice Elena Ioris Barddal, Anderson Castro Soares de Oliveira, Daniel Moura de Aguiar, Rísia Lopes Negreiros, and Richard de Campos Pacheco. 2018. "Seroprevalence, Spatial Analysis and Risk Factors of Infection with Neospora Caninum in Cattle in Brazil's Northern Pantanal Wetland." *Revista Brasileira de Parasitologia Veterinária* 27 (4): 455–63. https://doi.org/10.1590/s1984-296120180058.

Selim, Abdelfattah, Hanem Khater, and Hamdan I. Almohammed. 2021. "A Recent Update about Seroprevalence of Ovine Neosporosis in Northern Egypt and Its Associated Risk Factors." *Scientific Reports*. https://doi.org/10.1038/s41598-021-93596-9.

Serrano-Martínez, E., I. Ferre, K. Osoro, G. Aduriz, R. A. Mota, A. Martínez, I. del-Pozo, C. O. Hidalgo, and L. M. Ortega-Mora. 2007. "Intrauterine Neospora Caninum Inoculation of Heifers and Cows Using Contaminated Semen with Different Numbers of Tachyzoites." *Theriogenology*. https://doi.org/10.1016/j.theriogenology.2006.10.004.

Serrano-Martínez, Enrique, Roberto R. Evaristo, Marco H. Quispe, and Elizabeth M. Hinostroza. 2018. "Seroprevalence Neospora Caninum in Bovines of Lima and Comparison between ELISA and IFAT." *Revista de Investigaciones Veterinarias Del Peru*. https://doi.org/10.15381/rivep.v29i3.14757.

Silva Andrade, Gislaine da, Fábio Raphael Pascoti Bruhn, Christiane Maria Barcellos Magalhães Rocha, Alessandro de Sá Guimarães, Aurora Maria Guimarães Gouveia, and Antônio Marcos Guimarães. 2012. "Seroprevalence and Risk Factors for Neospora Caninum in Sheep in the State Minas Gerais, Southeastern Brazil." *Veterinary Parasitology*. https://doi.org/10.1016/j.vetpar.2012.03.006.

Silva, Rodrigo, and Gustavo Machado. 2016. "Canine Neosporosis: Perspectives on Pathogenesis and Management." *Veterinary Medicine: Research and Reports*. https://doi.org/10.2147/vmrr.s76969.

Sinnott, Francine A., Leonardo G. Monte, Thais F. Collares, Bruno M. De Matos, Diene B. Pacheco, Sibele Borsuk, Renato Andreotti, and Cláudia P. Hartleben. 2014. "Blocking Elisa Using Recombinant Ncsrs2 Protein for Diagnosing Bovine Neosporosis." *Current Microbiology*. https://doi.org/10.1007/s00284-014-0737-y.

Sinnott, Francine Alves, Leonardo Garcia Monte, Thaís Farias Collares, Roberta Maraninchi Silveira, and Sibele Borsuk. 2017. "Review on the Immunological and

Molecular Diagnosis of Neosporosis (Years 2011–2016)." *Veterinary Parasitology*. https://doi.org/10.1016/j.vetpar.2017.04.008.

Snak, Alessandra, Felipe Gustavo Garcia, Arielle Aparecida Lara, Hilda Fátima Jesus Pena, and Silvia Cristina Osaki. 2018. "Neospora Caninum in Properties in the West Region of Paraná, Brazil: Prevalence and Risk Factors." *Revista Brasileira de Parasitologia Veterinária* 27 (1): 51–59. https://doi.org/10.1590/s1984-29612018001.

Souza, Giovanna Gati de, Lidiana Zanetti Amatti, Luana Venâncio Garcia, Letícia Ramos Costa, Ana Flávia Minutti, Thais Agostinho Martins, Alexey Leon Gomel Bogado, et al. 2022. "Neospora Caninum Infection and Reproductive Problems in Dairy Cows from Brazil: A Case-Control Study." *Veterinary Parasitology: Regional Studies and Reports* 28 (February): 100683. https://doi.org/10.1016/j.vprsr.2021.100683.

Topazio, J. P., A. Weber, G. Camillo, F. F. Vogel, G. Machado, A. Ribeiro, A. B. Moura, et al. 2014. "Seroprevalence and Risk Factors for Neospora Caninum in Goats in Santa Catarina State, Brazil." *Rev Bras Parasitol Vet* 23: 360–66. https://doi.org/10.1590/S1984-29612014062.

Trees, Alexander J., and Diana J. L. Williams. 2005. "Endogenous and Exogenous Transplacental Infection in Neospora Caninum and Toxoplasma Gondii." *Trends in Parasitology* 21 (12): 558–61. https://doi.org/10.1016/j.pt.2005.09.005.

Tuo, Wenbin, Xiaosheng Feng, Lili Cao, Bryan Vinyard, J. P. Dubey, Raymond Fetterer, and Mark Jenkins. 2021. "Vaccination with Neospora Caninum-Cyclophilin and -Profilin Confers Partial Protection against Experimental Neosporosis-Induced Abortion in Sheep." *Vaccine*. https://doi.org/10.1016/j.vaccine.2021.06.032.

Uzêda, R. S., G. Schares, L. M. Ortega-Mora, C. R. Madruga, A. Aguado-Martinez, L. G. Corbellini, D. Driemeier, and L. F. P. Gondim. 2013. "Combination of Monoclonal Antibodies Improves Immunohistochemical Diagnosis of Neospora Caninum." *Veterinary Parasitology*. https://doi.org/10.1016/j.vetpar.2013.07.008.

Valbuena-Carson, Roselyn, Robert Valeris, Egar Sánchez, Adelso Ramírez, Kelly Ochoa, David Uzcátegui, Everts Chacín, David Simoes, Roger Ramírez, and Francisco Angulo-Cubillánu. 2013. "Detección Serológica de Neospora Caninum (Apicomplexa, Sarcocystidae) En Búfalas (Bubalus Bubalis) Del Municipio Colón, Estado Zulia, Venezuela [*Serological Detection of Neospora Caninum (Apicomplexa, Sarcocystidae) In Buffaloes (Bubalus Bubalis) From Colón Municipality, Zulia State, Venezuela*]." *Revista Cientifica de La Facultad de Ciencias Veterina-rias de La Universidad Del Zulia* 23 (5): 396–402.

Venturoso, Poliana de Jesus Souza, Osvaldo Juliatti Venturoso, Gisele Glomba Silva, Maerle Oliveira Maia, Rute Witter, Daniel Moura Aguiar, Richard de Campos Pacheco, Elvino Ferreira, Alvimar José da Costa, and Thais Rabelo dos Santos-Doni. 2021. "Risk Factor Analysis Associated with Neospora Caninum in Dairy Cattle in Western Brazilian Amazon." *Revista Brasileira de Parasitologia Veterinária* 30 (1): e023020. https://doi.org/10.1590/s1984-296120201088.

Vieira, Maria Lucia Carneiro, Luciane Santini, Augusto Lima Diniz, and Carla de Freitas Munhoz. 2016. "Microsatellite Markers: What They Mean and Why They Are so Useful." *Genetics and Molecular Biology*. https://doi.org/10.1590/1678-4685-GMB-2016-0027.

Villa, Luca, Alessia Libera Gazzonis, Emanuele Fumagalli, Sergio Aurelio Zanzani, and Maria Teresa Manfredi. 2022. "The Utility of Serological Analysis for Neospora Caninum Infection in Dairy Cattle Farms Management: Serological Investigation and Evaluation of the Effects on Reproductive and Productive Performances in Two Study Herds in Northern Italy." *Animals* 12 (6): 786. https://doi.org/10.3390/ani12060786.

Villa, Luca, Pavlo Maksimov, Christine Luttermann, Mareen Tuschy, Alessia L. Gazzonis, Sergio A. Zanzani, Michele Mortarino, Franz J. Conraths, Maria Teresa Manfredi, and Gereon Schares. 2021. "Spatial Distance between Sites of Sampling Associated with Genetic Variation among Neospora Caninum in Aborted Bovine Foetuses from Northern Italy." *Parasites and Vectors*. https://doi.org/10.1186/s13071-020-04557-6.

Weber, Fred H., James A. Jackson, Brian Sobecki, Les Choromanski, Mary Olsen, Todd Meinert, Rodney Frank, Michael P. Reichel, and John T. Ellis. 2013. "On the Efficacy and Safety of Vaccination with Live Tachyzoites of Neospora Caninum for Prevention of Neospora-Associated Fetal Loss in Cattle." *Clinical and Vaccine Immunology*. https://doi.org/10.1128/CVI.00225-12.

Wei, Xin-Yu, Qi An, Nian-Yu Xue, Yu Chen, Ying-Yu Chen, Yuan Zhang, Quan Zhao, and Chu-Ren Wang. 2022. "Seroprevalence and Risk Factors of Neospora Caninum Infection in Cattle in China from 2011 to 2020: A Systematic Review and Meta-Analysis." *Preventive Veterinary Medicine* 203: 105620. https://doi.org/j.prevetmed.2022.105620.

Weston, J. F., C. Heuer, and N. B. Williamson. 2012. "Efficacy of a Neospora Caninum Killed Tachyzoite Vaccine in Preventing Abortion and Vertical Transmission in Dairy Cattle." *Preventive Veterinary Medicine*. https://doi.org/10.1016/j.prevetmed.2011.08.010.

Williams, D. J. L., C. S. Guy, R. F. Smith, J. Ellis, C. Björkman, M. P. Reichel, and A. J. Trees. 2007. "Immunization of Cattle with Live Tachyzoites of Neospora Caninum Confers Protection against Fetal Death." *Infection and Immunity*. https://doi.org/10.1128/IAI.00777-06.

Williams, D. J. L., C. S. Hartley, C. Björkman, and A. J. Trees. 2009. "Endogenous and Exogenous Transplacental Transmission of Neospora Caninum – How the Route of Transmission Impacts on Epidemiology and Control of Disease." *Parasitology* 136 (14): 1895–1900. https://doi.org/10.1017/S0031182009990588.

Chapter 8

Toxoplasmosis in Livestock Ruminants from South America

**João Luis Garcia*
Luiz Daniel de Barros
and Fernando de Souza Rodrigues**
Department of Preventive Veterinary Medicine,
Laboratory of Animal Protozoology,
State University of Londrina, Londrina, PR, Brazil

Introduction

Toxoplasmosis caused by the protozoan *Toxoplasma gondii* is quite common in warm-blooded animals worldwide, this parasite is obligate intracellular of the Phylum Apicomplexa, Class Conoidasida, Subclass Coccidia, Order Eucoccidiorida, Suborder Eimeriorina, and Family Sarcocystidae (Schoch et al. 2020). Felids are the definitive hosts, while humans and other animals are intermediate hosts. *T. gondii* was first identified in 1908 by Splendore, an Italian naturalized Brazilian researcher, in rabbits that he used in his research, at the Faculty of Medicine in the city of São Paulo, Brazil. In the same year, Nicolle and Manceaux, from the Pasteur Institute in Tunis, discovered the same parasite in an African rodent, *Ctenodactylus gundi*, and in the following year, in 1909, they named the new parasite found *Toxoplasma gondii* due to its arc shape (taxon = arc, plasma = shape) and in honor of the rodent in which it was found (Tenter, Heckeroth, and Weiss 2000).

* Corresponding Author's Email: jlgarcia@uel.br.

In: Infectious and Parasitic Diseases of Animals in Developing Countries
Editor: Selwyn Arlington Headley
ISBN: 979-8-88697-504-8

In livestock animals, the main signs are miscarriages, but in most infections, individuals are asymptomatic. Among the species of domestic animals most susceptible to infection and that usually develop clinical signs of the disease, we can highlight sheep and goats, with a smaller proportion of felines, dogs, and swine. Horses, cattle, and buffalo can also develop the disease, but several experimental studies have shown that these animals are more resistant and rarely present clinical forms, such as abortion. *Toxoplasma gondii* is one of the major causes of abortion in goats and sheep worldwide, which outbreaks occur frequently (Innes et al. 2009; Dubey 1981a). In spite of such, there is no description of the economic losses of toxoplasmosis in the sheep industry from Brazil. It was estimated about US $1.4 to $4.68 million/annually for the sheep industry in Uruguay (Freyre et al. 1999), where 27% of abortion were caused by *T. gondii*, higher than other causes of fetal losses (Dorsch et al., 2022).

The parasite is the second most commonly diagnosed cause of infectious abortion in sheep in the UK, accounting for 24% of the diagnosed cases. Neonatal losses due to ovine toxoplasmosis are estimated to be 1-2% in the UK national flock (Innes et al. 2009), resulting in losses of 0.5 million lambs every year. Goats are one of the most susceptible species for *T. gondii* (Dubey and Adams, 1990). Like sheep, the main clinical signs of infection are reproductive disorders. However, death in young and adult goats can occur (Dubey 1981a). Consumption of *T. gondii*-infected raw or undercooked goat and sheep meat, and unpasteurized goat milk containing bradyzoites and tachyzoites constitute a significant infection risk for people (Dubey et al. 1980; Chiari and Neves 1984; Dubey et al. 2014). A study showed that the burden of *T. gondii* in muscle samples of goats even in small quantities such as 5-10 g of meat has the potential for transmission if consumed raw or under-cooked (Rani et al. 2020).

Sheep and Goats

Epidemiology

T. gondii infection in sheep and goats occurs across the world, and seroprevalence studies from Brazil (Table 1) ranged from 9.2 to 56.9% for sheep(Garcia et al. 1999; Guimarães et al. 2013; Pinheiro et al. 2009; Sakata et al. 2012; Ogawa et al. 2003; Figliuolo et al. 2004; de Moraes et al. 2010;

Luciano et al. 2011; Lopes et al. 2010), and 17.0 to 44.7% for goats (Luciano et al. 2011; Santos et al. 2012; G. Garcia et al. 2012; Figliuolo et al. 2004; Anderlini et al. 2011; Sella et al. 1994; Reis et al. 2007; Lúcio et al. 2016; Moura et al. 2016).

Table 1. Seroprevalence of indirect immunofluorescence assay (IFA, cut-off ≥64) to *Toxoplasma gondii* from farm sheep in Brazil

Sheep		
Author	**State**	**%**
Garcia et al., 1999	Paraná	51.8
Ogawa et al., 2003	Paraná	47.8
Figlioulo et al., 2004	São Paulo	34.7
Romanelli et al., 2007	Paraná	51.5
Pinheiro et al., 2009	Alagoas	32.9
Ueno et al., 2009	Distrito Federal	35.4
Moraes et al., 2010	Pernambuco	9.2
Luciano et al., 2011	Rio de Janeiro	38.0
Rossi et al., 2011	Minas Gerais	46.5
Lopes et al., 2011	São Paulo	52.0
Sakata et al., 2012	Santa Catarina	56.9
Guimarães et al., 2013	Bahia	30.2
De Oliveira et al., 2016	Rio Grande do Sul	20.2
Goats		
Author	**State**	**%**
Sella et al., 1994	Paraná	30.7
Figlioulo et al., 2004	São Paulo	28.7
Reis et al., 2007	Paraná	44.7
Lima et al., 2008	Rio Grande do Norte	51.5
Luciano et al., 2011	Rio de Janeiro	29.1
Anderlini et al., 2011	Alagoas	39.0
Santos et al., 2012	Paraíba	18.1
Garcia et al., 2012	Paraná	36.0
Lucio et al., 2016	Pernambuco	25.8
Moura et al., 2016	Santa Catarina	33.0

We described in Table 1 only studies from Brazil that used indirect fluorescence assay (IFA) with cut-off ≥ 64, because when the results of prevalence studies are compared, caution needs to be taken since the observed differences might be directly related to the serological techniques employed, the cut-off values, the sample size, and the type of animal that is being investigated. However, how the seroprevalence studies from sheep and goats are scarce from other countries in South America, we did not take this into consideration. Thus, the prevalence of *T. gondii* in sheep from Argentina ranged from 10% (Hecker et al. 2018) to 17.3% (Hecker et al. 2013), both studies used IFA cut-off ≥ 50, in Uruguay Freyre et al. (Freyre et al. 1999) showed a 38.5% positivity by direct agglutination test (DA, cut-off ≥64), and Suzuki et al. (Suzuki et al. 2011) by a commercial ELISA 38.9%, finally Gorman et al. (Gorman et al. 1999) showed 28% seroprevalence in Chile (IFA, cut-off ≥ 16). The prevalence of *T. gondii* in goats from Argentina was 46.8% by IFA with a cut-off ≥ 100 (Gos et al. 2017), and in Colombia 18.4% by ELISA (Martínez-Rodriguez, Tafur-Gómez, and Guzman-Barragan 2020).

The main methods used to detect antibodies against *T. gondii* are IFA (indirect fluorescence assay), MAT (modified agglutination test), and ELISA (enzyme-linked immunosorbent assay). High antibody titers can be found in acute infections and in the case of reactivation of *T. gondii* (Robert, Chabasse, and Hocquet 1981). Therefore, an epidemic abortion in a herd associated with high titers of antibodies against *T. gondii* (≥ 1,024) could be indicative of *T. gondii* as the causative agent. However, there are also reports in which high titers of anti-*T. gondii* antibodies in goats were maintained for long periods, independently of the existence of clinical signs. Therefore, high titers in specific antibodies may not always be considered as a diagnostic marker of recent infection (Dubey 1981a).

The detection of *T. gondii* can be performed by different techniques, including molecular, histopathological, and either bioassay with mice or cats (Dubey 2010; Yan et al. 2010). For detecting viable tissue cysts, bioassay in cats is considered the gold standard; however, it is not viable, and mice are the most used (Dubey, Laurin, and Kwowk 2016). There is a strong agreement between mouse bioassay with the polymerase chain reaction (PCR) (Schares et al. 2018).

The most PCR targets used for *T. gondii* DNA amplification are ITS1, and B1 gene, repetitive 529 DNA fragment by either conventional PCR or qPCR. Generally, nested-PCR is more sensitive than conventional PCR, but it is not preferred in the diagnostic routine because it requires two PCR amplification stages, making it more laborious, expensive, and with a higher risk of contamination (Calderaro et al. 2006). The qPCR was more effective to detect *T. gondii* DNA, but the other markers had similar results (Minutti et al., 2021).

The Disease

Toxoplasma gondii is transmitted to ruminants through the consumption of sporulated oocysts either in food, water, or pasture or vertically from mother to fetus if a primary infection occurs. After ingestion, sporozoites from oocysts penetrate the intestinal tissues, transform into tachyzoites, multiply locally within cells, and are disseminated throughout the body via the blood and the lymph compartments. After several cycles, tachyzoites transform into bradyzoites contained within intracellular cysts localized in a variety of tissues. Bradyzoites can remain viable for extended periods of time and probably for the entire life of the host. After a primary infection goats and sheep develop immunity that can prevent any subsequent disease related to novel contaminations that would occur during following gestations (Buxton 1998). However, primary *T. gondii* infection occurring during gestation may lead to infection of the fetus, and depending on the stage of gestation, the result of infection may be variable.

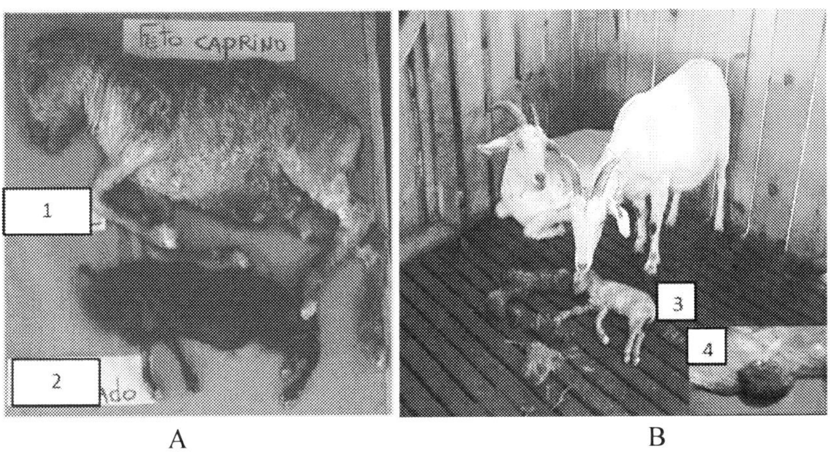

Source: O. Vidotto, I.T. Navarro, Freire, R.L., and Garcia, J.L.

Figure 1. Toxoplamosis infection in goats (A. Twin foetus; B. Stillborn and aborted foetus; 1. Foetus stillborn; 2. Mummified foetus; 3. Kid that born weak and died one hour after; 4. Cotyledon with macroscopic lesions caused by *Toxoplasma gondii*).

The outcome of *T. gondii* infection depends on the stage of gestation, in the early stage the damage for the fetus is severe once the ability to respond against the parasite is just achieved within 70 days of pregnancy, and *Toxoplasma* infection may result in fetal death and resorption; however, the clinical signs usually occurs when the animals are infected in the mid-stage of gestation, compared with infection during the late stage of pregnancy, when the fetal immunity is relatively well developed (Buxton 1998). Clinical signs include absorption, mummification, maceration, abortion, stillbirth, or the birth of a weak young that often will not survive over the first weeks of life, those that survive the first week generally grow normally to adulthood (Figure 1). Alternatively, offspring may be born infected but without any clinical signs.

Abortion or stillbirths caused by *T. gondii* in goats usually have a bimodal occurrence (Obendorf, Statham, and Munday 1990). After an initial exposure to the pathogen, animals may abort during the first four weeks. In this case, antibodies against the parasite may not be systematically detected. Goats may also abort or produce stillborn young, 8 weeks following infection. In this latter scenario, antibodies against *T. gondii* are detected. This bimodal occurrence of disease may result from acute toxoplasmosis (as in the first case described) and can lead to abortion without apparent infection of the fetus, or it may be due to congenital toxoplasmosis, as described in the second scenario (Obendorf, Statham, and Munday 1990).

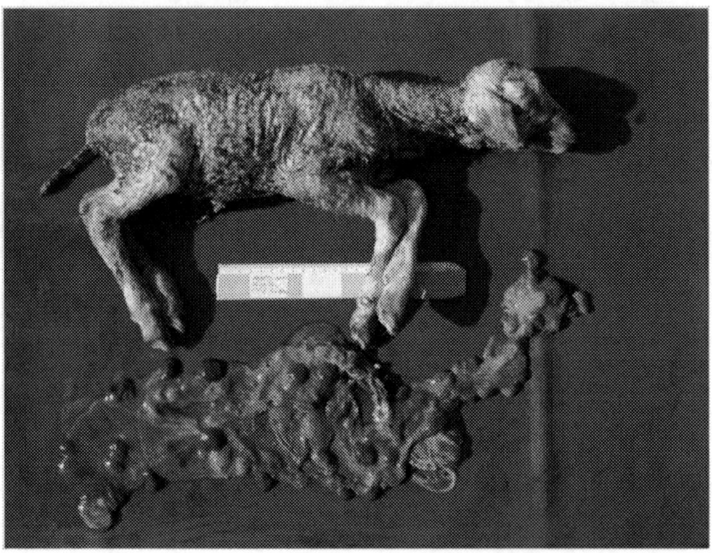

Source: Garcia, J.L.

Figure 2. Toxoplasmosis infection in sheep. (Pictured: a stillborn animal and placenta with macroscopic lesions caused by *Toxoplasma gondii*).

The main clinical signs in adult goats are reproductive disorders. However, some animals may present anorexia, prostration, fever, and mastitis. During an investigation of a *T. gondii* outbreak on a goat farm in southern Brazil, sixty-one (44.8%) out of 136 pregnant females were aborted (Silva

Filho et al. 2008). All abortions occurred during the third trimester of gestation, and aborted fetuses presented abnormalities including mummification, maceration, deformity, and stillbirth (Figure 1). Some young were born very weak and died shortly after birth. The dams' clinical signals were mainly anorexia, prostration, fever, and mastitis. One dam demonstrated severe symptoms and subsequently died. All dams from the herd were treated for five days with sulfadiazine (4 mg/kg) and trimethoprim (20 mg/kg) by the intramuscular route and the abortions ceased two weeks after treatment (Silva Filho et al. 2008).

Host-Pathogen Interaction

The most important host factor to determine the susceptibility to *T. gondii* is how fast the immune system can produce IFN-y, and there is a clear difference among the various host animal species (Innes et al. 2007). The severity of the disease may be related to the species, the host age, hormones, gestation, the immunological status, host nutritional condition, the parasite strain, parasite stages, the burden of infection, and concomitant infections (Dubey 1994; Dubey and Jones 2008; Garcia 2009; Liesenfeld et al. 2001). The mechanisms involved in host protection against infection involve components of both the humoral and cellular immune response.

One of the differences in *T. gondii* infection between sheep and goats is that the latter are more susceptible. The susceptibility of caprines to *T. gondii* is dose-dependent: doses as low as 10 sporulated oocysts (GT-1 strain) may produce abortion (Dubey 1989a); in addition, goats fed with 100 oocysts (GT-1 strain) may show lethargy, fever, and diarrhea while animals fed with 1,000 oocysts (GT-1 strain) may die between 7 and 20 days following infection (Dubey 1981d; 1981a; 1989b). In an experimental study, pregnant does were infected initially with oocysts of GT1 strain, all animals aborted, and in the next breed season these animals were re-infected with oocysts of homologous strain, and one out of six animals repeated transplacental transmission of *T. gondii* (Dubey 1981d). In contrast, in an experiment using 11 pregnant goats that aborted after a previously infection with TS-2 strain (25,000 oocysts) and were re-infected one year later during the next gestation with a combination of TS-2/TC177 strains (10,000 oocysts), none of the young borns had congenital toxoplasmosis (Obendorf, Statham, and Munday 1990). More studies are required to improve our understanding of the pathogenesis of congenital toxoplasmosis in goats and how the infected animals develop protective immune responses.

Control Strategies

The control of toxoplasmosis is similar in sheep, goats, and other livestock animals. Biosecurity measures should be conducted on farms to prevent contact between cats, rodents, and feed bins (Innes 2010; Innes et al. 2019). There is a commercial vaccine Toxovac® to help prevent congenital toxoplasmosis, which is prescribed to sheep and goats. The vaccine comprises live tachyzoites of the S48 strain of *T. gondii* that has lost the ability to differentiate into bradyzoites. This parasite strain thus only undergoes limited multiplication in the sheep and goats and does not persist. The S48 strain was developed in New Zealand, and it was found to be highly effective when administered before mating in protecting them against transmission of parasites to the fetus (O'Connell, Wilkins, and Punga 1988), it is advised to be administered at least 3 weeks before mating and has a meat and milk withdrawal period of six weeks following vaccination. Additionally, vaccination of sheep can protect against the establishment of tissue cysts following challenge with a complete strain of *T. gondii*, what could improve the safety of meat for human consumption (Katzer et al. 2014). Studies showed that protection by the S48 strain was reached through cell-mediated immune responses in sheep and that the duration of immunity following a primary immunization was at least 18 months(Buxton and Innes 1995; Buxton et al. 1993). As it is a live vaccine, there are problems associated with a short shelf life and care should be taken by those administering it as it is a zoonotic pathogen (Innes and Vermeulen 2006).

Different strategies have been used to test vaccine candidates against *T. gondii* in sheep. A vaccine with a total extract of *T. gondii* proteins (TE) associated with maltodextrin nanoparticles (DGNP) was evaluated to protect against latent and congenital toxoplasmosis in sheep (Ducournau et al. 2020). The authors tested either intranasal or intradermal route and showed a high level of protection against latent toxoplasmosis and its transplacental transmission in sheep by the intranasal route.

The microneme, rhoptry, and dense granules proteins were investigated as vaccine candidates in sheep (Hiszczynska-Sawicka, Li, et al. 2010; Hiszczynska-Sawicka, Akhtar, et al. 2010; Hiszczynska-Sawicka et al. 2012; Hiszczynska-Sawicka, Li, et al. 2011; Hiszczynska-Sawicka, Oledzka, et al.

2011). Those authors tested DNA vaccines associated with MIC3, GRA1, GRA4, GRA6, and GRA7 into liposomes, and ROP1 fused to ovine CD154 to sheep, and they a significant immune response against *T. gondii*, what could be candidates for vaccine.

A mutant RH *T. gondii* strain lacking the *mic1* and *mic3* genes (Mic1-3KO was tested in ewes after vaccination mild febrile and serum IgG antibodies were observed. Ewes were mated two months after vaccination and were orally challenged with the PRU strain which resulted in a slight febrile response, whereas unvaccinated ewes developed a more severe and longer fever. All unvaccinated ewes were aborted whereas 62%-91% of the lambs from vaccinated ewes were viable, with no clinical signs of infection (Mevelec et al. 2010).

There are few studies considering vaccines against *T. gondii* in goats. The S48 live vaccine (Toxovax) was tested in goats and protection was observed against abortion (Chartier and Mallereau 2001), however, 25% of the vaccinated group had stillbirths after challenge with a high dose (10,000) of sporulated oocysts (the strain was not informed). Two studies conducted to prevent toxoplasmosis used the closely related parasite *Hammondia* to immunize and protect them against congenital toxoplasmosis (Dubey 1981b; 1981c). The first study (Dubey 1981c) used oocysts of *H. hammondi and H. heydorni* to protect against a challenge with *T. gondii* oocysts, and just immunization with *H. hammondi* was able to protect goats against lethal challenges. In the second study (Dubey 1981b) the author used pregnant does vaccinated with 1 million oocysts of CR-4 *H. hammondi* strain to evaluate protection against GT-1 challenge (1,000 oocysts), the vaccine was able to prevent damage in fetuses from five does, but not fetal infection, and one doe had three dead kids.

Cattle

Seroepidemiological studies of. *T gondii* infection in cattle in Brazil varies from 3.4 to 71% (Costa and Costa 1978; Costa et al. 1978; Costa et al. 2012; Garcia et al. 1999; Gondim et al. 1999; Santos et al. 2009; Spagnol et al. 2009; de Souza et al. 2016; Moura et al. 2010; Santos et al. 2013; Carmo et al. 2017; Gomes et al. 2021) (Table 2). The first study carried out in Brazil to assess the prevalence of antibodies against *T. gondii* in cattle found 12% of seropositive in Poços de Caldas, Minas Gerais (Costa and Costa 1978), and in the same year, a prevalence of 32.3% was observed (Costa et al. 1978) in animals slaughtered in Jaboticabal, São Paulo. Since then, several studies have been carried out to evaluate the occurrence of antibodies against *T. gondii* in this species, as can be seen in Table 2. In Argentina the occurrence of anti-*T. gondii* antibodies in cattle was 91% (82/90) using IFA with a cut-off $\geq$25 (Moré et al. 2008). A meta-analysis study showed that the global seroprevalence of *T. gondii* by IFA in cattle is about 20.3% and ranges from 15.2 to 30.1% in America (Omonijo et al., 2022).

T. gondii can be transmitted transplacentally in cattle (Canada et al. 2002); however, this does not suggest that this parasite is an important abortifacient in bovine species. Wiengcharoen et al. (Wiengcharoen et al. 2011) described that *T. gondii* can be a cause of abortion in cows. These authors were based on an experimental study where heifers were infected with high doses (3 x 10^8) of RH strain tachyzoites subcutaneously. However, this form of infection does not mimic the natural route of infection in ruminants. In contrast, Costa et al. (Costa et al. 2011) infected pregnant cows with sporulated oocysts (high dose, 10^5) of *T. gondii* and did not observe any abortions or isolated *T. gondii* from their fetuses. In Argentina, no abortion caused by *T. gondii* was observed by the National Institute of Agrarian Technology from 1999 to 2007(Moore et al. 2008).

Since its description as transmissible by carnivorism (Weinman and Chandler 1954) *T. gondii* has been studied in different animal tissues to assess the risk of transmission to humans. Among the meats for consumption, beef has a prominent role, either because of its high consumption or because of the variable opinion among researchers about the risk it presents to the human population. Some described the low risk of infection, as they did not detect the parasite in the meats and tissues studied (Dubey and Streitel 1976; Passos, Lima, and Figueiredo 1984; Dubey et al. 2005) others, however, isolated the parasite from muscle, brain and/or bovine tissues. Jacobs et al. (Jacobs, Remington, and Melton 1960) investigated the presence of *T. gondii* cysts in meat from swine, sheep, and cattle in the USA through artificial digestion and inoculation of mice. Of the 60 bovine diaphragms examined, only one was positive in the bioassay. Mayer (Mayer 1965), in Argentina, isolated 46 samples of *T. gondii* from the retina of 304 cattle. The same author isolated nine strains from the retina and seven from the brain of over 27 cattle, concluding that the retina is the material of choice for the isolation of *T. gondii* in cattle. Jamra et al. (Jamra, Deane, and Guimarães 1969) were unable to isolate the parasite from the brain, liver, and beef from markets and butchers in the city of São Paulo. However, these authors detected 8.1% of seropositive mice in the bioassay after being infected with meat peptic digestion products.

Dubey et al. (2005) determined the prevalence of viable *T. gondii* cysts in 6,282 meat samples (2,094 each of beef, pork, and chicken) obtained from 698 retail meat stores in 28 major geographic areas of the United States. For that, pools of meat samples were administered to cats free of the parasite for three days and the feces were examined for identification of oocysts for 14 days. In all, seven cats fed a pool of pork samples shed oocysts. None of the cats that were fed chicken or beef samples shed oocysts. The author found that the prevalence of viable *T. gondii* cysts in meat and flaps was very low. However, consumers, especially pregnant women, should be aware that they can acquire *T. gondii* infection from eating undercooked meat, particularly pork.

Table 2. Seroprevalence of indirect immunofluorescence assay (IFA, cut-off ≥64) to *Toxoplasma gondii* from farm cattle in Brazil

Authors	State	n	%
Costa & Costa, 1978	Minas Gerais	350	12
Costa et al., 1978	São Paulo	204	32.3
Passos et al., 1984	Several States	991	9
Gondim et al., 1999	Bahia	194	1
Garcia et al., 1999	Paraná	400	25.8
Costa et al., 2001	São Paulo, and Minas Gerais	600	49.1
Albuquerque et al., 2005	Rio de Janeiro	589	14.8
Santos, 2008	Mato Grosso	2000	71
Spagnol et al., 2009	Bahia	600	11.8
De Moura et al., 2010	Paraná	250	30.8
Costa et al., 2012	Pernambuco	100	3
Santos et al., 2013	Rio Grande do Sul	121	17.4
Souza et al., 2016	Rondônia	1000	5.3
Carmo et al., 2017	Pará	500	40.6
Gomes et al., 2021	Goiás	1533	8.9

In Argentina, Moré et al. (Moré et al. 2008) performed a study to diagnose *T. gondii* by PCR samples of diaphragm, esophagus, and myocardium from 90 beef cattle, and the parasite was identified in the myocardium of only two animals.

Therefore, epidemiological studies of *T. gondii* in cattle are important because although we find conflicting information in the literature regarding the isolation of the parasite from the tissues of these animals, some authors have described that the risk of infection by *T. gondii* can be 2.5 to 5.5 times higher in pregnant women who consumed raw or undercooked beef (Laurence Baril 1999; Cook 2000). Additionally, 4 (9.5%) out of 42 outbreaks of *T.*

gondii from 1965-2020 in Brazil were caused by raw or undercooked beef (Balbino et al. 2022).

Conclusion

Toxoplasma gondii is spread in ruminant herds all over South America; the main problems are abortion, either in sheep or goats. There are few studies on ruminants outside Brazil in South America, which could be improved. There is no commercial vaccine available in our region either for use in sheep/goats or cats, what should be driven to avoid abortion, the production of tissue cysts for production animals, and oocysts in cats.

References

Anderlini, Giulliano Aires, Rinaldo Aparecido Mota, Eduardo Bento Faria, Erika Fernanda Torres Samico Fernandes Cavalcanti, Rômulo Menna Barreto Valença, José Wilton Pinheiro, Pedro Paulo Feitosa de Albuquerque, and Orestes Luiz de Souza Neto. 2011. "Ocorrência e Fatores de Risco Associados à Infecção Por *Toxoplasma gondii* Em Caprinos Do Estado de Alagoas. [*Occurrence and Risk Factors Associated with* Toxoplasma gondii *Infection in Goats in the State of Alagoas*]" *Revista Da Sociedade Brasileira de Medicina Tropical* 44 (2): 157–62. https://doi.org/10.1590/S0037-86822011005000017.

Balbino, Letícia Santos, Juliana Correa Bernardes, Winni Alves Ladeia, Felippe Danyel Cardoso Martins, Beatriz de Souza Lima Nino, Regina Mitsuka-Breganó, Italmar Teodorico Navarro, and Fernanda Pinto-Ferreira. 2022. "Epidemiological Study of Toxoplasmosis Outbreaks in Brazil." *Transboundary and Emerging Diseases* 69 (4): 2021–28. https://doi.org/10.1111/tbed.14214.

Buxton, D, and EA Innes. 1995. "A Commercial Vaccine for Ovine Toxoplasmosis." *Parasitology* 110 Suppl: S11-6.

Buxton, D, KM Thomson, S Maley, S Wright, and HJ Bos. 1993. "Experimental Challenge of Sheep 18 Months after Vaccination with a Live (S48) *Toxoplasma gondii* Vaccine." *Vet Rec* 133 (13): 310–12.

Buxton, David. 1998. "Protozoan Infections (*Toxoplasma gondii*, *Neospora caninum* and Sarcocystis Spp.) in Sheep and Goats: Recent Advances." *Veterinary Research* 29 (3–4): 289–310.

Calderaro, Adriana, Giovanna Piccolo, Chiara Gorrini, Simona Peruzzi, Laura Zerbini, Simona Bommezzadri, Giuseppe Dettori, and Carla Chezzi. 2006. "Comparison between Two Real-Time PCR Assays and a Nested-PCR for the Detection of *Toxoplasma gondii*." *Acta Biomedica de l'Ateneo Parmense*.

Canada, Nuno, Carla S Meireles, A Rocha, JM Correia da Costa, MW Erickson, and JP Dubey. 2002. "Isolation of Viable *Toxoplasma gondii* from Naturally Infected Aborted Bovine Fetuses." *Journal of Parasitology* 88 (6): 1247–48. https://doi.org/10.1645/0022-3395(2002)088[1247:iovtgf]2.0.co;2.

Carmo, Ediclei Lima do, Rafaela dos Anjos Pinheiro Bogoevich Morais, Michele de Souza Lima, Carla Cristina Guimarães de Moraes, George Rêgo Albuquerque, Aristeu Vieira da Silva, and Marinete Marins Póvoa. 2017. "Anti-*Toxoplasma gondii* Antibodies in Beef Cattle Slaughtered in the Metropolitan Region of Belém, Brazilian Amazon." *Revista Brasileira de Parasitologia Veterinária* 26 (2): 226–30. https://doi.org/10.1590/s1984-29612017012.

Chartier, C, and MP Mallereau. 2001. "Efficacité Vaccinale de La Souche S48 de *Toxoplasma gondii*vis-à-Vis d'une Infection Expérimentale Chez La Chèvre [*S48 Strain against an Experimental Infection in Goats*]. Vaccine Efficacy of *Toxoplasma gondii*" *Annales de Médecine Vétérinaire* 145 (1): 202–9.

Chiari, CA, and DP Neves. 1984. "Human Toxoplasmosis Acquired by Ingestion of Goat's Milk." *Memorias Do Instituto Oswaldo Cruz* 79 (3): 337–40. https://doi.org/10.1590/S0074-02761984000300007.

Cook, AJC. 2000. "Sources of Toxoplasma Infection in Pregnant Women: European Multicentre Case-Control Study Commentary: Congenital Toxoplasmosis---Further Thought for Food." *BMJ* 321 (7254): 142–47. https://doi.org/10.1136/bmj.321.7254.142.

Costa, AJ, and EP Costa. 1978. "Freqüência de Bovinos Reagentes à Reação de Imunofluorescência Indireta Para *Toxoplasma gondii* Em Poços de Caldas, MG, Brasil. [*Frequency of Cattle Reactive to the Indirect Immunofluorescence Reaction for* Toxoplasma gondii *in Poços de Caldas, MG, Brazil.*]" *Arquivos Da Escola de Veterinária Da Universidade Federal de Minas Gerais* 30 (1): 47–51.

Costa, AJ, N Kasai, AC Paulillo, MB Silva, and H Galesco. 1978. "Anticorpos Anti-Toxoplasma Em Soros de Bovinos Do Município de Jaboticabal, S.P., Brasil. [*Anti-Toxoplasma antibodies in bovine sera from the municipality of Jaboticabal, S.P., Brazil.*]" *Arquivos Do Instituto Biológico* 45 (4): 299–302.

Costa, DGC, Marvulo, MFV, Silva, JSA, Santana, SC, Magalhães, FJR, Filho, CDFL, Ribeiro, VO, Alves, LC, Mota, RA, Dubey, JP, & Silva, JCR. 2012. "Seroprevalence of *Toxoplasma gondii* in Domestic and Wild Animals from the Fernando de Noronha, Brazil." *Journal of Parasitology* 98 (3): 679–80. https://doi.org/10.1645/GE-2910.1.

Costa, Gustavo Henrique Nogueira, Alvimar José da Costa, Welber Daniel Zanetti Lopes, Katia Denise Saraiva Bresciani, Thais Rabelo dos Santos, César Roberto Esper, and Áureo Evangelista Santana. 2011. "*Toxoplasma gondii*: Infection Natural Congenital in Cattle and an Experimental Inoculation of Gestating Cows with Oocysts." *Experimental Parasitology* 127 (1): 277–81. https://doi.org/10.1016/j.exppara.2010.08.005.

de Souza, JBR, Soares, VE, Maia, MO, Pereira, CM, Ferraudo, AS, Cruz, BC, Pires Teixeira, WF, Felippelli, G, Maciel, WG, Gonçalves, WA, da Costa, AJ, & Zanetti Lopes, WD. 2016. "Spatial Distribution and Risk Factors for *Toxoplasma gondii* Seropositivity in Cattle Slaughtered for Human Consumption in Rondônia, North

Region, Brazil." *Veterinary Parasitology* 226 (August): 145–49. https://doi.org/10.1016/j.vetpar.2016.07.015.

Dubey, JP 1981d. "Toxoplasma-Induced Abortion in Dairy Goats." *Journal of the American Veterinary Medical Association* 178 (7): 671–74.

Dubey, JP, and DS Adams. n.d. "Prevalence of *Toxoplasma gondii* Antibodies in Dairy Goats from 1982 to 1984 - PubMed." *Journal of the American Veterinary Medical Association*. 1990 Jan;196(2):295-296. Accessed July 12, 2022. https://pubmed.ncbi.nlm.nih.gov/2298654/.

Dubey, JP, and JL Jones. 2008. "*Toxoplasma gondii* Infection in Humans and Animals in the United States." *Int J Parasitol* 38 (11): 1257–78. https://doi.org/10.1016/j.ijpara.2008.03.007.

Dubey, JP, and RH Streitel. 1976. "Prevalence of Toxoplasma Infection in Cattle Slaughtered at an Ohio Abattoir." *Journal of the American Veterinary Medical Association* 169 (11): 1197–99.

Dubey, JP, E Laurin, and OCH Kwowk. 2016. "Validation of the Modified Agglutination Test for the Detection of *Toxoplasma gondii* in Free-Range Chickens by Using Cat and Mouse Bioassay." *Parasitology* 143 (3): 314–19. https://doi.org/10.1017/S0031182015001316.

Dubey, JP, Hill, DE, Jones, JL, Hightower, AW, Kirkland, E, Roberts, JM, Marcet, PL, Lehmann, T, Vianna, MCB, Miska, K, Sreekumar, C, Kwok, OCH, Shen, SK, & Gamble, HR. 2005. "Prevalence of Viable *Toxoplasma gondii* in Beef, Chicken, and Pork from Retail Meat Stores in the United States: Risk Assessment to Consumers." *The Journal of Parasitology* 91 (5): 1082–93. https://doi.org/10.1645/GE-683.1.

Dubey, JP, SK Verma, LR Ferreira, S Oliveira, AB Cassinelli, Y Ying, OCH Kwok, W Tuo, OA Chiesa, and JL Jones. 2014. "Detection and Survival of *Toxoplasma gondii* in Milk and Cheese from Experimentally Infected Goats." *Journal of Food Protection* 77 (10): 1747–53. https://doi.org/10.4315/0362-028X.JFP-14-167.

Dubey, JP, SP Sharma, CW Lopes, JF Williams, CS Williams, and SE Weisbrode. 1980. "Caprine Toxoplasmosis: Abortion, Clinical Signs, and Distribution of Toxoplasma in Tissues of Goats Fed *Toxoplasma gondii* Oocysts." *American Journal of Veterinary Research* 41 (7): 1072–76.

Dubey, JP. 1981a. "Epizootic Toxoplasmosis Associated with Abortion in Dairy Goats in Montana." *J Am Vet Med Assoc* 178 (7): 661–70.

Dubey, JP. 1981b. "Prevention of Abortion and Neonatal Death Due to Toxoplasmosis by Vaccination of Goats with the Nonpathogenic Coccidium Hammondia Hammondi." *Am J Vet Res* 42 (12): 2155–57.

Dubey, JP. 1981c. "Protective Immunity against Clinical Toxoplasmosis in Dairy Goats Vaccinated with Hammondia Hammondi and Hammondia Heydorni." *Am J Vet Res* 42 (12): 2068–70.

Dubey, JP. 1989a. "Lesions in Goats Fed *Toxoplasma gondii* Oocysts." *Veterinary Parasitology* 32 (2–3): 133–44. https://doi.org/10.1016/0304-4017(89)90114-3.

Dubey, JP. 1989b. "Lesions in Goats Fed *Toxoplasma gondii* Oocysts." *Veterinary Parasitology* 32 (2–3): 133–44. https://doi.org/10.1016/0304-4017(89)90114-3.

Dubey, JP. 1994. "Toxoplasmosis." *J Am Vet Med Assoc* 205 (11): 1593–98.

Dubey, JP. 2010. "*Toxoplasma gondii* Infections in Chickens (Gallus Domesticus): Prevalence, Clinical Disease, Diagnosis and Public Health Significance." *Zoonoses and Public Health* 57 (1): 60–73. https://doi.org/10.1111/j.1863-2378.2009.01274.x.

Ducournau, Céline, Nathalie Moiré, Rodolphe Carpentier, Pauline Cantin, Clément Herkt, Isabelle Lantier, Didier Betbeder, and Isabelle Dimier-Poisson. 2020. "Effective Nanoparticle-Based Nasal Vaccine against Latent and Congenital Toxoplasmosis in Sheep." *Frontiers in Immunology* 11 (September). https://doi.org/10.3389/fimmu.2020.02183.

Figliuolo, LPC, N Kasai, AMA Ragozo, VSO de Paula, RA Dias, SLP Souza, and SM Gennari. 2004. "Prevalence of Anti-*Toxoplasma gondii* and Anti-*Neospora caninum* Antibodies in Ovine from São Paulo State, Brazil." *Veterinary Parasitology* 123 (3–4): 161–66. https://doi.org/10.1016/j.vetpar.2004.06.006.

Freyre, A, J Bonino, J Falcon, D Castells, O Correa, and A Casaretto. 1999. "The Incidence and Economic Significance of Ovine Toxoplasmosis in Uruguay." *Veterinary Parasitology* 81 (1): 85–88. https://doi.org/10.1016/S0304-4017(98)00215-5.

Garcia, Guilherme, Cristina Sotomaior, Aguinaldo José do Nascimento, Italmar Teodorico Navarro, and Vanete Thomaz Soccol. 2012. "*Toxoplasma gondii* in Goats from Curitiba, Paraná, Brazil: Risks Factors and Epidemiology." *Revista Brasileira de Parasitologia Veterinaria* 21 (1): 42–47. https://doi.org/10.1590/s1984-29612012000100009.

Garcia, JL. 2009. "Vaccination Concepts against *Toxoplasma gondii*." *Expert Rev Vaccines* 8 (2): 215–25. https://doi.org/10.1586/14760584.8.2.215.

Garcia, JL, Navarro, IT, Ogawa, L, and Oliveira, RC. 1999. "Seroprevalence of *Toxoplasma gondii* in Swine, Bovine, Ovine and Equine, and Their Correlation with Human, Felines and Canines, from Farms in North Region of Paraná State, Brazil." *Ciência Rural* 29 (1): 91–97.

Gomes, Daniella Ferreira Cordeiro, Lucas Andrade Mendes, Juliana Moraes Dias, Müller Ribeiro-Andrade, Pollyanne Raysa Fernandes de Oliveira, Rinaldo Aparecido Mota, Emmanuel Arnhold, Maria Clorinda Soares Fioravanti, and Cairo Henrique Sousa de Oliveira. 2021. "Seroprevalence, Spatial Distribution and Risk Factors Associated with *Toxoplasma gondii* Infection among Cattle in a Quilombola Community in the Brazilian Cerrado." *Revista Brasileira de Parasitologia Veterinaria* 30 (1). https://doi.org/10.1590/s1984-296120201080.

Gorman, Texia, Juan Pablo Arancibia, Myriam Lorca, David Hird, and Hector Alcaino. 1999. "Seroprevalence of *Toxoplasma gondii* Infection in Sheep and Alpacas (Llama Pacos) in Chile." *Preventive Veterinary Medicine* 40 (3–4): 143–49. https://doi.org/10.1016/S0167-5877(99)00044-6.

Gos, María Laura, Jorge Alberto Manazza, Ernesto J A Späth, Lais Pardini, María Andrea Fiorentino, Juan Manuel Unzaga, Gastón Moré, and María Cecilia Venturini. 2017. "Seroprevalence of *Toxoplasma gondii* and *Neospora caninum* Infections in Goats from Two Argentinean Provinces." *Open Veterinary Journal* 7 (4): 319–22. https://doi.org/10.4314/ovj.v7i4.5.

Guimarães, Luciana Afonso, Rodrigo Alves Bezerra, Daniele de Santana Rocha, and George Rêgo Albuquerque. 2013. "Prevalence and Risk Factors Associated with Anti-*Toxoplasma gondii* Antibodies in Sheep from Bahia State, Brazil." *Revista Brasileira de Parasitologia Veterinaria* 22 (2): 220–24. https://doi.org/10.1590/S1984-2961 2013000200041.

Hecker, Yanina P, Dadín P Moore, Jorge A Manazza, Juan M Unzaga, Ernesto JA Späth, Lais L Pardini, María C Venturini, José L Roberi, and Carlos M Campero. 2013. "First Report of Seroprevalence of *Toxoplasma gondii* and *Neospora caninum* in Dairy Sheep from Humid Pampa, Argentina." *Tropical Animal Health and Production* 45 (7): 1645–47. https://doi.org/10.1007/s11250-013-0396-1.

Hecker, Yanina P, Fernando Mogaburu Masson, Joaquín I Armendano, Juan Cora, Carlos Flores Olivares, Ignacio Gual, Lais Pardini, Dadín P Moore, Gastón Moré, and Germán J Cantón. 2018. "Evaluation of Frequency of Antibodies against *Toxoplasma gondii, Neospora caninum* and Sarcocystis Spp. and Transmission Routes in Sheep from Humid Pampa, Argentina." *Acta Parasitologica* 63 (2): 416–21. https://doi.org/ 10.1515/ap-2018-0048.

Hiszczynska-Sawicka, E, G Oledzka, L Holec-Gasior, H Li, J B Xu, R Sedcole, J Kur, R Bickerstaffe, and M Stankiewicz. 2011. "Evaluation of Immune Responses in Sheep Induced by DNA Immunization with Genes Encoding GRA1, GRA4, GRA6 and GRA7 Antigens of *Toxoplasma gondii.*" *Vet Parasitol* 177 (3–4): 281–89. https://doi.org/S0304-4017(10)00697-7 [pii] 10.1016/j.vetpar.2010.11.047.

Hiszczynska-Sawicka, E, H Li, J Boyu Xu, M Akhtar, L Holec-Gasior, J Kur, R Bickerstaffe, and M Stankiewicz. 2012. "Induction of Immune Responses in Sheep by Vaccination with Liposome-Entrapped DNA Complexes Encoding *Toxoplasma gondii* MIC3 Gene." *Pol J Vet Sci* 15 (1): 3–9.

Hiszczynska-Sawicka, E, H Li, JB Xu, G Oledzka, J Kur, R Bickerstaffe, and M Stankiewicz. 2010. "Comparison of Immune Response in Sheep Immunized with DNA Vaccine Encoding *Toxoplasma gondii* GRA7 Antigen in Different Adjuvant Formulations." *Exp Parasitol* 124 (4): 365–72. https://doi.org/10.1016/j.exppara.20 09.11.015.

Hiszczynska-Sawicka, E, H Li, JB Xu, L Holec-Gasior, J Kur, R Sedcole, R Bickerstaffe, and M Stankiewicz. 2011. "Modulation of Immune Response to *Toxoplasma gondii* in Sheep by Immunization with a DNA Vaccine Encoding ROP1 Antigen as a Fusion Protein with Ovine CD154." *Vet Parasitol* 183 (1–2): 72–78. https://doi.org/10.1016/ j.vetpar.2011.06.010.

Hiszczynska-Sawicka, E, M Akhtar, GW Kay, L Holec-Gasior, R Bickerstaffe, J Kur, and M Stankiewicz. 2010. "The Immune Responses of Sheep after DNA Immunization with, *Toxoplasma gondii* MAG1 Antigen-with and without Co-Expression of Ovine Interleukin 6." *Vet Immunol Immunopathol* 136 (3–4): 324–29. https://doi.org/S0165-2427(10)00090-5 [pii] 10.1016/j.vetimm.2010.03.018.

Innes, EA, 2010. "A Brief History and Overview of *Toxoplasma gondii.*" *Zoonoses and Public Health* 57 (1): 1–7. https://doi.org/10.1111/j.1863-2378.2009.01276.x.

Innes, EA, and AN Vermeulen. 2006. "Vaccination as a Control Strategy against the Coccidial Parasites Eimeria, Toxoplasma and Neospora." *Parasitology* 133 Suppl: S145-68. https://doi.org/10.1017/s0031182006001855.

Innes, EA, PM Bartley, D Buxton, and F Katzer. 2009. "Ovine Toxoplasmosis." *Parasitology* 136 (14): 1887–94. https://doi.org/10.1017/s0031182009991636.

Innes, EA, PM Bartley, SW Maley, SE Wright, and D Buxton. 2007. "Comparative Host-Parasite Relationships in Ovine Toxoplasmosis and Bovine Neosporosis and Strategies for Vaccination." *Vaccine* 25 (30): 5495–5503. https://doi.org/10.1016/j.vaccine.2007.02.044.

Innes, Elisabeth A, Clare Hamilton, Joao L Garcia, Andreas Chryssafidis, and David Smith. 2019. "A One Health Approach to Vaccines against *Toxoplasma gondii*." *Food and Waterborne Parasitology* 15 (June): e00053. https://doi.org/10.1016/j.fawpar.2019.e00053.

Jacobs, L, JS Remington, and ML Melton. 1960. "A Survey of Meat Samples from Swine, Cattle, and Sheep for the Presence of Encysted Toxoplasma." *J Parasitol* 46: 23–28.

Jamra, LF, MP Deane, and EC Guimarães. 1969. "On the Isolation of *Toxoplasma gondii* from Human Food and Animals Origin. Partial Results in the City of São Paulo (Brazil)." *Revista Do Instituto de Medicina Tropical de São Paulo* 11 (3): 169–76.

Katzer, F, G Canton, A Burrells, J Palarea-Albaladejo, B Horton, PM Bartley, Y Pang, F Chianini, EA Innes, and J Benavides. 2014. "Immunization of Lambs with the S48 Strain of *Toxoplasma gondii* Reduces Tissue Cyst Burden Following Oral Challenge with a Complete Strain of the Parasite." *Vet Parasitol* 205 (1–2): 46–56. https://doi.org/10.1016/j.vetpar.2014.07.003.

Laurence Baril, Thierry Ancelle, Vé. 1999. "Risk Factors for Toxoplasma Infection in Pregnancy: A Case-Control Study in France." *Scandinavian Journal of Infectious Diseases* 31 (3): 305–9. https://doi.org/10.1080/00365549950163626.

Liesenfeld, O, TA Nguyen, C Pharke, and Y Suzuki. 2001. "Importance of Gender and Sex Hormones in Regulation of Susceptibility of the Small Intestine to Peroral Infection with *Toxoplasma gondii* Tissue Cysts - PubMed." *J. Parasitology* 87(6). 2001. https://pubmed.ncbi.nlm.nih.gov/11780848/.

Lopes, Welber Daniel Zanetti, Thaís Rabelo dos Santos, Ricardo dos Santos da Silva, Walter Matheus Rossanese, Fernando Augusto de Souza, Joana D Ark de Faria Rodrigues, Rafael Paranhos de Mendonça, Vando Edésio Soares, and Alvimar José da Costa. 2010. "Seroprevalence of and Risk Factors for *Toxoplasma gondii* in Sheep Raised in the Jaboticabal Microregion, São Paulo State, Brazil." *Research in Veterinary Science* 88 (1): 104–6. https://doi.org/10.1016/j.rvsc.2009.06.006.

Luciano, DM, RC Menezes, LC Ferreira, JL Nicolau, LB das Neves, RM Luciano, MA Dahroug, and MR Amendoeira. 2011. "Occurrence of Anti-*Toxoplasma gondii* Antibodies in Cattle and Pigs Slaughtered, State of Rio de Janeiro." *Rev Bras Parasitol Vet* 20 (4): 351–53.

Lúcio, EC, SMS Clemente, JL Pimentel, JMB Oliveira, JL Silva Júnior, PPF Albuquerque, RA Mota, and JW Pinheiro Junior. 2016. "Epidemiological Analysis of *Toxoplasma gondii* Infection in Goats in Pernambuco, Brasil." *Brazilian Journal of Veterinary Medicine* 38 (1): 13–18.

Martínez-Rodriguez, Lorena C, Gabriel Andres Tafur-Gómez, and Blanca Lisseth Guzman-Barragan. 2020. "*Toxoplasma gondii* in Small Ruminants in Northeastern Areas of Colombia: Seroprevalence and Risk Factors." *Parasite Epidemiology and Control* 10 (August): e00147. https://doi.org/10.1016/j.parepi.2020.e00147.

Mayer, H. 1965. "Investigaciones Sobre Toxoplasmosis." *Boletin de La Oficina Sanitaria Panamericana* 58 (6): 485–97.

Mevelec, MN, C Ducournau, A Bassuny Ismael, M Olivier, E Seche, M Lebrun, D Bout, and I Dimier-Poisson. 2010. "Mic1-3 Knockout *Toxoplasma gondii* Is a Good Candidate for a Vaccine against T. Gondii-Induced Abortion in Sheep." *Vet Res* 41 (4): 49. https://doi.org/10.1051/vetres/2010021.

Moore, DP, Regidor-Cerrillo, J, Morrell, E, Poso, MA, Cano, DB, Leunda, MR, Linschinky, L, Odeón, AC, Odriozola, E, Ortega-Mora, LM, & Campero, CM. 2008. "The Role of *Neospora caninum* and *Toxoplasma gondii* in Spontaneous Bovine Abortion in Argentina." *Veterinary Parasitology* 156 (3–4): 163–67. https://doi.org/10.1016/J.VETPAR.2008.06.020.

Moraes, Érica Paes Barreto Xavier de, André Mariano Batista, Eduardo Bento Faria, Roberta Lemos Freire, Antonio Carlos Freitas, Maria Angélica Ramos Silva, Valdir A. Braga, and Rinaldo Aparecido Mota. 2010. "Experimental Infection by *Toxoplasma gondii* Using Contaminated Semen Containing Different Doses of Tachyzoites in Sheep." *Veterinary Parasitology* 170 (3–4): 318–22. https://doi.org/10.1016/j.vetpar.2010.02.017.

Moré, G, W Basso, D Bacigalupe, MC Venturini, and L Venturini. 2008. "Diagnosis of Sarcocystis Cruzi, *Neospora caninum*, and *Toxoplasma gondii* Infections in Cattle." *Parasitology Research* 102 (4): 671–75. https://doi.org/10.1007/S00436-007-0810-6.

Moura, Anderson Barbosa de, André Ribeiro, Antonio Pereira de Souza, Marcio Orides da Silva, Gustavo Machado, Vanderlei Klauck, Rafael Pazinato, and Aleksandro Schafer da Silva. 2016. "Seroprevalence and Risk Factors for *Toxoplasma gondii* Infection in Goats in Southern Brazil." *Acta Scientiae Veterinariae* 44 (1): 7–8. https://doi.org/10.22456/1679-9216.81073.

Moura, Anderson Barbosa de, Silvia Cristina Osaki, Dauton Luiz Zulpo, João Luís Garcia, and Everton Borba Teixeira. 2010. "Detecção De Anticorpos Contra *Toxoplasma gondii* Em Bovinos De Corte Abatidos Em Guarapuava, Pr, Brasil. [*Detection of Antibodies against* Toxoplasma gondii *in Beef Cattle Slaughtered in Guarapuava, PR, Brazil*]" *Archives of Veterinary Science* 15 (2). https://doi.org/10.5380/avs.v15i2.14779.

O'Connell, E, MF Wilkins, and WA te Punga. 1988. "Toxoplasmosis in Sheep. II. The Ability of a Live Vaccine to Prevent Lamb Losses after an Intravenous Challenge with *Toxoplasma gondii*." *N Z Vet J* 36 (1): 1–4. https://doi.org/10.1080/00480169.1988.35461.

Obendorf, DL, P Statham, and BL Munday. 1990. "Resistance to Toxoplasma Abortion in Female Goats Previously Exposed to Toxoplasma Infection." *Australian Veterinary Journal* 67 (6): 233–34. https://doi.org/10.1111/J.1751-0813.1990.TB07773.X.

Ogawa, Liza, Italmar Teodorico Navarro, Roberta Lemos Freire, Rosângela Claret de Oliveira, and Odilon Vidotto. 2003. "Ocorrência de Anticorpos Anti-*Toxoplasma gondii* Em Ovinos Da Região de Londrina No Estado Do Paraná. [*Occurrence of Anti-*Toxoplasma gondii *Antibodies in Sheep from Londrina Region, Paraná State*]" *Semina: Ciências Agrárias* 24 (1): 57. https://doi.org/10.5433/1679-0359.2003v24n1p57.

Passos, LMF, JD Lima, and BL Figueiredo. 1984. "Determinação Da Infecção Por *Toxoplasma gondii* Em Bovinos Abatidos Em Belo Horizonte (MG) Através Da Freqüência de Anticorpos e Tentativa de Isolamento a Partir de Musculatura

Diafragmática. Determination of *Toxoplasma gondii* Infection in Cattle Slaughtered in Belo Horizonte (MG) Through Antibody Frequency and Attempted Isolation from Diaphragmatic Musculature." *Arquivo Brasileiro de Medicina Veterinária e Zootecnia* 36: 581–89.

Pinheiro, José Wilton, Rinaldo Aparecido Mota, Andréa Alice da Fonseca Oliveira, Eduardo Bento Faria, Luis Fernando Pita Gondim, Aristeu Vieira da Silva, and Giulliano Aires Anderlini. 2009. "Prevalence and Risk Factors Associated to Infection by *Toxoplasma gondii* in Ovine in the State of Alagoas, Brazil." *Parasitology Research* 105 (3): 709–15. https://doi.org/10.1007/s00436-009-1472-3.

Pita Gondim, LF, Hv Barbosa, CHA Ribeiro Filho, and H Saeki. 1999. "Serological Survey of Antibodies to *Toxoplasma gondii* in Goats, Sheep, Cattle and Water Buffaloes in Bahia State, Brazil." *Veterinary Parasitology* 82 (4): 273–76. https://doi.org/10.1016/S0304-4017(99)00033-3.

Rani, Surabhi, Camila K Cerqueira-Cézar, Fernando HA Murata, Oliver CH Kwok, Jitender P Dubey, and Abani K Pradhan. 2020. "Distribution of *Toxoplasma gondii* Tissue Cysts in Shoulder Muscles of Naturally Infected Goats and Lambs." *Journal of Food Protection* 83 (8): 1396–1401. https://doi.org/10.4315/JFP-20-024.

Reis, CR, FMR Lopes, DB Gonçalves, RL Freire, JL Garcia, and IT Navarro. 2007. "Occurrence of Anti-*Toxoplasma gondii* Antibodies in Caprines from Pitanga City, Paraná State, Brazil." *Brazilian Journal Vet. Res. Anim. Sci.* 44 (5): 358–63.

Robert, R, D Chabasse, and P Hocquet. 1981. "Antitoxoplasma IgM Studied by Indirect Immunofluorescence and Hemagglutination: Elimination of False Positives and Negatives by Adsorption of IgG on Immobilized Protein A - PubMed." *Biomedicina.* 1981. https://pubmed.ncbi.nlm.nih.gov/7020782/.

Sakata, Francine Bragagnolo Liz Stefen, Valdomiro Bellato, Amélia Aparecida Sartor, Anderson Barbosa de Moura, Antonio Pereira de Souza, and Juliana Antunes Farias. 2012. "*Toxoplasma gondii* Antibodies Sheep in Lages, Santa Catarina, Brazil, and Comparison Using IFA and ELISA." *Revista Brasileira de Parasitologia Veterinaria* 21 (3): 196–200. https://doi.org/10.1590/s1984-29612012000300004.

Santos, Carolina de Sousa Américo Batista, Sérgio Santos de Azevedo, Herbert Sousa Soares, Severino Silvano Dos Santos Higino, Hilda Fátima de Jesus Pena, Clebert José Alves, and Solange Maria Gennari. 2012. "Risk Factors Associated with *Toxoplasma gondii* Seroprevalence in Goats in the State of Paraíba, Brazil." *Revista Brasileira de Parasitologia Veterinaria* 21 (4): 399–404. https://doi.org/10.1590/s1984-29612012005000002.

Santos, F, Laura, Maria Damé, Beatris Cademartori, Nilton Cunha Filho, Nara R Farias, and Jerônimo Ruas. 2013. "Occurrence of Antibodies to *Toxoplasma gondii* in Water Buffaloes and Meat Cattle in Rio Grande Do Sul State, Southern Brazil." *Acta Parasitologica* 58 (3). https://doi.org/10.2478/s11686-013-0148-4.

Santos, TR, AJ Costa, GH Toniollo, MCR Luvizotto, AH Benetti, RR Santos, DH Matta, WDZ Lopes, JA Oliveira, and GP Oliveira. 2009. "Prevalence of Anti-*Toxoplasma gondii* Antibodies in Dairy Cattle, Dogs, and Humans from the Jauru Micro-Region, Mato Grosso State, Brazil." *Veterinary Parasitology* 161 (3–4): 324–26. https://doi.org/10.1016/j.vetpar.2009.01.017.

Schares, G, Koethe, M, Bangoura, B, Geuthner, AC, Randau, F, Ludewig, M, Maksimov, P, Sens, M, Bärwald, A, Conraths, FJ, Villena, I, Aubert, D, Opsteegh, M, & Van der Giessen, J. 2018. "*Toxoplasma gondii* Infections in Chickens – Performance of Various Antibody Detection Techniques in Serum and Meat Juice Relative to Bioassay and DNA Detection Methods." *International Journal for Parasitology*. 48(9–10), 751–762.https://doi.org/10.1016/j.ijpara.2018.03.007.

Schoch, CL, Ciufo, S, Domrachev, M, Hotton, CL, Kannan, S, Khovanskaya, R, Leipe, D, Mcveigh, R, O'Neill, K, Robbertse, B, Sharma, S, Soussov, V, Sullivan, JP, Sun, L, Turner, S, & Karsch-Mizrachi, I. 2020. "NCBI Taxonomy: A Comprehensive Update on Curation, Resources and Tools." *Database* 2020. https://doi.org/10.1093/DATABASE/BAAA062.

Sella, MZ, IT Navarro, O Vidotto, RL Freire, and PN Shida. 1994. "Epidemiologia Da Toxoplasmose Caprina, Levantamento Sorológico Do *Toxoplasma gondii* Em Caprinos Leiteiros Na Micro Região de Londrina, Paraná, Brasil. Epidemiology of Caprine Toxoplasmosis, Serological Survey of *Toxoplasma gondii* in Dairy Goats in the Micro Region of Londrina, Paraná, Brazil." *Brazilian Journal of Veterinary Parasitology* 3 (1): 13–16.

Silva Filho, MF, E Erzinger, IAL Cunha, FM Bugni, FN Hamada, ERM Marana, RL Freire, JL Garcia, and IT Navarro. 2008. "*Toxoplasma gondii*: Abortion Outbreak in a Goatherd from Southern Brazil." *Semina: Ciências Agrárias* 29 (4): 887–94.

Spagnol, Fernando H, Elisson B Paranhos, Laura Lucia dos S Oliveira, Simoni M de Medeiros, Carlos Wilson G Lopes, and George R Albuquerque. 2009. "Prevalência de Anticorpos Anti-*Toxoplasma gondii* Em Bovinos Abatidos Em Matadouros Do Estado Da Bahia, Brasil. Prevalence of Anti-*Toxoplasma gondii* Antibodies in Cattle Slaughtered in Slaughterhouses in the State of Bahia, Brazil" *Revista Brasileira de Parasitologia Veterinaria* 18 (2): 42–45. https://doi.org/10.4322/rbpv.01802009.

Suzuki K, Corva SG, Traveria G, Cattaneo M, Puentes R, Martinicorena M, Moreno J, Furtado A, Freyre A, Satragno D, Acevedo C, Nunez R, Bermudez J. 2011. "Seroprevalence of *Toxoplasma gondii* and *Neospora caninum* in Sheep in Uruguay." *Analecta Veterinaria* 31 (2): 28–32.

Weinman, D, and AH Chandler. 1954. "Toxoplasmosis in Swine and Rodents; Reciprocal Oral Infection and Potential Human Hazard." *Proceedings of the Society for Experimental Biology and Medicine* 87 (1): 211–16.

Wiengcharoen, J, RCA Thompson, C Nakthong, P Rattanakorn, and Y Sukthana. 2011. "Transplacental Transmission in Cattle: Is *Toxoplasma gondii* Less Potent than *Neospora caninum*?" *Parasitology Research* 108 (5): 1235–41. https://doi.org/10.1007/s00436-010-2172-8.

Yan, C, CL Yue, ZG Yuan, RQ Lin, Y He, CC Yin, MJ Xu, HQ Song, and XQ Zhu. 2010. "Molecular and Serological Diagnosis of *Toxoplasma gondii* Infection in Experimentally Infected Chickens." *Veterinary Parasitology* 173 (3–4): 179–83. https://doi.org/10.1016/j.vetpar.2010.07.011.

Chapter 9

Tritrichomonosis in Livestock Ruminants from Latin America

Fernando de Souza Rodrigues*
Luiz Daniel de Barros
and João Luis Garcia
Department of Preventive Veterinary Medicine,
Laboratory of Animal Protozoology,
State University of Londrina, Londrina, PR, Brazil

Introduction

Tritrichomonas foetus is an extracellular agellated protozoan parasite that is often found in the urogenital tract of the bovine hosts (Ondrak 2016). *T. foetus* infection in cattle cause Tritrichomonosis or Tritrichomoniasis which is a notifiable disease by the World Organisation for Animal Health (OIE). Transmission occurs mainly during coitus (Parsonson, Clark, and Dufty 1976). In bulls, *T. foetus* is usually clinically asymptomatic. However, in cows *T. foetus* can cause genital infection, which can result in embryonic death and abortion. The effect of genital infection can cause economic losses due to reproduction problems and productive (D O Rae 1989; Michi et al. 2016; Yao 2021). This chapter describes the aspects related to the etiologic agent, life cycle, epidemiology, pathogenesis, immune response, diagnosis, treatment, and control of tritrichomonosis in cattle.

---

* Corresponding Author's Email: fernando.rodriguesvet@gmail.com.

In: Infectious and Parasitic Diseases of Animals in Developing Countries
Editor: Selwyn Arlington Headley
ISBN: 979-8-88697-504-8

Etiologic Agent and Life Cycle

The trichomonads (Metamonada, Parabasalia) are extracellular parasites of the phylum *Parabasalia*, order *Tritrichomonadida*, and family *Tritrichomonadidae* (Adl et al. 2019). Trichomonads are a group of flagellates that are characterized by having hydrogenosomes (modified mitochondria), a typical arrangement of mastigont set of kinetosomes and their associated appendages, a parabasal apparatus (Cepicka, Hampl, and Kulda 2010).

Morphologically, *T. foetus* has a trophozoite and pseudocyst form (Pereira-Neves and Benchimol 2009). Trophozoites of *T. foetus* are pyriform-shaped approximately 20x10 μm long and 5-15 μm wide with a rounded anterior end and generally a pointed posterior. *T. foetus* has a single nucleus and four flagella. The flagella arise from the kinetosome complex at the anterior end. Three of the flagella are free anteriorly, and the fourth flagellum runs towards the undulating membrane around ¾ of the body (D Owen Rae and Crews 2006). *T. foetus* has a well-developed cytoskeleton composed of an axostyle, costa, and pelta (Dąbrowska et al. 2019).

Pseudocysts form is rounded shape, with internalized flagella, without motility, and does not have a true cyst wall. Changes in physicochemical characteristics of the environment can activate their defense mechanism (resistance), leave the vegetative form (trophozoite) and assume a rounded shape (pseudocysts) (Benchimol 2004).

Reproduction of the trophozoite form of *T. foetus* is achieved asexually by cryptopleuromitosis, a special type of closed mitosis, characteristic of the trophozoite form that results in two identical daughter cells (Pereira-Neves and Benchimol 2009).

T. foetus occurs mainly in the urogenital tract of cattle but also infects the domestic cat and swine. Different from that in cattle, the predilection site of feline infection is the gastrointestinal tract which can results in chronic diarrhea (Yao and Köster 2015). The feline strain differs from its bovine counterpart by one base pair of the ITS-2 sequence (Yao 2013; Yao and Ketzis 2018). Although differences were detected in other genes, the majority of these were less than 1% except for the cysteine protease 2 and 6 genes (Slapeta et al. 2012; Yao and Ketzis 2018). A different species, *T. blagburni*, was proposed for the protozoan of the feline host, but the name has not been accepted (Walden et al. 2013).

Additionally, *Tritrichomonas* spp. was described in swine. *T. suis* is commonly found in the nasal cavity, stomach, cecum, and colon of swine as a commensal organism, molecular data had suggested this species is a synonym of *T. foetus* (Slapeta et al. 2012; Sun, Stack, and Šlapeta 2012; Tachezy et al. 2002). Furthermore, it was suggested that the bovine, feline, and swine isolates should be known as *T. foetus* (Slapeta et al. 2012). Moreover, the *T. foetus* bovine isolate was occasionally reported in humans (Yao 2012; Yao and Ketzis 2018).

Epidemiology

Tritrichomonosis is a notifiable disease by the OIE and was reported in six continents including North America, South America, Europe, Asia, Africa and Oceania (BonDurant et al. 1990; D Owen Rae et al. 2004; Filho et al. 2018; Jesús A Mendoza-Ibarra et al. 2012; Jesús Alberto Mendoza-Ibarra et al. 2013; Mardones et al. 2008; Martín-Gómez et al. 1998; McCool et al. 1988; Pefanis et al. 1988; Szonyia et al. 2012). In Latin America, the protozoan was reported in most countries with a triving cattle industry. The occurrence of *T. foetus* in cattle from Central and South America is summarized in Table 1.

Table 1. Occurrence of *Tritrichomonas foetus* in cattle from Latin America (1955 to 2021)

Country	Occurrence (%)	Diagnostic method	References
Brazil	9.09	Direct exam	Rabello 1955
Brazil	14.6	Culture	Guida et al. 1972
Colombia	13.7	Culture	Griffiths et al. 1984
Brazil	1.88	Culture	Gomes et al. 1991
Costa Rica	7.2	Culture	Perez et al. 1992
Argentina and Uruguay**	0.8	Culture	Fernández et al. 2007
Brazil	2.63	Culture	Silva et al. 2009
Colombia	61.8	Culture	González-Carmona et al. 2012
Argentina	1.1	Culture	Molina et al. 2013
Brazil	33.4	PCR	De Oliveira et al. 2015
St. Kitts	0.0	Culture	Coker et al. 2018
Brazil	3.7	PCR	Filho et al. 2018
Uruguay	2.25	PCR	Silveira et al. 2020

*Not reported that use of a culture diagnostic method.

** One sample was from Uruguay

The mode of transmission occurs during coitus, where the parasite passes from the infected bull to a susceptible cow and conversely. *T. foetus* is more effectively transmitted from an infected male to a susceptible female than from a cow to a bull. Susceptible heifers may be infected after a single copulation with *T. foetus* positive bull, with the rate of transmission up to 95% (Parsonson, Clark, and Dufty 1976).

T. foetus is capable of surviving temperatures used to preserve semen for artificial insemination (AI). Semen contaminated with this organism at the time of cryopreservation could lead to transmission of the trichomonads by AI (Yao 2013). Another transmission mode of less importance is iatrogenic transmission (Goodger and Skirrow 1986).

The age of the animal appears to have importance in the development of a chronic infection compared to a transient infection in the bull. In different studies, younger bulls (<3 years) were less infected than older bulls (BonDurant et al. 1990; D Owen Rae et al. 2004). Most of the bulls with 1-2 years were refractory to infection. Alterations in mucosa folds and deeper crypts in the preputial and penile epithelia of older bulls, probably cause a reduced oxygen environment that increase the susceptibility to infection with *T. foetus*. Bull infected with *T. foetus* can become a chronic carrier (Parsonson, Clark, and Dufty 1974; Yao 2013).

In cows the elimination of *T. foetus*, normally occur between 90–95 days of sexual repose (Mancebo et al. 1995), however, the duration of infection is variable, with reported varying of 13 weeks to 22 months after infection (S. Skirrow 1987; S. Z. Skirrow and BonDurant 1990a).

Risk factors for tritrichomonosis detected in different experiments were the presence of older bulls in the herd, many bulls per breeding group, the presence of disease in the previous year, continuous breeding season, neighbouring a positive herd(s), commingling with other herds, grazing on public allotments, elapsed time taken to fix a broken fence(s) a week or longer, greater bull-to-cow ratio, and lack of knowledge of the disease (D Owen Rae et al. 2004; Jesús A Mendoza-Ibarra et al. 2012; Jin et al. 2014; Mardones et al. 2008; Molina et al. 2018; Perez et al. 1992). No breed predilections to tritrichomonosis have been established for bull (Abbitt and Meyerholz 1979; BonDurant et al. 1990; D Owen Rae et al. 2004).

Economic losses caused by tritrichomonosis mainly consist of prolonged breeding season, reduced uniformity in calf weights, costs of testing bulls and veterinary expenses, as well as the culling and replacement of *T. foetus*-infected bulls and cows. Besides, the parasite can cause 5% to 12% reduction in weight gain during the sucking/growing period, 4% to 10% reduction in weaning weights, 4% to 10% reduction in monetary returns per calf born, 14% to 50% reduction in annual calf crop, and 5% to 35% reduction in financial returns per cow, compared to those exposed to a fertile bull (D O Rae 1989; Michi et al. 2016; Yao 2021).

Pathogeny and Immune Response

T. foetus parasites the epithelium of the prepuce, penis, and occasionally the urethral orifice of bulls. The location of the protozoan facilitates the evasion of the immune responses so *T. foetus* can persist in the genital tract of bulls Eduardo R Cobo, Corbeil, and BonDurant 2011). Antibody responses to *T. foetus* infection in the genital tract of the bulls were incapable of eliminating genital infection. Surface antigen-specific IgG1, IgA, and IgM antibodies in the smegma of bulls naturally infected with *T. foetus* occurred concurrently with *T. foetus*–positive smegma cultures (Rhyan et al. 1999).

T. foetus seems to be resistant or does not induce pathogen-specific inflammation in bulls, because it infects the lower genital tract without causing clinical symptoms. Experimentally or naturally, *T. foetus* genital infections in bulls are clinically asymptomatic without any gross pathological changes (Parsonson, Clark, and Dufty 1974). The histologic response in the prepuce and penis of bulls infected with *T. foetus* is limited to infiltration of intraepithelial lymphocytes, subepithelial lymphocytes, and plasma cells (Parsonson, Clark, and Dufty 1974; Rhyan et al. 1999). Additionally, it was shown that bulls with *T. foetus* did not have more inflammation than unaffected bulls (Flower et al. 1983).

After infection of cows, the agent penetrates the cells of the vaginal and uterine epithelium and placenta and colonizes the oviduct. Inflammation causes an adverse intrauterine environment (Givens 2006). In cows, *T. foetus* causes irregular early abortions, heat cycles, pyometra, and temporary subfertility. Most fetal loss occurs within the first 5 months of gestation followed by a 2- to 6-month period of infertility as the immune system clears the parasite from the reproductive tract (BonDurant 1997).

Cows infected with *T. foetus* induced antigen-specific antibody response in the vagina. Infected nonpregnant heifers with *T. foetus* induced *T. foetus* cell-specific IgG1 and IgA antibodies in vaginal secretions (Anderson et al. 1996; L B Corbeil et al. 1998; L B Corbeil et al. 2001; S. Z. Skirrow and BonDurant 1990b). IgA persists for 24 weeks after infection or until genital clearance (Ikeda, BonDurant, and Corbeil 1995). In heifers, genital infections were limited to 13 to 28 weeks (Anderson et al. 1996; L B Corbeil et al. 2001; L B Corbeil et al. 2005; S. Z. Skirrow and BonDurant 1990b).

IgA has not been shown to eliminate *T. foetus*, but it does immobilize and prevent adherence to the mucosa (Robert H Bondurant 2005). Complement opsonization and killing are consiedered mediated by IgG1 (L B Corbeil et al. 1998). The extracellular location of *T. foetus* initiates a humoral response from the host and, thus, short-term immunity (L B Corbeil et al. 1998). The immunity to natural infections is short with females becoming susceptible within one year and consequently to the next breeding season (Robert H Bondurant 2005).

The nonprotective genital antibody response against *T. foetus* might be affected by parasite factors. Virulent factors of *T. foetus* include secreted extracellular cysteine proteinases (Thomford et al. 1996). *In vitro* cysteine proteinases digest IgG1 and IgG2 antibodies, fibrinogen, fibronectin, albumin, and lactoferrin (Talbot, Nielsen, and Corbeil 1991), the third component of complement (C3) (Kania et al. 2001). The virulent factor possibly affects local immunity by covering antigens or digesting proteins involved in innate and/or acquired immunity (Michi et al. 2016)

Diagnosis

A definitive diagnosis must be made based on epidemiological data, clinical signs, and laboratory tests. Samples of choice to detect *T. foetus* are preputial smegma, semen, placenta, vaginal secretion, and fetal fluid (Alves, Stynen, and Miranda 2011; Givens 2006).

Material collected must be inoculated and transported in selected media. Different selected media such as Diamond's (Sarah Parker, Campbell, and Gajadhar 2003) and InPouch TF (Biomed Diagnostics, San Jose, CA, USA) were developed to maintain the parasite viable for detection. Samples are incubated at 37°C and examined 1, 3, 5, and 7 days after sampling by placing a drop on a glass slide and examining by light microscopy at magnifications of 40x to 100x. Samples are considered positive when living trichomonads with size, shape, rapid and irregular movement of the protozoan body compatible with *T. foetus* are observed (Bondurant et al., 1999).

The presence of non-pathogenic trichomonads like *Tetratrichomonas* spp. that are commensals of the bovine gastrointestinal tract can create false positive results and the time for culture results has resulted in the development of molecular-based testing (Bondurant et al., 1999; Campero et al. 2003; Eduardo Rubén Cobo et al. 2003; Sarah Parker et al. 2003).

PCR is considered as the gold standard and is the preferred diagnostic test due to the high sensitivity and specificity (McMillen and Lew 2006; Schaut et al. 2017; Szonyi et al. 2012). PCR should be performed to differentiate *T. foetus* from other protozoa that may occasionally be present in the samples submitted for diagnosis (Campero et al. 2003). PCR techniques and Real-time PCR are also used successfully for the direct diagnosis of *T. foetus* infection in clinical material (McMillen and Lew 2006; Oyhenart et al. 2013; S Parker, Lun, and Gajadhar 2001;).

A direct RT-qPCR exhibited 100% diagnostic sensitivity and 100% specificity, and a qPCR (culture qPCR), which utilizes cultured samples, exhibited 95% diagnostic sensitivity and 100% specificity. The agreement between direct RT-qPCR and culture qPCR was 98%. Direct RT-qPCR enables simplified sample collection, elimination of culture medium, faster results, applicability in cows, and lower cost than culture qPCR (Ginter Summarell et al. 2018).

A combination of *in vitro* culture methods and confirmation of the diagnostic status of the positive cultures with an appropriate PCR assay can provide a useful approach to the diagnosis of this disease (D Owen Rae and Crews 2006).

Serologic tests to detect the antibody or antigen resulting from exposure to *T. foetus* have been limited application (R H Bondurant et al. 1996). Anti-*T. foetus* monoclonal antibodies have been tested by immunofluorescence assay (L B Corbeil et al. 2008). Latex beads conjugated assay was developed to detect *T. foetus* antigens that could be used as a screening tool. The detection of parasite antigens may provide earlier detection and is a viable option for detecting infection throughout under field conditions (Schaut et al. 2017).

Treatment/Prevention

Therapy for bulls infected with *T. foetus* can be performed with imidazole derivatives suca as metronidazole and ipronidazole (Love et al. 2017; S. Z. Skirrow and Bondurant 1988). Metronidazole (5mg/ml) at a dosage of 60 mg/Kg with two doses with an interval of 24 hours showed potential for treating the protozoan in bulls (Love et al. 2017).

Prevention of *T. foetus* in cattle herds involves the application of basic cattle husbandry practices. One of the main control strategies of tritrichomonosis is the implantation in the cattle farm of an artificial insemination program with quality semen since this will prevent the most important way of transmission of the disease, sexual contact (Robert H Bondurant 2005).

Other strategies include the replacement of older bulls for virgin bulls (less than 3 years), seasonal separation of bulls and cows (Molina et al. 2018), sexual rest for 3-4 cycles for the recovery of females, limited breeding season (60-90 days), and the culling of *T. foetus* positive bull (D Owen Rae and Crews 2006).

It is necessary to test cows with a history of abortion and no pregnant cows, especially in suspected herds for the protozoan (Yao 2021). In Wyoming, testing all bulls and culling *T. foetus*-positive animals led to a gradual and steady decrease in bovine prevalence from 2.69% in 1999 to 0.21% by 2010 (Yao et al. 2011).

Producers should avoid public grazing that allows for a significant increase in both males and females becoming infected through coitus (Gay, Ebel, and Kearley 1996) and preventing the introduction of infected animals (male and female) into the herd, for this control measure, good fencing is necessary (Ondrak 2016).

Vaccination has been shown to be very effective in preventing estrus repetitions and abortions caused by *T. foetus,* especially in areas with natural breeding (Robert H Bondurant 2005). Experimental vaccines based on killed *T. foetus* cells have been shown to improve reproductive health, reduce the losses and number of infected cows, and by increasing the percentage of pregnancy in comparison to non-vaccinated animals (Eduardo Rubén Cobo et al. 2004; Edmondson et al. 2017; Kvasnicka et al. 1989).

A vaccine based on killed-*T. foetus* in different adjuvants had different median times for clearance of infection. In non-immunized animals, the median time for clearance of infection was 69 days, 55 days in animals treated with aluminium hydroxide, 41 days with oil-in-water or saponin-based vaccines or with a commercial vaccine and 27 days in animals treated with saponin plus aluminium hydroxide (Fuchs et al. 2017).

Conclusion

Tritrichomonosis can cause abortion and reproductive failures in cows. The disease has a low frequency in Latin America and the main transmission mode is during coitus. Additionally, molecular testing is one of the best options for the diagnosis of tritrichomonosis. The prevention/control of the disease involves basic cattle husbandry practices with the use of AI with quality semen (without the protozoan), replacing older bull,s and the diagnosis of cases of abortion and reproductive failures.

References

Abbitt, B., and Meyerholz, G. W. (1979). "*Trichomonas fetus* Infection of Range Bulls in South Florida." *Veterinary Medicine, Small Animal Clinician: VM, SAC*, 74 (9), 1339–42.

Adl, Sina, M., David Bass, Christopher E. Lane, Julius Lukeš, Conrad L. Schoch, Alexey Smirnov, Sabine Agatha, et al. (2019). "Revisions to the Classification, Nomenclature, and Diversity of Eukaryotes." *Journal of Eukaryotic Microbiology*, 66 (1), 4–119. https://doi.org/10.1111/jeu.12691.

Alves, Telma, M., Ana Paula R Stynen, and Karina L Miranda. (2011). "Campilobacteriose Genital Bovina e Tricomonose Genital Bovina : Epidemiologia, Diagnóstico e Controle [*Bovine genital campylobacteriosis and bovine genital trichomonosis: epidemiology, diagnosis and control*]" *Pesquisa Veterinária Brasileira*, 31 (4), 336–44.

Anderson, M. L., BonDurant, R. H., Corbeil, R. R., and Corbeil, L. B. (1996). "Immune and Inflammatory Responses to Reproductive Tract Infection with *Tritrichomonas foetus* in Immunized and Control Heifers." *The Journal of Parasitology*, 82 (4), 594–600.

Benchimol, and Marlene. (2004). "Trichomonads under Microscopy." *Microscopy and Microanalysis : The Official Journal of Microscopy Society of America, Microbeam Analysis Society, Microscopical Society of Canada*, 10 (5), 528–50. https://doi.org/10.1017/S1431927604040905.

Bondurant, and Robert, H. (2005). "Venereal Diseases of Cattle: Natural History, Diagnosis, and the Role of Vaccines in Their Control." *The Veterinary Clinics of North America. Food Animal Practice*, 21 (2), 383–408. https://doi.org/10.1016/j.cvfa.2005.03.002.

BonDurant, R. H. (1997). "Pathogenesis, Diagnosis, and Management of Trichomoniasis in Cattle." *The Veterinary Clinics of North America. Food Animal Practice*, 13 (2), 345–61. https://doi.org/10.1016/s0749-0720(15)30346-7.

BonDurant, R. H., Anderson, M. L., Blanchard, P., Hird, D., Danaye-Elmi, C., Palmer, C., Sischo, W. M., Suther, D., Utterback, W., and Weigler, B. J. (1990). "Prevalence of Trichomoniasis among California Beef Herds." *Journal of the American Veterinary Medical Association*, 196 (10), 1590–93.

BonDurant, R. H., Gajadhar, A., Campero, C. M., Johnson, E., Lun, Z. R., Nordhausen, R. W., Van Hoosear, K. A., Villanueva, M. R., and Walker, R. L. (1999). "Preliminary Characterization of a *Tritrichomonas foetus*-Like Protozoan Isolated from Preputial Smegma of Virgin Bulls". *The Bovine Practitioner*, 33 (2), 124-27. https://doi.org/10.21423/bovine-vol33no2p124-127.

Bondurant, R. H., van Hoosear, K. A., Corbeil, L. B., and Bernoco, D. (1996). "Serological Response to *in Vitro*-Shed Antigen(s) of *Tritrichomonas foetus* in Cattle." *Clinical and Diagnostic Laboratory Immunology*, 3 (4), 432–37. https://doi.org/10.1128/cdli.3.4.432-437.1996.

Campero, C. M., Rodriguez Dubra, C., Bolondi, A., Cacciato, C., Cobo, E., Perez, S., Odeon, A., Cipolla, A., and BonDurant, R. H. (2003). "Two-Step (Culture and PCR) Diagnostic Approach for Differentiation of Non-*T. foetus* Trichomonads from Genitalia of Virgin Beef Bulls in Argentina." *Veterinary Parasitology*, 112 (3), 167–75. https://doi.org/10.1016/s0304-4017(02)00423-5.

Cepicka, Ivan, Vladimír Hampl, and Jaroslav Kulda. (2010). "Critical Taxonomic Revision of Parabasalids with Description of One New Genus and Three New Species." *Protist*, 161 (3), 400–433. https://doi.org/10.1016/j.protis.2009.11.005.

Cobo, Eduardo Rubén, Carlos Manuel Campero, Rafael Meyer Mariante, and Marlene Benchimol. (2003). "Ultrastructural Study of a Tetratrichomonad Species Isolated from Prepucial Smegma of Virgin Bulls." *Veterinary Parasitology*, 117 (3), 195–211. https://doi.org/10.1016/j.vetpar.2003.07.026.

Cobo, Eduardo Rubén, Claudia Morsella, Dora Cano, Ana Cipolla, and Carlos Manuel Campero. (2004). "Immunization in Heifers with Dual Vaccines Containing *Tritrichomonas foetus* and *Campylobacter fetus* Antigens Using Systemic and Mucosal Routes." *Theriogenology*, 62 (8), 1367–82. https://doi.org/10.1016/j.theriogenology.2003.12.034.

Cobo, Eduardo, R., Lynette B Corbeil, and Robert H BonDurant. (2011). "Immunity to Infections in the Lower Genital Tract of Bulls." *Journal of Reproductive Immunology*, 89 (1), 55–61. https://doi.org/10.1016/j.jri.2011.02.002.

Coker, Kimberly, E., Joseph J Lim, Rebecca L Schleisman, Christopher Vosloo, Hilari M French, Juan C Samper, John J Callanan, Robert O Gilbert, Fortune Sithole, Chaoqun Yao, and Aspinas Chapwanya. (2018). "Freedom from Tritrichomonas Foetus Infection in Cattle in St . Kitts," *Tropical Animal Health and Production*, 1171–73.

Corbeil, L. B., Anderson, M. L., Corbeil, R. R., Eddow, J. M., and BonDurant, R. H. (1998). "Female Reproductive Tract Immunity in Bovine Trichomoniasis." *American Journal of Reproductive Immunology (New York, N.Y.: 1989)*, 39 (3), 189–98. https://doi.org/10.1111/j.1600-0897.1998.tb00353.x.

Corbeil, L. B., Campero, C. M., Rhyan, J. C., Anderson, M. L., Gershwin, L. J., Agnew, D. W., Munson, L., and Bondurant, R. H. (2005). "Uterine Mast Cells and Immunoglobulin-E Antibody Responses during Clearance of Tritrichomonas Foetus." *Veterinary Pathology*, 42 (3), 282–90. https://doi.org/10.1354/vp.42-3-282.

Corbeil, L. B., Munson, L., Campero, C., and BonDurant, R. H. (2001). "Bovine Trichomoniasis as a Model for Development of Vaccines against Sexually-Transmitted Disease." *American Journal of Reproductive Immunology (New York, N.Y. : 1989)*, 45 (5), 310–19. https://doi.org/10.1111/j.8755-8920.2001.450507.x.

Corbeil, Lynette, B., Carlos M Campero, Karen Van Hoosear, and Robert H Bondurant. (2008). "Detection of Trichomonad Species in the Reproductive Tracts of Breeding and Virgin Bulls." *Veterinary Parasitology*, 154 (3–4), 226–32. https://doi.org/10.1016/j.vetpar.2008.03.014.

Dąbrowska, Joanna, Jacek Karamon, Maciej Kochanowski, Jacek Sroka, Jolanta Zdybel, and Tomasz Cencek. (2019). "*Tritrichomonas foetus* as a Causative Agent of Tritrichomonosis in Different Animal Hosts." *Journal of Veterinary Research*, 63 (4), 533–41. https://doi.org/10.2478/jvetres-2019-0072.

De Oliveira, Júnior Mário Baltazar, Gesika Maria, Pollyanne Raysa, Fernandes De Oliveira, and Daniel Friguglietti Brandespim. (2015). "Prevalence and Risk Factors Associated with Bovine Genital Campylobacteriosis and Bovine Trichomonosis in the State of Pernambuco, Brazil." *Tropical Animal Health Production*, 549–55. https://doi.org/10.1007/s11250-015-0761-3

Edmondson, Misty, A., Kellye S Joiner, Jennifer A Spencer, Kay P Riddell, Soren P Rodning, Julie A Gard, and Daniel Givens, M. (2017). "Impact of a Killed Tritrichomonas Foetus Vaccine on Clearance of the Organism and Subsequent Fertility of Heifers Following Experimental Inoculation." *Theriogenology*, 90 (March), 245–51. https://doi.org/10.1016/j.theriogenology.2016.09.056.

Fernández, M. E., Campero, C. M., Morrell, E., Cantón, G. J., Moore, D. P., Cano, A., Malena, R., Odeón, A. C., Paolicchi, F., Odriozola, E. R. (2007). "Pérdidas Reproductivas En Bovinos Causadas Por Abortos, Muertes Prematuras, Natimortos y Neonatos : Casuística Del Período 2006-2007. (Bovine reproductive losses due to abortion, premature deliveries, stillbirth and neonatal losses: case report 2006-2007)" *Revista de Medicina Veterinária*, 88, 246–54.

Filho, Ruy Brayner de Oliveira, Karla Campos Malta, Jonas de Melo Borges, Pollyanne Raysa Fernandes de Oliveira, Givanildo Jacinto Dos Santos Filho, Glaucia Grazielle Nascimento, Rinaldo Aparecido Mota, and José Wilton Pinheiro Júnior. (2018). "Prevalence and Risk Factors Associated with *Tritrichomonas foetus* Infection in Cattle in the State of Paraíba, Brazil." *Acta Parasitologica*, 63 (2), 346–53. https://doi.org/10.1515/ap-2018-0039.

Flower, P. J., Ladds, P. W., Thomas, A. D., and Watson, D. L. (1983). "An Immunopathologic Study of the Bovine Prepuce." *Veterinary Pathology*, 20 (2), 189–202. https://doi.org/10.1177/030098588302000206.

Fuchs, Lumila I, Marcelo C Fort, Dora Cano, Carina M Bonetti, Hugo D Giménez, Pablo M Vázquez, Diana Bacigalupe, Javier D Breccia, Carlos M Campero, and Jorge A Oyhenart. (2017). "Clearance of *Tritrichomonas foetus* in Experimentally Infected Heifers Protected with Vaccines Based on Killed-T. Foetus with Different Adjuvants." *Vaccine*, 35 (9), 1341–46. https://doi.org/10.1016/j.vaccine.2016.12.030.

Gay, J. M., Ebel, E. D., and Kearley, W. P. (1996). "Commingled Grazing as a Risk Factor for Trichomonosis in Beef Herds." *Journal of the American Veterinary Medical Association*, 209 (3), 643–46.

Ginter Summarell, Carly, C., Thomas B Hairgrove, Megan E Schroeder, Robert Conley, and Mangkey A Bounpheng. (2018). "Improvements in *Tritrichomonas foetus* Molecular Testing." *Journal of Veterinary Diagnostic Investigation : Official Publication of the American Association of Veterinary Laboratory Diagnosticians, Inc*, 30 (4), 603–8. https://doi.org/10.1177/1040638718767943.

Givens, and Daniel, M. (2006). "A Clinical, Evidence-Based Approach to Infectious Causes of Infertility in Beef Cattle." *Theriogenology*, 66 (3), 648–54. https://doi.org/10.1016/j.theriogenology.2006.04.021.

Gomes, M. J. P., Fernandes, J. C., Silva, C. E., and Sousa, S. T. B. (1991). "Identificação de Tritrichomonas foetus em bovinos do Estado do Rio Grande do Sul, Brasil. [*Identification of Tritrichomonas foetus in cattle from the State of Rio Grande do Sul, Brazil.*]" *Arquivos da Faculdade de Veterinária UFRGS*, 19, 103-111.

González-Carmona, L. C., Sánchez-Ladino, M. J., Castañeda-Salazar, R., Pulido-Villamarín, A. D. P., Guáqueta-Munar, H., Aranda-Silva, M., and Rueda Varón, M. J. (2012). "Determination of presence of Tritrichomonas foetus in uterine lavages from cows with reproductive problems." *Revista Brasileira de Parasitologia Veterinária*, 21, 201-205.

Goodger, W. J, and Skirrow, S. Z. (1986). "Epidemiologic and Economic Analyses of an Unusually Long Epizootic of Trichomoniasis in a Large California Dairy Herd." *Journal of the American Veterinary Medical Association*, 189 (7), 772–76.

Griffiths, I. B., Gallego, M. I., and de Leon, L. S. (1984). "Levels of some Reproductive Diseases in the Dairy Cattle of Colombia." *Tropical Animal Health Production*, 16, 219-223. DOI: 10.1515/ap-2018-0039.

Guida, H. G., Ramos, A. A., Coelho, N. M., Ramos, J. A., and Mendonza, T. R. (1972). "Incidência de Trichomonas foetus em Reprodutores Bovinos da Região Centro-Sul do Brasil. (Incidence of Trichomonas foetus in Cattle Breeders in the Center-South Region of Brazil.)" *Pesquisa Agropecuária Brasileira*, 7, 23-25.

Ikeda, J. S., BonDurant, R. H., and Corbeil, L. B. (1995). "Bovine Vaginal Antibody Responses to Immunoaffinity-Purified Surface Antigen of Tritrichomonas foetus." *Journal of Clinical Microbiology*, 33 (5), 1158–63. https://doi.org/10.1128/ jcm.33. 5.1158-1163.1995.

Jin, Yinzhu, Brant Schumaker, Jim Logan, and Chaoqun Yao. (2014). "Risk Factors Associated with Bovine Trichomoniasis in Beef Cattle Identified by a Questionnaire." *Journal of Medical Microbiology*, 63 (Pt 6), 896–902. https://doi.org/10.1099/jmm.0. 074971-0.

Kania, S. A., Reed, S. L., Thomford, J. W., BonDurant, R. H., Hirata, K., Corbeil, R. R., North, M. J., and Corbeil, L. B. (2001). "Degradation of Bovine Complement C3 by Trichomonad Extracellular Proteinase." *Veterinary Immunology and Immunopathology*, 78 (1), 83–96. https://doi.org/10.1016/s0165-2427(00)00256-7.

Kvasnicka, W. G., Taylor, R. E., Huang, J. C., Hanks, D., Tronstad, R. J., Bosomworth, A., and Hall, M. R. (1989). "Investigations of the Incidence of Bovine Trichomoniasis in Nevada and of the Efficacy of Immunizing Cattle with Vaccines Containing Tritrichomonas foetus." *Theriogenology*, 31 (5), 963–71. https://doi.org/10.1016/ 0093-691x(89)90479-2.

Love, David, Virginia R Fajt, Thomas Hairgrove, Meredyth Jones, and James A Thompson. (2017). "Metronidazole for the Treatment of Tritrichomonas foetus in Bulls." *BMC Veterinary Research*, 13 (1), 107. https://doi.org/10.1186/s12917-017-0999-2.

Mancebo, O. A., Russo, A. M., Carabajal, L. L., and Monzon, C. M. (1995). "Persistence of Tritrichomonas foetus in Naturally Infected Cows and Heifers in Argentina." *Veterinary Parasitology*, 59 (1), 7–11. https://doi.org/10.1016/0304-4017(94)00734-t.

Mardones, F. O., Perez, A. M., Martínez, A., and Carpenter, T. E. (2008). "Risk Factors Associated with *Tritrichomonas foetus* Infection in Beef Herds in the Province of

Buenos Aires, Argentina." *Veterinary Parasitology*, 153 (3–4), 231–37. https://doi.org/10.1016/j.vetpar.2008.01.038.

Martín-Gómez, S., González-Paniello, R., Pereira-Bueno, J., and Ortega-Mora, L. M. (1998). "Prevalence of *Tritrichomonas foetus* Infection in Beef Bulls in Northwestern Spain." *Veterinary Parasitology*, 75 (2–3), 265–68. https://doi.org/10.1016/s0304-4017(97)00189-1.

McCool, C. J., Townsend, M. P., Wolfe, S. G., Simpson, M. A., Olm, T. C., Jayawardhana, G. A., and Carney, J. V. (1988). "Prevalence of Bovine Venereal Disease in the Victoria River District of the Northern Territory: Likely Economic Effects and Practicable Control Measures." *Australian Veterinary Journal*, 65 (5), 153–56. https://doi.org/10.1111/j.1751-0813.1988.tb14445.x.

McMillen, Lyle, and Ala E Lew. (2006). "Improved Detection of *Tritrichomonas foetus* in Bovine Diagnostic Specimens Using a Novel Probe-Based Real Time PCR Assay." *Veterinary Parasitology*, 141 (3–4), 204–15. https://doi.org/10.1016/ j.vetpar.2006.06.012.

Mendoza-Ibarra, Jesús Alberto, Luis Miguel Ortega-Mora, Susana Pedraza-Díaz, Silvia Rojo-Montejo, Jose Antonio Ruiz-Santa-Quiteria, Francisco Javier García-Peña, Vanesa Navarro-Lozano, María Del Carmen Cuevas-Martín, Koldo Osoro, and Esther Collantes-Fernández. (2013). "Differences in the Prevalence of *Tritrichomonas foetus* Infection in Beef Cattle Farmed under Extensive Conditions in Northern Spain." *Veterinary Journal (London, England: 1997)*, 196 (3), 547–49. https://doi.org/10.1016/j.tvjl.2012.10.026.

Mendoza-Ibarra, Jesús, A., Susana Pedraza-Díaz, Francisco J García-Peña, Silvia Rojo-Montejo, Jose A Ruiz-Santa-Quiteria, Elena San Miguel-Ibáñez, Vanesa Navarro-Lozano, Luis M Ortega-Mora, Koldo Osoro, and Esther Collantes-Fernandez. (2012). "High Prevalence of *Tritrichomonas foetus* Infection in Asturiana de La Montaña Beef Cattle Kept in Extensive Conditions in Northern Spain." *Veterinary Journal (London, England: 1997)*, 193 (1), 146–51. https://doi.org/10.1016/ j.tvjl.2011.09.020.

Michi, Aubrey, N., Pedro H Favetto, John Kastelic, and Eduardo R Cobo. (2016). "A Review of Sexually Transmitted Bovine Trichomoniasis and Campylobacteriosis Affecting Cattle Reproductive Health." *Theriogenology*, 85 (5), 781–91. https://doi.org/10.1016/j.theriogenology.2015.10.037.

Molina, L. L., Angón, E., García, A., Caballero-Villalobos, J., Giorgis, A. O., Moralejo, R. H., and Perea, J. (2018). "A Retrospective Epidemiological Analysis of Shared Risk Factors for Bovine Trichomoniasis and Bovine Genital Campylobacteriosis in La Pampa Province (Argentina)." *Preventive Veterinary Medicine*, 161 (December), 109–14. https://doi.org/10.1016/j.prevetmed.2018.10.022.

Ondrak, and Jeff, D. (2016). "*Tritrichomonas foetus* Prevention and Control in Cattle." *The Veterinary Clinics of North America. Food Animal Practice*, 32 (2), 411–23. https://doi.org/10.1016/j.cvfa.2016.01.010.

Oyhenart, Jorge, Florencia Martínez, Rosana Ramírez, Marcelo Fort, and Javier D Breccia. (2013). "Loop Mediated Isothermal Amplification of 5.8S RDNA for Specific Detection of *Tritrichomonas foetus*." *Veterinary Parasitology*, 193 (1–3), 59–65. https://doi.org/10.1016/j.vetpar.2012.11.034.

Parker, S., Lun, Z. R., and Gajadhar, A. (2001). "Application of a PCR Assay to Enhance the Detection and Identification of *Tritrichomonas foetus* in Cultured Preputial Samples." *Journal of Veterinary Diagnostic Investigation: Official Publication of the American Association of Veterinary Laboratory Diagnosticians, Inc*, 13 (6), 508–13. https://doi.org/10.1177/104063870101300609.

Parker, Sarah, John Campbell, and Alvin Gajadhar. (2003). "Comparison of the Diagnostic Sensitivity of a Commercially Available Culture Kit and a Diagnostic Culture Test Using Diamond's Media for Diagnosing *Tritrichomonas foetus* in Bulls." *Journal of Veterinary Diagnostic Investigation: Official Publication of the American Association of Veterinary Laboratory Diagnosticians, Inc*, 15 (5), 460–65. https://doi.org/10.1177/104063870301500510.

Parker, Sarah, John Campbell, Kathy McIntosh, and Alvin Gajadhar. (2003). "Diagnosis of Trichomoniasis in 'virgin' Bulls by Culture and Polymerase Chain Reaction." *The Canadian Veterinary Journal*, 44 (9), 732–34.

Parsonson, I. M., Clark, B. L., and Dufty, J. (1974). "The Pathogenesis of *Tritrichomonas foetus* Infection in the Bull." *Australian Veterinary Journal*, 50 (10), 421–23. https://doi.org/10.1111/j.1751-0813.1974.tb06861.x.

Parsonson, I. M., Clark, B. L., and Dufty, J. H. (1976). "Early Pathogenesis and Pathology of *Tritrichomonas foetus* Infection in Virgin Heifers." *Journal of Comparative Pathology*, 86 (1), 59–66. https://doi.org/10.1016/0021-9975(76)90028-1.

Pefanis, S. M., Herr, S., Venter, C. G., Kruger, L. P., Queiroga, C. C., and Amaral, L. (1988). "Trichomoniasis and Campylobacteriosis in Bulls in the Republic of Transkei." *Journal of the South African Veterinary Association*, 59 (3), 139–40.

Pereira-Neves, Antonio, Carlos Manuel Campero, Alfredo Martínez, and Marlene Benchimol. (2011). "Identification of *Tritrichomonas foetus* Pseudocysts in Fresh Preputial Secretion Samples from Bulls." *Veterinary Parasitology*, 175 (1–2), 1–8. https://doi.org/10.1016/j.vetpar.2010.10.007.

Pereira-Neves, Antonio, and Marlene Benchimol. (2009). "*Tritrichomonas foetus*: Budding from Multinucleated Pseudocysts." *Protist*, 160 (4), 536–51. https://doi.org/10.1016/j.protis.2009.05.001.

Perez, Enrique, Patricia A Conrad, David Hird, Ana Ortuno, Jorge Chacon, Robert BonDurant, and Jos Noordhuizen. (1992). "Prevalence and Risk Factors for *Trichomonas foetus* Infection in Cattle in Northeastern Costa Rica." *Preventive Veterinary Medicine*, 14 (3), 155–65. https://doi.org/https://doi.org/10.1016/0167-5877(92)90013-6.

Rabello, E. X. (1955). "Incidência da *Trichomonas foetus* Riedmüller, 1928, em touros usados para inseminação artificial no estado de São Paulo. [*Incidence of* Trichomonas feotus *Riedmüller, 1928, in bulls used for artificial insemination in the state of São Paulo*]" *Revista da Faculdade Medicina Veterinária de São Paulo*, 5 (3), 539-550.

Rae, D. O. (1989). "Impact of Trichomoniasis on the Cow-Calf Producer's Profitability." *Journal of the American Veterinary Medical Association*, 194 (6), 771–75.

Rae, Owen, D., and John E Crews. (2006). "*Tritrichomonas foetus*." *The Veterinary Clinics of North America. Food Animal Practice*, 22 (3), 595–611. https://doi.org/10.1016/j.cvfa.2006.07.001.

Rae, Owen, D., John E Crews, Ellis C Greiner, and Arthur Donovan, G. (2004). "Epidemiology of *Tritrichomonas foetus* in Beef Bull Populations in Florida." *Theriogenology*, 61 (4), 605–18. https://doi.org/10.1016/s0093-691x(03)00236-x.

Rhyan, J. C., Wilson, K. L., Wagner, B., Anderson, M. L., BonDurant, R. H., Burgess, D. E., Mutwiri, G. K., and Corbeil, L. B. (1999). "Demonstration of *Tritrichomonas foetus* in the External Genitalia and of Specific Antibodies in Preputial Secretions of Naturally Infected Bulls." *Veterinary Pathology*, 36 (5), 406–11. https://doi.org/10.1354/vp.36-5-406.

Schaut, Robert, G., Lynette B Corbeil, Courtney N Blake, and Matthew T Brewer. (2017). "Development of a Bead-Agglutination Assay for Rapid Detection of *Tritrichomonas foetus*." *Veterinary Parasitology*, 243 (August), 188–91. https://doi.org/10.1016/j.vetpar.2017.06.025.

Silva, A. S., Zanette, R. A., Oliveira, C. B., Gallio, M., Pereira, P. L., Fernandes, M. B., Tonin, A. A., Badke, M. R. T., and Monteiro, S. G. (2009). "Leptospirose e tritricomonose: isolamento em propriedade com problemas reprodutivos no sul do Brasil. [*Leptospirosis and tritrichomonosis: isolation in a property with reproductive problems in southern Brazil*]" *Arquivos de Ciências Veterinárias e Zoologia da UNIPAR*, 12, 87-90.

Silveira, Caroline da Silva, Martín Fraga, Cecilia Monesiglio, Rafael Delpiazzo, Melissa Macías-rioseco, Federico Giannitti, and Franklin Riet-correa. (2020). "Detección de *Tritrichomonas foetus* por PCR en Esmegma Prepucial de Toros en Uruguay. [*Detection of Tritrichomonas foetus by PCR in preputial smegma of bulls in Uruguay*]", 56 (213), 1–7. https://doi.org/10.29155/VET.56.213.7.

Skirrow, S. (1987). "Identification of Trichomonad-Carrier Cows." *Journal of the American Veterinary Medical Association*, 191 (5), 553–54.

Skirrow, S. Z., and Bondurant, R. H. (1988). "Treatment of Bovine Trichomoniasis with Ipronidazole." *Australian Veterinary Journal*, 65 (5), 156. https://doi.org/10.1111/j.1751-0813.1988.tb14446.x.

Skirrow, S. Z., and Bondurant, R. H. (1990a). "Induced *Tritrichomonas foetus* Infection in Beef Heifers." *Journal of the American Veterinary Medical Association*, 196 (6), 885–89.

Skirrow, S. Z., and Bondurant, R. H. (1990b). "Immunoglobulin Isotype of Specific Antibodies in Reproductive Tract Secretions and Sera in Tritrichomonas Foetus-Infected Heifers." *American Journal of Veterinary Research*, 51 (4), 645–53.

Slapeta, Jan, Norbert Müller, Colin M Stack, Giselle Walker, Ala Lew-Tabor, Jan Tachezy, and Caroline F Frey. (2012). "Comparative Analysis of *Tritrichomonas foetus* (Riedmüller, 1928) Cat Genotype, *T. Foetus* (Riedmüller, 1928) Cattle Genotype and Tritrichomonas Suis (Davaine, 1875) at 10 DNA Loci." *International Journal for Parasitology*, 42 (13–14), 1143–49. https://doi.org/10.1016/ j.ijpara.2012.10.004.

Sun, Zichen, Colin Stack, and Jan Šlapeta. (2012). "Sequence Differences in the Diagnostic Region of the Cysteine Protease 8 Gene of *Tritrichomonas foetus* Parasites of Cats and Cattle." *Veterinary Parasitology*, 186 (3–4), 445–49. https://doi.org/10.1016/j.vetpar.2011.12.001.

Szonyi, Barbara, Indumathi Srinath, Andy Schwartz, Alfonso Clavijo, and Renata Ivanek. (2012). "Spatio-Temporal Epidemiology of *Tritrichomonas foetus* Infection in Texas

Bulls Based on State-Wide Diagnostic Laboratory Data." *Veterinary Parasitology*, 186 (3–4), 450–55. https://doi.org/10.1016/j.vetpar.2011.11.075.

Tachezy, Jan, Ruth Tachezy, Vladimír Hampl, Miroslava Sedinová, Stepánka Vanacová, Martin Vrlík, Marc Van Ranst, Jaroslav Flegr, and Jaroslav Kuldaa. (2002). "Cattle Pathogen *Tritrichomonas foetus* (Riedmüller, 1928) and Pig Commensal Tritrichomonas Suis (Gruby & Delafond, 1843) Belong to the Same Species." *The Journal of Eukaryotic Microbiology*, 49 (2), 154–63. https://doi.org/10.1111/j.1550-7408.2002.tb00360.x.

Talbot, J. A., Nielsen, K., and Corbeil, L. B. (1991). "Cleavage of Proteins of Reproductive Secretions by Extracellular Proteinases of *Tritrichomonas foetus*." *Canadian Journal of Microbiology*, 37 (5), 384–90. https://doi.org/10.1139/m91-062.

Thomford, J. W., Talbot, J. A., Ikeda, J. S., and Corbeil, L. B. (1996). "Characterization of Extracellular Proteinases of *Tritrichomonas foetus*." *The Journal of Parasitology*, 82 (1), 112–17.

Walden, Heather Stockdale, Christine Dykstra, Allen Dillon, Soren Rodning, Daniel Givens, Richard Bird, Joseph Newton, and David Lindsay. (2013). "A New Species of Tritrichomonas (Sarcomastigophora: Trichomonida) from the Domestic Cat (Felis Catus)." *Parasitology Research*, 112 (6), 2227–35. https://doi.org/10.1007/s00436-013-3381-8.

Yao, and Chaoqun. (2012). "Opportunistic Human Infections Caused by Tritrichomonas Species: A Mini-Review." *Clinical Microbiology Newsletter*, 34 (16), 127–31. https://doi.org/https://doi.org/10.1016/j.clinmicnews.2012.07.004.

Yao, and Chaoqun. (2013). "Diagnosis of *Tritrichomonas foetus*-Infected Bulls, an Ultimate Approach to Eradicate Bovine Trichomoniasis in US Cattle?" *Journal of Medical Microbiology*, 62 (Pt 1), 1–9. https://doi.org/10.1099/jmm.0.047365-0.

Yao, and Chaoqun. (2021). "Control and Eradication of Bovine Trichomonosis in Wyoming, USA by Testing and Culling Positive Bulls." *Veterinary Research*, 52 (1), 129. https://doi.org/10.1186/s13567-021-00996-w.

Yao, Chaoqun, and Jennifer K Ketzis. (2018). "Aberrant and Accidental Trichomonad Flagellate Infections: Rare or Underdiagnosed?" *Transactions of the Royal Society of Tropical Medicine and Hygiene*, 112 (2), 64–72. https://doi.org/10.1093/ trstmh/ try027.

Yao, Chaoqun, and Liza S Köster. (2015). "*Tritrichomonas foetus* Infection, a Cause of Chronic Diarrhea in the Domestic Cat." *Veterinary Research*, 46 (1), 35. https://doi.org/10.1186/s13567-015-0169-0.

Yao, Chaoqun, Katherine D Bardsley, Elizabeth A Litzman, Mariah L Hall, and Mark R Davidson. (2011). "*Tritrichomonas foetus* Infection in Beef Bull Populations in Wyoming" *Journal of Bacteriology and Parasitology*, 2 (5). https://doi.org/10.4172/ 2155-9597.1000117.

Chapter 10

General Aspects of Anthelmintic Resistance: Phytotherapy as a Non-Chemical Alternative for Parasite Control

Javier Hernán Schapiro[1,2*]
and Sergio Ivan Jorge Lobayan[3,†]
[1] Institute of Pathobiology-IPVET, CICVyA,
National Institute of Agricultural Technology (INTA)
Castelar, Buenos Aires, Argentina
[2] School of Veterinary Medicine,
Faculty of Agricultural and Veterinary Sciences,
University of Salvador (USAL), Buenos Aires, Argentina
[3] School of Veterinary Medicine,
Faculty of Agricultural and Veterinary Sciences,
University of Salvador (USAL), Corrientes, Argentina

Introduction

Verminous gastroenteritis is one of the most frequent parasitic diseases and causes important economic losses in ruminant production worldwide. It is caused by parasitic nematodes that belongs to several families and genera that affect the abomasum and small and large intestines, among which Trichostrongylidae (*Haemonchus, Teladorsagia, Trichostrongylus* and *Cooperia*), Molineidae (*Nematodirus*), Ancylostomatidae (*Bunostomum*) and Strongylidae (*Chabertia* and *Oesophagostomum*) stand out (Cordero del Campillo and Rojo-Vázquez 1999). They usually occur in a mixed or

[*] Corresponding Author's Email: hernan.schapiro@usal.edu.ar.
[†] Corresponding Author's Email: sergio.lobayan@usal.edu.ar.

In: Infectious and Parasitic Diseases of Animals in Developing Countries
Editor: Selwyn Arlington Headley
ISBN: 979-8-88697-504-8

pluriospecific form, i.e., each host can simultaneously harbor more than one parasitic species. Direct losses are related to the loss of meat, wool, and milk production, and in extreme cases, death of severely affected animals (Kaplan et al. 2004). Currently, anthelmintics continue to be the main input for the control of gastrointestinal nematodes (GIN). They are grouped into different chemical groups: benzimidazoles (fenbendazole, albendazole, ricobendazole), imidazothiazoles (levamisole), macrocyclic lactones (ivermectin, doramectin, abamectin and moxidectin), aminoacetonitrile derivatives (monepantel), salicinalides (closantel), spiroindoles (derquantel) and organophosphates (Lanusse 1993; Steffan et al. 2011). Strategically, an ideal control should also contemplate combined strategies that include animal and pasture management (Steffan et al. 2005; Suárez 2007). The absence of concrete control measures that are not based on the use of anthelmintics contributed to an almost exclusive dependence on the use of anthelmintics in recent decades, which contributed to the emergence of the phenomenon of Anthelmintic Resistance (AR) (Nari 2002; FAO 2003; 2004; Caracostantogolo et al. 2005; Suárez and Cristel 2011).

Anthelmintic Resistance

The resistance of parasitic nematodes to anthelmintic drugs is considered one of the most important problems facing the production of large and small ruminants worldwide. It was defined as the ability of a parasitic population to decrease its sensitivity to the action of one or more anthelmintic drugs, expressed through a significant increase of resistant individuals capable of tolerating doses proven lethal for the majority of the normal (susceptible) population of the same species. It has a heritable nature, that is, the progeny of resistant parasites will also present this characteristic (Melo and Bevilaqua 2002; FAO 2004).

Main Factors Contributing to the Development of Anthelmintic Resistance

It can be considered as a multicausal phenomenon involving factors related to animal and parasite management. The first are those that are under man control, and are linked to the intensive and indiscriminate use of drugs without considering epidemiological criteria of the disease, on many occasions in the absence of a diagnosis that determines the real need to carry out the treatment, with erroneous calculated dosages, and absent or inadequate rotation of active principles. In reference to the last point, it generates an increase in the selection pressure on the parasite species, where those that are genetically resistant will be selected and will transmit this characteristic to their offspring. For this reason, it is recommended to rotate annually with antiparasitics that have different mode of action in order to eliminate the individuals selected as resistant by the previous drug. This mismanagement inevitably led to the selection of resistant nematode populations (Anziani 2001; Caracostantogolo et al. 2005; Caracostantogolo et al. 2012).

Parasite-linked factors include genetic aspects, degree of dominance of heterozygotes, mutation rate at which resistant alleles are produced, and the reproductive potential of these individuals. The rate at which a parasite develops resistance will depend on the selection pressure to which it is subjected, and this is directly related to the frequency of treatments. Once resistance to a given drug has been developed, resistance to other products of the same chemical group is usually established as well (FAO 2004). The following sections are the 3 phases in the development of anthelmintic resistance.

Establishment of Resistant Genes

Nematodes undergo random gene modifications that give them some resistance to treatments in the early stages. After successive dewormings using the same drug, the mostly susceptible population initially dies and only those resistant individuals survive. After several treatments (selection pressure), the latter increase their population and transmit resistant alleles from generation to generation, inevitably leading to the AR phenomenon. Köhler in 2001 (FAO 2003) proposed that the main mechanism that helminths use to acquire resistance is through modifications in the receptors for the drug, with the consequent decrease or loss of affinity to them.

Diffusion of Resistant Genes

Resistant parasites spread in a hidden way from the place where the establishment of the mutation occurred to other areas through the movement of infested animals.

Emergency or Clinical Appearance of Resistance

The failure of antiparasitic efficacy becomes visible when the proportion of resistant parasites in a population reaches values close to 25% (Fiel et al. 2001).

History of Anthelmintic Resistance

This is not a new problem, since there is a documented history of this phenomenon since 1957, when it was initially reported in the United States with resistant strains of *Haemonchus contortus* to phenothiazine, followed by other reports also from the USA in 1964 of resistance of *Haemonchus contortus* to thiabendazole, and in 1968 of *Teladorsagia circumcincta* to organophosphates (Márquez Lara 2003; Kaplan 2004). In some South American countries, it has been proven that this is an increasingly worrying problem, especially in Argentina, Brazil, Paraguay and Uruguay, where simultaneous resistance to different chemical groups (multiple resistance) has reached important levels that make sheep activity inefficient (Prichard 1994; Echevarria et al, 1996; Eddi et al. 1996; Maciel et al. 1996; Nari et al. 1996; Waller 1996; Molento and Prichard 2001; Bonino and Mederos 2003; Anziani 2004; Caracostantogolo et al. 2005; Torres-Acosta et al. 2012; Cristel et al. 2017).

Particularly in Argentina, Romero et al. (1992) reported the first evidence of resistance to oxfendazole in sheep in the province of Buenos Aires, Eddi et al. in 1996 carried out a study of the prevalence of AR, and Romero et al. (1998) found that in Mesopotamia 90% of flocks showed resistance to benzimidazoles. In cattle, the first reports were made by O. Anziani and C. Fiel in 2000 (Anziani 2001). From that moment, a significant number of cases of AR began to be reported in several cattle farms in the country.

Early Detection of Anthelmintic Resistance Phenomenon

In order to establish a rational parasite control and preserve the useful life of antiparasitics, it is vitally important to achieve an early detection of this phenomenon. Anthelmintics must be properly chosen based on tests that determine their real efficacy, which should be carried out at least once a year.

The obtained information will contribute to establish a specific control program for each livestock establishment. There are two types of tests:

In vitro, they are little used because they are not properly standardized yet and there is a lack of repeatability of the results between the different laboratories. Table 1 describes the main ones:

Table 1. Main *in vitro* methods and chemical group in which anthelmintic resistance is detected

Method	Detects resistance to
Egg hatching	Benzimidazoles
Egg paralysis	Levamisol
Larval paralysis	Levamisol and morantel
Binding to tubulin	Benzimidazoles
Larval development tests	Various groups

In vivo, they are widely used in the field, which are briefly described below:

Faecal Egg Count Reduction Test (F.E.C.R.T.)

This estimates anthelmintic efficacy by comparing egg counts per gram of faeces (EPG) before and after treatment compared to an undosed control group. This methodology is widely used because it is the most convenient due to its practicality and the possibility of evaluating several anthelmintics at the same time, determining which ones have an effect and which ones do not. As a disadvantage, it presents low sensitivity in the initial stages of AR, but it does offer reliable results when the proportion of resistant parasites in the population is higher than 25% (Coles et al. 1992).

Controlled Efficacy Test

It is considered the gold standard test to evaluate the efficacy of anthelmintic drugs. It is the most reliable and accurate method since it compares parasite burden in treated animals versus control animals. It is not widely used due to its main disadvantage, which is its high cost, because it requires animal necropsy (Wood 1995).

The latest research work carried out in Argentina confirms that this phenomenon is widely distributed and installed in production systems. In 2004, the first national survey was carried out through a Technical Cooperation Project sponsored by FAO with the participation of INTA and different universities. The prevalence of AR was studied in the main cattle and sheep production areas of the country. In the former, out of a total of 69 farms sampled, the results showed that only 41% had parasitic nematodes susceptible to treatment with all the drugs evaluated, and in the remaining 59% there was 10% resistance to benzimidazoles, 7% to levamisole, 55% to ivermectin, and 13% multiple resistance. For its part, in the study carried out on 35 sheep production establishments, it was observed that only 38% had parasitic nematodes susceptible to treatment with all the drugs evaluated, and in the remaining 62% there was 53% resistance to benzimidazoles, 25% to levamisole, 50% to ivermectin and 16% of *Haemonchus contortus* resistant to closantel.

Almost a decade later (Cristel et al. 2017), carried out a new national survey of AR prevalence in 62 cattle breeding establishments. Strikingly, it was observed that only 5% of the establishments had parasites sensitive to the drugs evaluated, while the remaining 95% presented anthelmintic resistance. The observed results were 94% resistance to ivermectin, 7% to fenbendazole, 28% to ricobendazole, 26% to the combination of ricobendazole + ivermectin, 33% multiple resistance (ivermectin + benzimidazole) and no establishments were found with parasites resistant to levamisole. The diagnostic technique used in all the cases was F.E.C.R.T.

Current Trends for Resistance Control

Based on the above, and due to the wide distribution of AR and the alarming levels it reaches in certain places (in cattle only 5% of the sampled establishments can still use all the drugs evaluated), as well as to prolong the useful life of those anthelmintics that still have efficacy, it is a priority to propose changes in the way of use of anthelmintics as well as to promote the search for new alternative or complementary tools to the pharmacological control of these helminthiases, it is a priority to propose changes in the way anthelmintics are used, as well as to promote the search for new alternative or complementary tools to the pharmacological control of these helminthiases aimed at developing a sustainable control of the parasitic disease. The idea is to reduce the exclusive dependence on the use of commercial anthelmintics, so that fewer animals are dewormed per year and the refuge is preserved (refuge: all those parasitic stages that are sheltered from antiparasitic treatments, such as larvae from the environment and animals that do not receive antiparasitic treatment). In Veterinary Parasitology, alternative control methodologies went from being a strictly academic field to become a discipline that acquired relevance in search of a diversification of control strategies (Molento et al. 2013).

The following are brief descriptions of some of the current trends that are in the research stage, and finally a more detailed description of phytomedicine:

Genetic Selection of Resistant Animals

There are some sheep breeds that are genetically resistant to infection by gastrointestinal nematodes such as Gulf Coast Native, Suffolk, Dorset and Rambouillet (Miller et al. 1998; Amarante et al. 1999; 2009) and others such as Scottish Blackface, Red Maasai, Barbados Blackbelly, Florida Native and St. Croix, Gulf Coast Native and Suffolk sheep in which resistance to *Haemonchus contortus* was specifically demonstrated (Castells 2002; Shakya et al. 2011). This variability of susceptibility to parasites is called Parasite Resistance, and it is the ability to resist the establishment and subsequent development of parasitic infection, where the individual controls with its immune processes the parasite burden (FAO 2003; Romero 2005). It is expressed with lower EPG values in relation to similar infestations of other animals. These animals require a minimum number of antiparasitic treatments and can be used in sustainable control strategies (FAO 2003; Romero 2005).

Biological Control with Nematophagous Fungi

Although a great variety of *Arthrobotrys, Dactylaria, Dactylella, Monacrosporium* species have been isolated, the best results were obtained with *Duddingtonia flagrans*. It basically consists in the administration of spores that pass through the gastrointestinal tract unchanged, and the control is exerted in the faeces where the hyphal net produces the capture and predation of infective larvae prior to their migration to pastures. It is still in research stages (Mendoza and Vazquez-Prats 1994; Larsen et al. 1997; 1998; Faedo et al. 1997; Larsen 1999; Saumell and Fernandez 2000; Mendoza de Gives et al. 2006).

Pharmacology: Combination of Drugs without Anthelmintic Effect

It is a strategy that can have different objectives: 1- modify the pharmacokinetics and pharmacodynamics of antiparasitic drugs, 2- combination of drugs that can achieve synergism, and 3- combination with other substances (plant extracts) that can improve the initial activity of the antiparasitic drug. The combination of drugs with different mechanisms of action is proposed as an alternative to delay the appearance of AR or to control parasite populations with diagnosed resistance. As a precondition for their use, there should be no cross-resistance between the components of the combination (Lanusse and Prichard 1993; FAO 2003; Molento et al. 2004; Molento et al. 2013).

Vaccines

For the development of vaccines against *H. contortus*, trials were carried out with irradiated larvae, larval extracts, secretion/excretion antigens, somatic fractions and hidden antigens. The latter are those that, under natural conditions, are not exposed to the host's immune system, are more immunogenic than conventional antigens and possibly cause more detrimental immune response to the parasite (FAO 2003; Jackson and Miller 2006). The development of a vaccine against GIN would solve some of the problems related to chemical control. The main strengths of its use are based on its safety without any additional risk to the environment, and that it does not leave chemical residues in the food (FAO 2003).

Silvopastoral Systems

They can contribute to reduce GIN infestations in the context of an integrated management of parasite control. The relationship between the decomposition process of faeces and the parasitological dynamics of nematodes is one of the most determining factors in the general behavior of this parasitosis in these systems. It is noteworthy that in these production systems the development of an edaphic fauna represented mainly by coprophagous beetles that actively participate in the processes of decomposition of fecal matter with the consequent decrease in the number of eggs and infective GIN larvae, thus decreasing the contamination and infectivity of pastures (Soca 2000; Mendonca et al. 2014; Schapiro et al. 2018).

Use of Medicinal Plants for Parasite Control (Phytotherapy)

The term phytotherapy derives from Greek ("phytós": plant or vegetable, and "therapeia": therapy) and is a type of millenary alternative medicine based on the use of plants or their extracts for the prevention and treatment of diseases. Preparations obtained from the infusion or cooking of plant substances were the first treatments used to control infectious and parasitic diseases in humans and animals (Waller et al. 2001). They are currently a complementary alternative to traditional medicine (Gobbo-Neto et al. 2007; Avello et al. 2010).

Despite advances in biotechnology for the development of new drugs, nature maintains a preponderant role as a source for new pharmaceutical compounds. Scientific development has led to interest in medicinal plants, since a great variety of plants and their extracts contain chemical compounds with the capacity to produce different therapeutic effects. In this sense, the research of plant extracts for parasite control in veterinary medicine has had a notorious growth in the last 30 years and since then there is a marked interest to consider it within the non-chemical strategies for parasite control. The trend is the search for drugs of plant origin, based in the concept that what is natural is healthy, free of side effects and chemical residues in food, and do not contaminate the environment (Hernández-Orduño 2008; Rochfort et al. 2008). It is estimated that less than 10% of the nearly 250,000 plant species worldwide have been investigated for their pharmacological properties, which constitutes a vast untapped reservoir of potential new antiparasitic drugs (Anthony et al. 2005).

Most of the scientific reports on plants with anthelmintic properties in sheep parasitized with trichostrongylid nematodes come from the African continent, Southeast Asia, Central America, and Brazil (Hammond et al. 1997; Niezen et al. 2002; Hördegen et al. 2003; Paolini et al. 2003; Nguyen et al. 2005). Many of them belong mainly to legumes that, due to their nutritional properties and their high content of secondary metabolites (SM), were shown to function as nutraceutical foods. These medicinal plants are called bioactive as they contain chemical compounds with the ability to produce various preventive or therapeutic effects, among which their capacity as nematodicides were reported (Athanasiadou et al. 2001; Niezen et al. 2002; Githiori et al. 2006; Molan & Faraj 2010). These SM are involved in plant defense mechanisms against pathogens and protection against solar radiation. The proportion of these is unique for each plant species, because their biosynthesis is related to plant genetics, physiology, stress, and geographic location. These compounds can be synthesized through different metabolic pathways obtaining flavonoids, terpenes, saponins, essential oils, alkaloids, among others. Research work is still needed to solve several questions about the active principles of plants, such as:

- Studying possible seasonal variations.
- To verify the efficacy for all animal species (ruminants and monogastrics) and against all species of parasites.
- To evaluate the frequency of administration and the possibility of its inclusion in animal diets.
- Determine its efficacy, dosage, modes of action and possible adverse effects.

Among the most studied plants are the polyphenolic ones (*Lotus* spp., *Sulla*, among others) or the bark of certain trees (Eucalyptus, Pine, Acacia, Quebracho, among others) that contain different concentrations of condensed tannins (CT) in their composition. It is precisely on these secondary plant metabolites that many research works have focused due to their beneficial effects on animal nutrition and health, obtaining improvements in productive parameters mainly due to a better utilization of dietary protein and a greater absorption of amino acids in the intestine (Avello et al. 2010).

Tannins

General Information and Classification

The term *tannin* is quite old and derives from the word "tanning," which refers to the vegetable components responsible for converting animal hides into leather by forming stable complexes with skin collagen (Bennick 2002; Waghorn 2008). According to their chemical structure, they are classified into two major groups: hydrolyzable tannins (HT) and condensed tannins (CT) (Figure 1) (Athanasiadou et al. 2001a; Barbehenn and Constabel 2011).

Condensed tannins are a group of polyphenolic compounds (also known as proanthocyanidins) of varying molecular weight (between 1000 to 20000 Dalton) and are named after their condensed chemical structure. Through their hydroxyl groups they can form bonds with polysaccharides (cellulose, hemicellulose and pectin), amino acids, alkaloids, minerals and proteins, with important effects on animal nutrition (Hagerman, 1992; Reed 1995; Frutos et al. 2000; Schofield et al. 2001; Hagerman 2011).

Hydrolyzable tannins (Gallotannins and Ellagitanins)

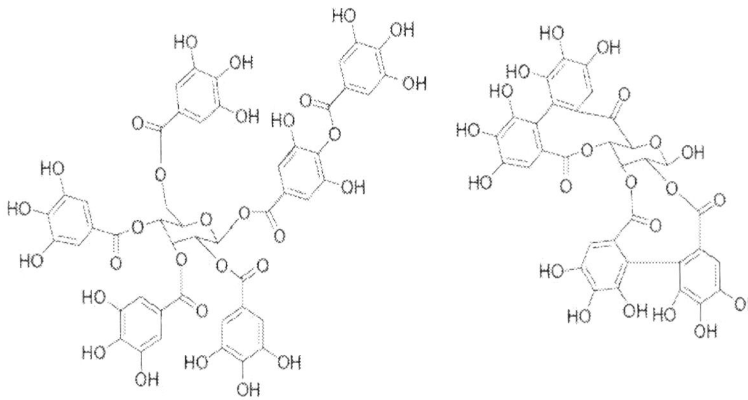

Condensed tannins (Proanthocyanidins)

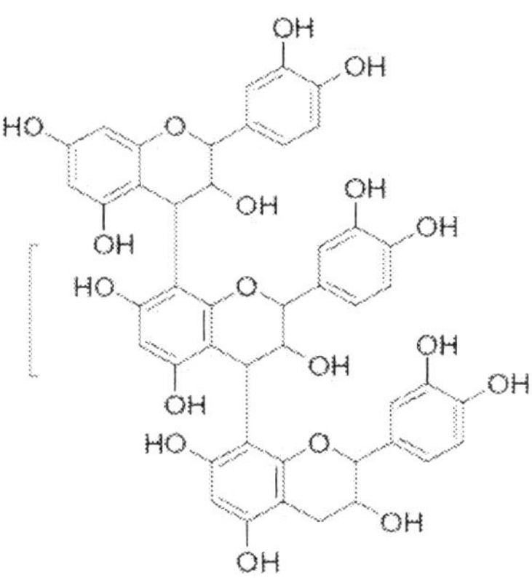

Figure 1. Structural schemes of hydrolyzable tannins and condensed tannins (adapted from Rochfort et al., 2008).

They have the property of binding most proteins through hydrogen bonds, forming tannin-protein complexes. This affinity is based on the large number of phenolic groups that constitute the bond points with the carbonyl groups of the peptides.

Distribution in Nature

The condensed tannins are synthesized by plants and form their defensive system against environmental stress factors, and against animal consumption due to their astringent properties and bitter taste (Wink, 1987; Montellano, 2010). They are secondary metabolites widely distributed in the plant kingdom, especially forage legumes commonly used in pastoral production systems (Niezen et al. 1998a; 1998b; Marley et al. 2003; Waghorn and McNabb, 2003; Otero et al. 2004; Waghorn G. 2008; Barbehenn and Constabel 2011). They are located in cell walls or vacuoles within living cells of stems, bark, leaves, flowers, and seeds, and are released during the chewing process (Ramos et al. 1998; Barry and McNabb 1999).

Effects of Tannins on Nutrition, Production and Animal Health

The effect of tannins is directly related to the concentration in which it is found in the food. Thus, the consumption of forage plants with moderate concentrations of TC (2% to 4.5% of dry matter (DM)) has beneficial effects on protein metabolism in ruminants. In these cases, ruminal proteolysis is reduced and consequently amino acid absorption in the small intestine is increased, which contributes to improved production rates (Aerts et al. 1999; Barry and McNabb 1999).

Conversely, when CTs are in high concentrations in the diet (6% to 10% of DM), they produce negative effects on voluntary consumption, rumen function and digestion, due to low palatability and destruction of the rumen microbiota (Barry et al. 1999; Frutos et al. 2000; Schofield et al. 2001; Nguyen et al. 2005). The decrease in food palatability is due to a direct reaction of CTs with salivary glycoproteins and with taste receptors leading to increased salivation and a sensation of astringency that decreases voluntary food intake (Reed 1995; Bennick 2002; Frutos et al. 2004).

It was observed that the consumption of forage plants such as *Lotus corniculatus* and *Sulla* that present moderate concentrations of CT can be used to optimize digestive efficiency in grazing sheep. This is reflected in improvements in wool growth (Douglas et al. 1995), in milk production (Frutos et al. 2004), and in higher ovulation rates with high lambing percentages. These improvements in productive parameters are due to a better use of dietary protein and increased amino acid absorption in the intestine

(Waghorn et al. 1998; 1999; Min et al. 1999; Athanasiadou et al. 2001a; 2001b; Min et al. 2003b).

Barry and McNabb (1999a) and Hoste (2006) observed different physiological effects in animals according to the percentage of CT consumed in the diet (Table 2).

The potential benefits of obtaining improvements in production levels and feed utilization efficiency were the basis for considering the incorporation of CTs as additives in ruminant diets (Waghorn et al. 1999).

Table 2. Effects of different concentrations of condensed tannins in the diet on nutrition and productive parameters in sheep (Barry and McNabb 1999a; Hoste et al. 2006).

CT content (DM) in the diet	Physiological effect on animals	Effects
Low (<2%)	Low or null	No effect on voluntary intake
Moderate (3 a 6%)	Beneficial	Increases amino acid absorption Increases wool production Increases milk production Increases ovulation rate Increases growth rate Prevention of tympanism
High (>7%)	Adverse	Decreases voluntary intake Decreases amino acid absorption Decreases wool production Decreases growth rate

DM: dry material.

Anthelmintic Effect

Since the 1990s, the nematodicidal activity of certain tannin-rich plant (TRP) began to be reported, and since then there has been a marked interest in considering them among the non-chemical alternatives for antiparasitic control (Niezen 1998a; 1998b; Min and Hart 2003). An improvement in body condition and production levels was observed in animals affected with gastrointestinal parasitosis when CTs were consumed at moderate concentrations (2% to 5%).

Mechanisms of Anthelmintic Action of Condensed Tannins

The mechanisms by which the consumption of certain bioactive plants or their extracts affect the viability, motility and fecundity of parasites are not fully elucidated, but would be related to a direct effect of CTs on GIN, and indirectly by enhancing the host immune response by increasing the availability of proteins (by-pass protein) (Bennick 2002; Githiori et al. 2006; Hoste et al. 2006; Ketzis et al. 2006).

Direct Effect on NGI

It was observed that the direct effect of CTs is due to their action in the gastrointestinal tract and in the faeces. In the first place, by binding with the proteins of the nematode wall, which affects their normal physiology and can even inactivate them. This is reflected in a reduction of the parasite burden and in the HPG values. In faeces it interferes with egg hatching and L3 development, viability and motility (Figures 2, 3 and 4) (Athanasiadou et al. 2001a; Min and Hart 2003; Paolini et al. 2003; Ketzis et al. 2006; Iqbal et al. 2007; Hoste et al. 2011).

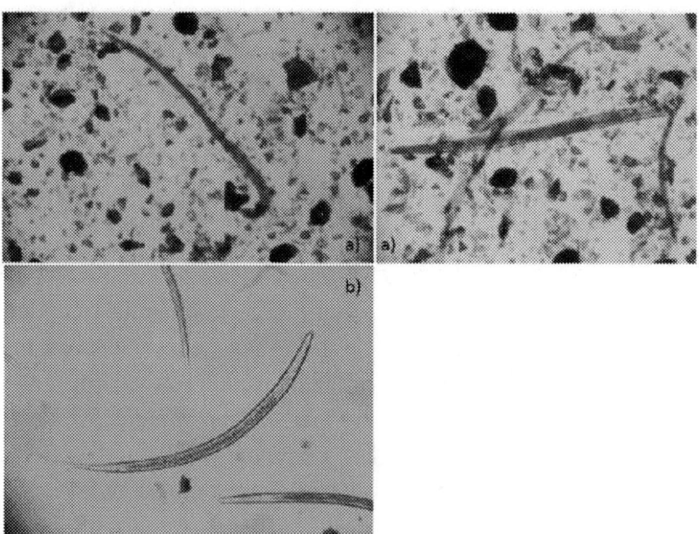

Source: Javier Schapiro.

Figure 2. (a) Images of infective larvae showing cuticle alteration (100X); (b) Infective larvae obtained from the untreated Control group.

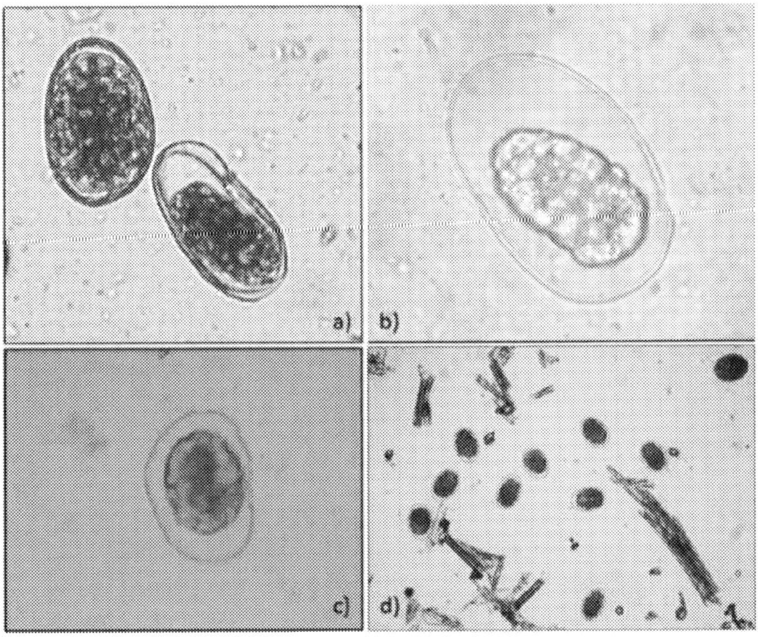

Source: Javier Schapiro.

Figure 3. (a-c) Microscopic observation (100X) of GIN eggs that were in contact with condensed tannins; (d) NGI eggs (40X) belonging to the Control group that retained their normal structure.

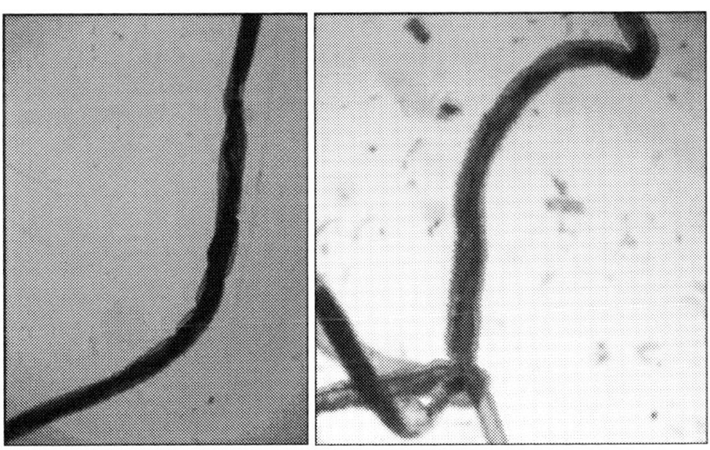

Source: Javier Schapiro.

Figure 4. Image of GIN in contact with CT of Quebracho (100X). Alteration of its cuticle is observed.

Indirect Effect on Gastrointestinal Nematodes

Condensed tannins improve protein nutrition by preventing their microbial degradation at the rumen level (pH 5 to 7.5) since they remain bounded to the CTs. During curdling (pH 2 to 3), a dissociation of the complex occurs, releasing the proteins that will be available for absorption as amino acids at the intestinal level (by-pass protein) (Hagerman et al. 1992; Coop and Kyriazakis 1999; Bennick 2002). This increase in the protein level compensates for the protein losses caused by gastrointestinal parasitism and at the same time stimulates the host´s immune system improving resilience and resistance against GIN (Paolini et al. 2003; Min and Hart 2003; Nguyen et al. 2005; Iqbal et al. 2007; Hoste et al. 2011).

Undoubtedly, most research work with plants in search of new anthelmintic drugs as alternatives to commercial chemical antiparasitics focused on CT-rich plants also called bioactive plants (Nguyen et al. 2005; Barbehenn and Constabel 2011). There is a significant amount of in vitro and *in vivo* work supporting their antiparasitic properties (Niezen et al. 1998a; 1998b; Athanasiadou et al. 2001; Waghorn and McNabb, 2003). The CT sources used were forage legumes such as Sulla (*Hedysarum coronarium*), Esparceta (*Onobrychis viciifolia*), Lotus (*Lotus corniculatus* and *L. pedunculatus*) and Achicoria (*Cichorium intybus*), and extracts obtained from Quebracho (*Schinopsis* spp.) and tropical legumes such as Acacia and Leucaena (Hoste et al. 2006; Waghorn 2008; Alonso-Díaz et al. 2010).

In Vitro Assays with Condensed Tannins from Quebracho (*Schinopsis balansae*)

The main *in vitro* assays used to demonstrate the nematodicidal activity of CT extracts were the egg hatching test (EHA) and the larval migration inhibition assay (LMIA) (Molan et al. 1999; 2000; Coles et al. 2005; 2006).

The first is a modification of the EHA used to evaluate anthelmintic resistance to benzimidazoles (Coles et al. 1992; 2005; 2006), and consists of incubating a known number of GIN eggs a few hours old (fresh, not larvae) against serial concentrations of a CT extract with potential anthelmintic activity.

The LMIA was developed by Wagland et al. (1992) and modified by Rabel et al. (1994), and its principle is based on measuring the migratory capacity of L3 through a 28 μm mesh after incubation with serial concentrations of a CT extract with potential anthelmintic activity. Infective larvae are used because this is the first parasitic stage that CTs are confronted with when they are consumed by the host.

Our Research

One of the main lines of research that is being carried out in the Parasitology Area of the Institute of Pathobiology-IPVET belonging to the Center for Research in Veterinary and Agronomic Sciences (CICVyA) of INTA Castelar (Buenos Aires, Argentina) is linked to determine the *in vitro* and *in vivo* anthelmintic effect of different concentrations of condensed tannins added to the animals' diet, as well as to the elaboration and evaluation of plant extracts from native plants. With these, *in vitro* methodologies are carried out to determine the activity on egg and on infective larvae stages of parasites in search of alternatives that can be added to the control of parasites.

One of the tests carried out was to determine the anthelmintic activity of different concentrations of a CT extract of Quebracho on the egg and larval stages of a pure strain of *Haemonchus contortus* by means of the egg hatching test (EHA) and the larval migration inhibition assay (LMIA).

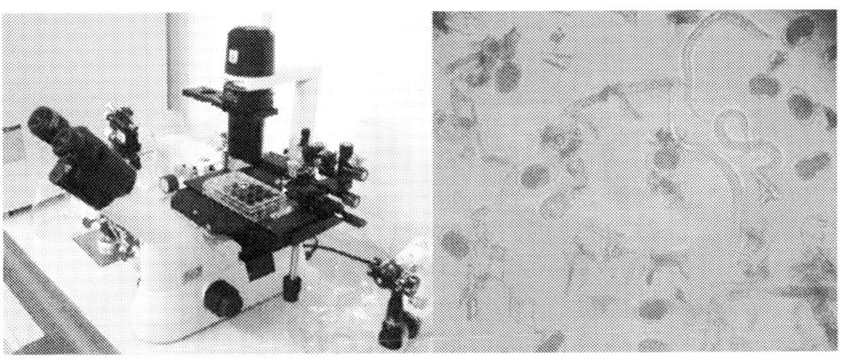

Source: Javier Schapiro.

Figure 5. Egg hatching inhibition test (left); Inverted microscope observation of a well with eggs confronted with a 50 mg/ml solution of CT (right).

As shown in Figures 5 and 6, nine concentrations of Quebracho CT dissolved in distilled water (50 mg/ml; 25 mg/ml; 12.5 mg/ml; 6.25 mg/ml;

3.12 mg/ml; 1.56 mg/ml; 0.78 mg/ml; 0.39 mg/ml and 0.19 mg/ml) were evaluated with 4 replicates each, in addition to a negative control (eggs in distilled water) which was analyzed in quadruplicate simultaneously.

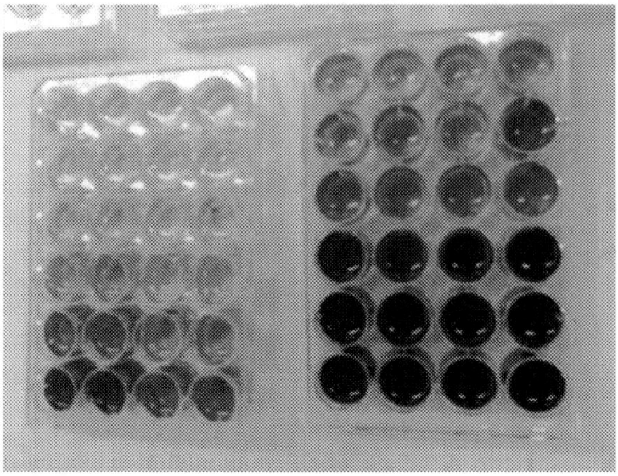

Source: Javier Schapiro.

Figure 6. Incubation plates with the different dilutions of condensed tannins from Quebracho and eggs from *Haemonchus contortus.*

Quebracho CTs shown to have *in vitro* action on the development of eggs and on the mobility of *Haemonchus contortus* larvae. They act directly on the eggs affecting their cover and consequently altering their normal hatching. They also inhibit the development, viability, and mobility of the larval stages. These actions would contribute to reduce contamination and infectivity of pastures.

It was observed that the inhibition of egg hatching was dose-dependent, i.e., the highest inhibition percentages (82.12%) were produced in those wells where the eggs were exposed to the highest concentrations of CT (50 mg/ml). This value decreased as the concentrations decreased until reaching a minimum value of 13.53% at the lowest concentration evaluated (0.19 mg/ml).

The results obtained in the LMIA technique (Figure 7) showed that the inhibition of larval migration was also dependent on the CT concentration, with a strong inhibition of larval migration (40%) at the highest CT concentrations, accompanied by a large proportion of dead larvae and a decrease in their mobility. Evidently, the L3 managed to migrate through the mesh but were affected by direct contact with the CT of the medium.

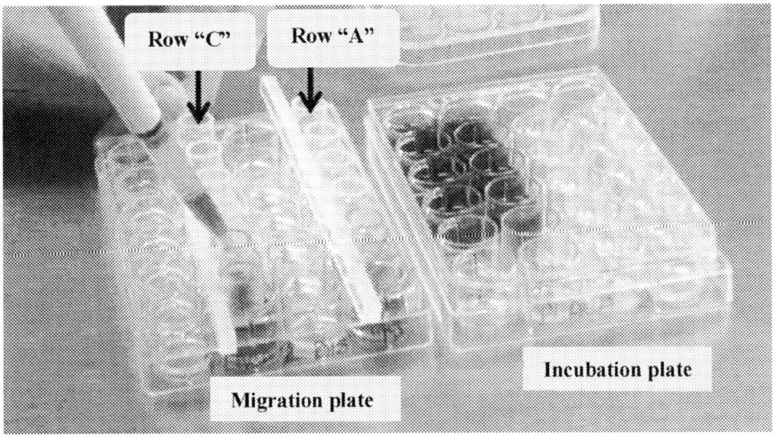

Source: Javier Schapiro.

Figure 7. Transfer of the contents from the incubation plate (right) to the migration plate (left) through the filters located in rows A and C.

Conclusion

Due to the obtained results, *in vivo* evaluations should be continued to confirm these preliminary results. It is encouraging to think about including Quebracho CTs in parasitic control programs, especially in those farms where resistance to anthelmintics has been diagnosed and constitutes one of the sanitary and productive problems to be solved.

The challenge is posed. Our mission is to demonstrate to the scientific community in general that these alternatives are sustainable for the integral control of gastrointestinal parasitism and anthelmintic resistance, and that they can be transferred as soon as possible to the productive sector. And for this we must all be together: research centers, universities, veterinarians, and livestock producers.

References

Aerts R. J., Barry T. N., McNabb W. C., 1999. Polyphenols and agriculture: beneficial effects of proanthocyanidins in forages. *Agriculture, Ecosystems & Environment* 75: 1-12.

Alonso-Díaz M. A., Torres-Acosta J. F. J., Sandoval-Castro C. A., Hoste H., 2010. Tannins in tropical tree fodders to small ruminants: A friendly foe? *Small Ruminant Research* 89: 164-173.

Amarante A. F. T., 2009. Actual standing and perspectives for the sustainable use and development of parasite resistant or tolerant breeds in Brazil. In *Animal Genetic Resources and Their Resistance.* Editores: Gauly M., Besbes B., Leyden B. and Pinard-van der Laan M. H. A Joint FAO/INRA Workshop: 44-46.

Amarante A. F. T., Craig T. M., Ramsey W. S., El-Sayed N. M., Desouki A. Y., Bazer F. W., 1999. Comparison of naturally acquired parasite burdens among Florida Native, Rambouillet and crossbreed ewes. *Veterinary Parasitology* 85: 61-69.

Anthony, J. P., Fyle, S, Smith, H., 2005. Plant active components - a resource for antiparasitic agents? *Trends in Parasitology*. Volume 21, Issue 10, Pages 462-468.

Anziani O. & Fiel C., 2004. Estado actual de la resistencia antihelmíntica (nematodos gastrointestinales) en bovinos de la Argentina. [*Current status of anthelmintic resistance (gastrointestinal nematodes) in cattle in Argentina*]. *Vet. Arg.* 21: 86-101.

Anziani O., Guglielmone A., Zimmermann G., Vázquez R. & Suárez V., 2001. Avermectin resistance to Cooperia pectinata in cattle in Argentina. *Vet. Rec.* 149: 58-59.

Athanasiadou S., Kyriazakis I., Jackson F., Coop R. L., 2001a. Direct anthelmintic effects of condensed tannins towards different gastrointestinal nematodes of sheep: in vitro and in vivo studies. *Veterinary Parasitology* 99: 205-219.

Athanasiadou S., Kyriazakis I., Jackson F., Coop R. L., 2001b. The effects of condensed tannins supplementation of foods with different protein content on parasitism, food intake and performance of sheep infected with Trichostrongylus colubriformis. *British Journal of Nutrition* 86: 697-706.

Avello, M., Cisternas, I., 2010. Phytotherapy, its origins, characteristics and status in Chile. *Revista Médica Chile*, 138, 1288-1293.

Barbehenn R. V. and ConSTABEL C. P., 2011. Tannins in plant-herbivore interactions. *Phytochemistry* 72: 1551-1565.

Barry T. N. and McNabb W. C., 1999. The implications of condensed tannins on the nutritive value of temperate forages fed to ruminants. *British Journal of Nutrition* 81: 263-272.

Barry T. N., McNabb W. C., Kemp P. D., Waghorn G. C., Min B. R. and Luque A., 1999. The effect of condensed tannins in Lotus corniculatus upon reproductive efficiency and wool production in sheep during late summer and autumn. *Proceedings of the New Zealand Grassland Association* 61: 51-55.

Bassetto, C. C., Silva, B. F., Fernandes, S., Amarante, A. F. T., 2009. Contaminação da pastagem com larvas infectantes de nematóides gastrintestinais após o pastejo de ovelhas resistentes ou suscetíveis à verminose. [*Contamination of pasture with infective gastrointestinal nematode larvae after grazing by worm-resistant or susceptible sheep*]. *Revista Brasileira de Parasitologia Veterinária*, v. 18, n. 4, p. 63-68.

Bennick, A., 2002. Interaction of plant polyphenols with salivary proteins. *Critical Reviews in Oral Biology and Medicine* 13: 184-196.

Bonino J., Mederos A., 2003. Resistencia antihelmíntica en ovinos. [*Anthelmintic resistance in sheep*]. *Revista del Plan Agropecuario* N° 107: 42-44.

Caracostantogolo J., Castaño R., Cutullé CH., Cetrá B., Lamberti R., Olaechea F., Ruiz M., Schapiro J., Martínez M., Balbiani G., Castro M., 2005. Evaluación de la resistencia a los antihelmínticos en rumiantes en Argentina. [*Evaluation of anthelmintic resistance in ruminants in Argentina*]. In: Eddi C., Vargas Terán M. (Editores). *Resistencia a los Antiparasitarios Internos en Argentina*. FAO Producción y Sanidad Animal, Roma: 7-34.

Caracostantogolo, J. L., Anziani, O., Romero, J., Suárez, V., y Fiel, C., 2012. Resistencia a los antihelmínticos en Argentina. En: Fiel, C. y Nari, A. Eds. Enfermedades parasitarias de importancia clínica y productiva en rumiantes [*Resistance to anthelmintics in Argentina*]. In: Fiel, C. and Nari, A. Eds. *Parasitic diseases of clinical and productive importance in ruminants. Epidemiological fundamentals for their prevention and control)*. Edit. Hemisferio Sur ISBN: 978-9974-674-35-6. Cap. 11, Pag 255-282.

Castells D., 2002. New approach in parasitic control of sheep. In: *Gastrointestinal Parasitosis of Sheep: Current Status and Research Advances*. INIA Uruguay: 14-22.

Coles G. C., 2005. Anthelmintic resistance - looking to the future: a UK perspective. *Research in Veterinary Science* 78: 99-108.

Coles, G. C., Bauer, C., Borgsteede, F., Geerts, S., Klei, T. R., Taylor, M. A., Waller, P, 1992. Word Association for the Advancement of Veterinary Parasitology (WAAVP). Methods for detection of anthelmintic resistance in nematodos of veterinary importance. *Veterinary Parasitology* 44: 35-44.

Coles, G. C., Jackson F., Pomroy W. E., Prichard R. K., Samson-Himmelstjerna G., Silvestre A., Taylor M. A., Vercruysse J., 2006. The detection of anthelmintic resistance in nematodes of veterinary importance. *Veterinary Parasitology* 136: 167-185.

Coop R. L. and Kyriazakis I., 1999. Nutrition-parasite interaction. *Veterinary Parasitology* 84: 187-204.

Cordero del Campillo M., Rojo Vázquez F. A., 1999. *Parasitología Veterinaria* [*Veterinary Parasitology*]. Editorial McGraw-Hill. Interamericana: 237-252.

Cristel, S., Fiel, C., Anziani, O., Descarga, C., Cetrá, B., Romero, J., Fernández, S., LLoberas, M., Medus, D., Steffan, P., 2017. Anthelmintic resistance in grazing beef cattle in central and northeastern areas of Argentina-An update. Veterinary Parasitology: *Regional Studies and Reports*. Volume 9, 2017, Pages 25-28.

Douglas G. B., Wang Y., Waghorn G. C., Barry T. N., Purchas R. W., Foote A G., Wilson G. F., 1995. Liveweight gain and wool production of sheep grazing Lotus corniculatus and Lucerne (Medicago sativa). *New Zealand Journal of Agricultural Research*, Volume 38: 95-104.

Echevarria F., Borba M. F. S., Pinheiro A. C., Waller P. J., Hansen J. W., 1996. The prevalence of anthelmintic resistance in nematode parasites of sheep in Southern Latin America: Brazil. *Veterinary Parasitology* 62: 199-206.

Eddi, C., Caracostantogolo, J., Peña, M., Schapiro, J., Marangunich, L., Waller, P. J. and Hansen, J. W., 1996. The prevalence of anthelmintic resistance in nematode parasites of sheep in Southern Latin America: Argentina. *Vet. Parasitol*. 62: 189-197.

Faedo, M., Larsen M. and Waller P. J., 1997. The potential of nematophagous fungi to control the free-living stages of nematode parasites of sheep: Comparison between

Australian isolates of Arthrobotrys spp. and Duddingtonia flagrans. *Veterinary Parasitology* 72: 149-155.

FAO Animal Production and Health Division, 2003. Resistencia a los antiparasitarios Estado actual con énfasis en América Latina. [*Antiparasitic resistance. Current status with emphasis on Latin America*]. In: *Estudio FAO producción y sanidad animal* 157. ISSN 1014-1200. Roma, Italia: 1-51.

FAO Animal Production and Health Division, 2004. CD, *Resistance managment and integrated parasited control in ruminants. Guidelines.*

Fiel C., Anziani O., Suárez V., Vázquez R., Eddi C., Romero J. R., Caracostantogolo J., Saumell C., Mejía M., Costa J. y Steffan P., (2001). Resistencia antihelmíntica en bovinos: causas, diagnóstico y profilaxis. (Anthelmintic resistance in cattle: causes, diagnosis and prophylaxis). *Veterinaria Argentina Volumen XVIII* 171: 21-33.

Frutos P., Hervas G., Giraldez F. J., Fernandez M. and Mantecon A. R., 2000. Digestive utilization of quebracho-treated soya bean meals in sheep. *Journal of Agricultural Science*, Cambridge 134: 101-108.

Frutos P., Hervas G., Giraldez F. J. and Mantecon A. R., 2004. Review. Tannins and ruminant nutrition. *Spanish Journal of Agricultural Research* 2 (2): 191-202.

Githiori J. B., Athanasiadou S., Thamsborg S. M., 2006. Use of plants in novel approaches for control of gastrointestinal helminths in livestock with emphasis on small ruminants. *Veterinary Parasitology* 139: 308-320.

Gobbo-Neto, L., Lopes, N. P., 2007. Medicinal plants: factors influencing the content of secondary metabolites. *Química Nova*, v. 30, n. 2, p. 374-381.

Hagerman A. E., 2011. Tannin Chemistry. *The Tannin Handbook*. Disponible en URL: http://www.users.muohio.edu/hagerman.

Hagerman A. E., Robbins C. T., Weerasuriya Y., Wilson T. C., McArthur C., 1992. Tannin chemistry in relation to digestion. *Journal of Range Management* 45: 57-62.

Hammond J. A., Fielding D. and Bishop S. C., 1997. Prospects for plant anthelmintics in tropical Veterinary Medicine. *Veterinary Research Communications* 21: 213-228.

Hernández-Orduño G., Torres-Acosta J. F. J., Sandoval-Castro C. A., Aguilar-Caballero A. J., Reyes-Ramirez R. R., Hoste H., Calderón-Quintal J. A., 2008. In vitro anthelmintic effect of Acacia gaumeri, Havardia albicans and Quebracho tannin extracts on a mexican strain of Haemonchus contortus L3 larvae. *Tropical and Subtropical Agroecosystems* 8: 191-197.

Hördegen P., Hertzberg H., Heilmann J., Langhans W., Maurer V., 2003. The anthelmintic efficacy of five plant products against gastrointestinal trichostrongylids in artificially infected lambs. *Veterinary Parasitology* 117: 51-60.

Hoste H., Jackson F., Athanasiadou S., Thamsborg S. M., Hoskin S. O., 2006. The effects of tannin-rich plants on parasitic nematodes in ruminants. *Trends in Parasitology* 22: 253-261.

Hoste H., Manolaraki F., Brunet S., Arroyo López C., Martínez-Ortiz de Montellano C., Sotiraki S., Torres Acosta F., 2011. The anthelmintic properties of tannin-rich legume forages: from knowledge to exploitation in farm conditions. *Options Méditerranéennes*, A N° 99: 295-304.

Iqbal Z., Sarwar M., Jabbar A., Ahmed S., Nisa M., Sajid M. S., Khan M. N., Mufti K. A., Yaseen M., 2007. Direct and indirect anthelmintic effects of condensed tannins in sheep. *Veterinary Parasitology* 144: 125-131.

Jackson F., Miller J., 2006. Alternative approaches to control-Quo vadit?. *Veterinary Parasitology* 139: 371-384.

Kaplan R. M., 2004. Drug resistance in nematodes of veterinary importance: a status report. Trends in Parasitology Vol. 20 N° 10: 477-481.

Ketzis J. K., Vercruysse J., Stromberg B. E., Larsen M., Athanasiadou S., Houdijk J. G. M., 2006. Evaluation of efficacy expectations for novel and non-chemical helminth control strategies in ruminants. *Veterinary Parasitology* 139: 321-335.

Köhler, P. 2001. The biochemichal basis of anthelmintic action and resistance. *International Journal for Parasitology* 31.

Lanusse C. and Prichard R., 1993. Relationship between pharmacological properties and clinical efficacy of rumiants anthelmintics. *Veterinary Parasitology* 49: 123-158.

Larsen M., 1999. Biological control of helminthes. *International Journal for Parasitology* 29: 139-146.

Larsen M., Faedo M., Waller P. J. and Hennessy D. R., 1998. The potential of nematophagous fungi to control the free-living stages of nematode parasites of sheep: Studies with Duddingtonia flagrans. *Veterinary Parasitology* 76: 121-128.

Larsen M., Nansen P., Grønvold J., Wolstrup J., Henriksen S. A., 1997. Biological control of gastro-intestinal nematodes - facts, future, or fiction? *Veterinary Parasitology* 72: 470-492.

Maciel S., Gimenez M., Gaona C., Waller P. J., Hansen J. W., 1996. The prevalence of anthelmintic resistance in nematode parasites of sheep in Southern Latin America: Paraguay. *Veterinary Parasitology* 62: 207-212.

Marley C. L., Cook R., Keatinge R., Barrett J., Lampkina N. H., 2003. The effect of birdsfoot trefoil (Lotus corniculatus) and chicory (Cichorium intybus) on parasite intensities and performance of lambs naturally infected with helminth parasites. *Veterinary Parasitology* 112: 147-155.

Márquez Lara, 2003. Resistencia a los antihelmínticos: origen, desarrollo y control. [*Anthelmintic resistance: origin, development and control*]. *Revista Corpoica*, VOL 4, N°1.

Melo Ana Carolina, Fonseca Lindoso y Bevilaqua C. M. L., 2002. Resistência anti-helmíntica em nematóides de pequenos ruminantes: uma revisão. [*Anthelmintic resistance in nematodes of small ruminants: a review*]. *Ciência animal*, 12 (1): 35-45.

Mendonca R. M. A., Leite R. C., Lana A. M. Q., Costa J. O., Toth G. 2014. Parasitic helminth infection in young cattle raised on silvopasture and open-pasture in Southeastern Brazil. *Agroforestry systems*, 88(1), 53-62.

Mendoza de Gives P. and Vazquez-Prats V. M., 1994. Reduction of Hamonchus contortus infective larvae by three nematophagous fungi in sheep faecal cultures. *Veterinary Parasitology* 55: 197-203.

Mendoza de Gives P., Zapata Nieto C., Hernández E. L., Arellano M. E., Rodríguez D. H., Garduño R. G., 2006. Biological control of gastrointestinal parasitic nematodes using Duddingtonia flagrans in sheep under natural conditions in Mexico. *Annals of the New York Academy of Science* 1081: 355-359.

Miller J. E., Bahirathan M., Lemarie S. L., Hembry F. G., Kearney M. T., Barras S. R., 1998. Epidemiology of gastrointestinal nematode parasitism in Suffolk and Gulf Coast Native sheep with special emphasis on relative susceptibility to Haemonchus contortus infection. *Veterinary Parasitology* 74: 55-74.

Min B. R., Barry T. N., Attwood G. T., McNabb W. C., 2003b. The effect of condensed tannins on the nutrition and health of ruminants fed fresh temperate forages: a review. *Animal Feed Science and Technology* 106: 3-19.

Min B. R. and Hart S. P., 2003a. Tannins for suppression of internal parasites. *Journal of Animal Science* 81: E102-E109.

Min B. R., McNabb, Barry T. N., Kemp P. D., Waghorn G. C. and McDonald M. F., 1999. The effect of condensed tannins in Lotus corniculatus upon reproductive efficiency and wool production in sheep during late summer and autumn. *The Journal of Agricultural Science*, Volume 132, 03: 323-334.

Molan A. L. and Faraj A. M., 2010. The effects of condensed tannins extracted from different plant species on egg hatching and larval development of Teladorsagia circumcincta (Nematoda: Trichostrongylidae). *Folia Parasitológica* 57[1]: 62-68.

Molan A. L., Waghorn G. C. and McNabb W. C., 1999. Condensed tannins and gastro-intestinal parasites in sheep. *Proceedings of the New Zealand Grassland Association* 61: 57-61.

Molan A. L., Waghorn G. C., Min B. R. and McNabb W. C., 2000. The effect of condensed tannins from seven herbages on Trichostrongylus colubriformis larval migration in vitro. *Folia Parasitologica* 47: 39-44.

Molento, M. B., Lifschitz, A., Sallovitz, J., Lanusse, C., Prichard, R. 2004. Influence of verapamil on the pharmacokinetics of the antiparasitic drugs ivermectin and moxidectin in sheep. *Parasitology Research*, v. 92, p. 121-127.

Molento M. B. and Prichard R. K., 2001. Effect of multidrug resistance modulators on the activity of ivermectin and moxidectin against selected strains of Haemonchus contortus infective larvae. *Pesquisa Veterinária Brasileira* 21(3): 117-121.

Molento M. B., Veríssimo C. J., Amarante A. T., Van Wyk J. A., Chagas A. C. S., Araújo J. V. de, Borges F. A., 2013. Alternatives for the control of gastrointestinal nematodes of small ruminants. . *Arq. Inst. Biol.*, São Paulo, v. 80, n. 2, abr/jun p. 253-263.

Montellano Martínez Ortíz Cintli, 2010. Thesis: Mecanismos de acción de las plantas ricas en taninos sobre la población adulta de nematodos gastrointestinales de los pequeños rumiantes. [*Thesis: Mechanisms of action of tannin-rich plants on the adult population of gastrointestinal nematodes of small ruminants*]: 1-129.: 1-129.

Nari A., Eddi C., 2002. Control de la resistencia a los antiparasitarios a la luz de los conocimientos actuales. [*Control of resistance to antiparasitic drugs in the light of current knowledge*]. *Sitio Argentino de Producción Animal*: 1-14.

Nari A., Salles J., Gil A., Waller P. J., Hansen J. W., 1996. The prevalence of anthelmintic resistance in nematode parasites of sheep in Southern Latin America: Uruguay. *Veterinary Parasitology* 62: 213-222.

Nguyen T. M., Binh D. V., Orskov E. R., 2005. Effect of foliages containing condensed tannins and on gastrointestinal parasites. *Animal Feed Science and Technology* 121: 77-87.

Niezen J. H., Charleston W. A. G., Robertson H. A., Shelton D., Waghorn G. C., Green R., 2002. The effect of feeding Sulla (Hedysarum coronarium) or Lucerne (Medicago sativa) on lamb parasite burdens and development of immunity to gastrointestinal nematodes. *Veterinary Parasitology* 105: 229-245.

Niezen J. H., Robertson H. A., Waghorn G. C. & Charleston W. A., 1998b. Production, faecal egg counts and worm burdens of ewe lambs which grazed six contrasting forages. *Veterinary Parasitology* 80: 15-27.

Niezen J. H., Waghorn G. C. and Charleston W. A., 1998a. Establishment and fecundity of Ostertagia circumcincta and Trichostrongylus colubriformis in lambs fed lotus (Lotus pedunculatus) or perennial ryegrass (Lolium perenne). *Veterinary Parasitology* 78: 13-21.

Otero M. J., Hidalgo L. G., 2004. Taninos condensados en especies forrajeras de clima templado: efectos sobre la productividad de rumiantes afectados por parasitosis gastrointestinales (una revisión). [*Condensed tannins in temperate forage species: effects on productivity of ruminants affected by gastrointestinal parasitosis (a review)*]. *Livestock Research for Rural Development* 16 (2): 1-11.

Paolini V., Frayssines A., De La Farge F., Dorchies P., Hoste H., 2003. Effects of condensed tannins on established populations and on incoming larvae of Trichostrongylus colubriformis and Teladorsagia circumcincta in goats. *Veterinary Research* 34: 1-9.

Prichard R., 1994. Anthelmintic resistance. *Veterinary Parasitology* 54 (1-3): 259-268.

Rabel B., McGregor R., Douch P. G. C., 1994. Improved bioassay for estimation of inhibitory effects of ovine gastrointestinal mucus and anthelmintics on nematode larval migration. *International Journal of Parasitology* 24: 671-676.

Ramos G. P., Frutos F. J., Giráldez y Mantecón A. R., 1998. Los compuestos secundarios de las plantas en la nutrición de los herbívoros. [*Secondary plant compounds in herbivore nutrition*]. Estación Agrícola Experimental CSIC, León (España). *Archivos de Zootecnia* 47: 597-620.

Reed J. D., 1995. Nutritional toxicology of tannins and related polyphenols in forage legumes. *Journal Animal Science* 73: 1516-1528.

Rochfort S., Parker A. J., Dunshea F. R., 2008. Plant bioactives for ruminant health and productivity. *Phytochemistry* 69: 299-322.

Romero J. R., Boero C., Vázquez R., Aristizábal M. T., Baldo A., 1998. Estudio de resistencia a antihelmínticos en majadas de la Mesopotamia. [*Study of anthelmintic resistance in Mesopotamian herds*]. *Revista de Medicina Veterinaria* 79 (5): 342-346.

Romero J. R., Espinosa G., Valera A. R., 1992. Demostración de Resistencia al Oxfendazole en Trichostrongylidos de ovinos de la Zona deprimida del Salado. [*Demonstration of Resistance to Oxfendazole in Trichostrongylidae of sheep from the Salado Depressed Zone*]. *Revista de Medicina Veterinaria* 73 (2): 82-86.

Saumell C. A. y Fernández A. S., 2000. Hongos nematófagos para el control biológico de nematodos parásitos de rumiantes. [*Nematophagous fungi for biological control of ruminant parasitic nematodes*]. *Revista de Medicina Veterinaria* 81: 270-273.

Schapiro J., Pantiu A. 2018. Capítulo 2: Manejo sostenible del parasitismo gastrointestinal en bovinos en sistemas silvopastoriles. 67-85. En: El suelo como reactor de los procesos de regulación funcional de los agroecosistemas. [*Chapter 2: Sustainable management of gastrointestinal parasitism in cattle in silvopastoral systems*]. In: *Soil as a reactor of functional regulation processes in agroecosystems.* INTA Ediciones. Colección: Investigación, Desarrollo e Innovación.

Schofield P., Mbugua D. M., PelL A.N., 2001. Analysis of condensed tannins: a review. *Animal Feed Science and Technology* 91: 21-40.

Shakya K. P., Miller J. E., Lomax L. G., Burnett, D. D., 2011. Evaluation of immune response to artificial infections of Haemonchus contortus in Gulf Coast Native compared with Suffolk lambs. *Veterinary Parasitology* 181: 239-247.

Soca M., Simón L. y Francisco A. G., 2000. Comportamiento de las nematodosis gastrointestinales de bovinos jovenes en un sistema silvopastoril. [*Behavior of gastrointestinal nematodes in young cattle in a silvopastoral system*]. *Pastos y Forrajes*, 23(4).

Steffan P. E., Fiel C. A., Saumell C. A., Fusé C. A., Iglesias L. E., 2005. El uso de antihelmínticos en los programas de control y el riesgo potencial de resistência. [*The use of anthelmintics in control programs and the potential risk of resistance*]. In: Eddi C., Vargas Terán M. (Editores), *Resistencia a los Antiparasitarios Internos en Argentina. FAO Producción y Sanidad Animal*, Roma: 85-94.

Steffan P., Sánchez E., Entrocasso C., Fiel C., LLoberas M., Riva E. y Guzmán M., 2011. Eficacia de Monepantel contra Nematodes de Ovinos con Resistencia Antihelmíntica Múltiple en la Región Templada de Argentina. [*Efficacy of Monepantel against Sheep Nematodes with Multiple Anthelmintic Resistance in the Temperate Region of Argentina*]. *Veterinaria Argentina* - Volumen XXVIII, Nº 273: 1-12.

Suárez V., 2007. Epidemiología y control de los nematodes gastrointestinales en el oeste de la Región Pampeana [*Epidemiology and control of gastrointestinal nematodes in the western Pampean Region*]. In: *Enfermedades parasitarias de los ovinos y otros rumiantes menores en el cono sur de América.* Suárez V., Olaechea F., Romero J., Rossanigo C. (Editores). EEA INTA Anguil: 43-62.

Suárez, V. & Cristel, S., 2011. Risk factors for the development of bovine anthelmintic resistance in Argentina. *Resúmenes de 23rd International Conference (WAAVP) of the World Assoc. for the Advancement of Veterinary Parasitology*, 21-24-08-2011, Buenos Aires, Argentina, 50 pp.

Torres-Acosta J. F. J., Mendoza de Gives P., Aguilar-Caballero A. J., Cuéllar Ordaz J. A., 2012. Anthelmintic resistance in sheep farms: Update of the situation in the American continent. *Veterinary Parasitology* 189: 89-96.

Waghorn G. C., Douglas G. B., Niezen J. H., McNabb W. C. and Foote A. G., 1998. Forages with condensed tannins - their management and nutritive value for ruminants. *Proceedings of the New Zealand Grassland Association* 60: 89-98.

Waghorn G. C., Reed J. D., Ndlovu L. R., 1999. Condensed tannins and herbivore nutrition. Sección 8- Tannins Plant Breeding and Animal Effects. In *Proceedings of the XVIIth International Grasslands Congress* 3: 153-156.

Waghorn G., 2008. Beneficial and detrimental effects of dietary condensed tannins for sustainable sheep and goat production-Progress and challenges. *Animal Feed Science and Technology* 174: 116-139.

Waghorn G., McNabb W. C., 2003. Consequences of plant phenolic compounds for productivity and health of ruminants. *Proceedings of Nutrition Society* 62: 383-392.

Wagland B. M., Jones W. O., Hribar L., Bendixsen T., Emery D. L., 1992. A new simplified assay for larval migration inhibition. *International Journal of Parasitology* 22: 1183-1185.

Waller P. J., Knox M. R., Faedo M., 2001. The potential of nematophagous fungi to control the free-living stages of nematode parasites of sheep: feeding and block studies with Duddingtonia flagrans. *Veterinary Parasitology* 102: 321-330.

Wink M., 1987. Plant breeding: importance of plant secondary metabolites for protection against pathogens and herbivores. *Theoretical and Applied Genetics* 75: 225-233.

Wood I. B., Amaral N. K., Bairden K., Duncan J. L., Kassai T., MAlone J. B., Pankavich J. A., Reinecke R. K., Slocombe O., Taylor S. M., Vercruysse, J., 1995. World Association for the Advancement of Veterinary Parasitology (W.A.A.V.P.). Second edition of guidelines for evaluating the efficacy of anthelmintics in ruminants (bovine, ovine, caprine). *Veterinary Parasitology* Volume 58, Issue 3. 181–213.

Chapter 11

Equine Neurological Diseases in Brazil

Fabrício Moreira Cerri, DVM
Rogério Martins Amorim, PhD
and Alexandre Secorun Borges*, PhD
Department of Veterinary Clinical Science (DCV),
School of Veterinary Medicine and Animal Science (FMVZ),
São Paulo State University (UNESP), Botucatu, São Paulo, Brazil

Introduction

Neurological diseases in horses in Brazil are frequently diagnosed and have clinical and epidemiological importance. In this chapter we will present a historical context of its description in Brazil. Establishing the diagnosis is essential for treatment and preventive measures to be adopted, minimizing the losses resulting from these processes. During neurological evaluation, it is always important to locate the lesion within the central nervous system and, along with the history and evolution of the process, establish a list of differential diagnosis and choose the most indicated complementary exams. Post-mortem examination and the collection of tissues to confirm the diagnosis are essential. It should be highlighted that rabies is still the most important neurological disease of horses in Brazil and is diagnosed throughout the country.

In this chapter, we describe the research papers and case reports published in Brazil dealing with neurological diseases resulting from the direct action of infectious or parasitic agents in horses. We also include tetanus, leukoence-

* Corresponding Author's Email: alexandre.s.borges@unesp.br.

In: Infectious and Parasitic Diseases of Animals in Developing Countries
Editor: Selwyn Arlington Headley
ISBN: 979-8-88697-504-8

phalomalacia and botulism here to complement the descriptions of diseases caused by the actions of bacteria or fungi.

Botulism

Botulism is a disease caused by the toxin produced by *Clostridium botulinum*. *C. botulinum* strains produce neurotoxins that cause flaccid paralysis. The toxin prevents the release of acetylcholine at the neuromuscular junction. The toxins produced by *C. botulinum* are classified from A to H (Lindström and Korkeala, 2006). Cases of botulism in horses are often related to toxins A and B in North America, but cases related to toxins C and D have been described in different parts of the world (Doutre 1969; Kinde et al. 1991; Ostrowski et al. 2012; Shnaiderman-Torban et al. 2018; Uzal et al. 2022). In horses, the toxin is usually ingested with feed (contaminated silage or hay) or water (Whitlock and McAdams 2006). The clinical signs observed are related to decreased muscle tone; initially, progressive weakness is observed, with fasciculations, paresis, reduced tongue tone, dysphagia and recumbency (Kelly et al. 1984; Ricketts et al. 1984; Haagsma et al. 1990; Johnson et al. 2010; Johnson et al. 2015).

Confirmation of botulism is based on physical examination, epidemiological data, and the detection of botulinum neurotoxin in the patient. The identification of botulinum toxin (BoNTs) in water, food, feces, gastric and intestinal contents must be carried out, and the standard method used is based on a mouse lethality assay followed by neutralization of the toxin with specific antitoxins (Lindström and Korkeala, 2006; Cai et al. 2007).

Although diagnosed in cattle in different regions of Brazil, laboratory confirmation of suspected cases in horses is uncommon. Suspected cases of botulism are generally described, but only three reports have confirmed the diagnosis and the detection of botulinum toxin in affected animals from Brazil. The first report of botulism in horses from Brazil (Midwest) described seven animals that presented locomotary difficulties (weakness), muscle tremors, tongue protrusion, and pelvic limb paresis followed by lateral recumbency. The mouse bioassay was positive (stomach contents) and associated with toxin neutralization, confirming the presence of botulinum toxin type C (Coelho et al. 2000). The second outbreak occurred in Southern Brazil (Argenta et al. 2017). *C. botulinum* type C was also identified, and as in the other description, it was not possible to identify the source of infection. In both cases, all affected animals died, demonstrating the high lethality of this disease, especially when patients are not intensively monitored in a hospital (Coelho et al. 2000; Argenta et al. 2017).

The first confirmed description of toxin type D causing botulism in horses was recently described in the state of São Paulo, Southeastern Brazil, with the disease being observed in eight horses from the same farm (Valim et al. 2022). The main clinical findings were flaccid paresis, inability to stand up, decreased tongue and tail tone, dysphagia, discharge of saliva from the nostrils and fasciculations. Three animals were referred to a Veterinary Hospital; one died, and the other animals were discharged up to 42 days of hospitalization. A sample of cecal contents was positive for the presence of botulinum toxin type D (mouse bioassay and toxin neutralization tests).

Tetanus

Tetanus is a disease caused by the action of toxins produced by *Clostridium tetani*. Neurological signs are due to tetanospasmin (TeTN), which prevents the release of inhibitory neurotransmitters in the central nervous system (Uzal et al. 2022). For the development of signs, previous contamination with the spores of *C. tetani* is usually described and under anaerobic conditions, spores germinate. (Popoff 2020). The main situations in which tetanus occurs in equines are cutaneous wounds, hoof injuries, castration, dental procedures, and umbilical infections in foals (Reichamann et al. 2008; Pimentel et al. 2009; Di Filippo et al. 2016, Ribeiro et al. 2018). Initially, there is the release of tetanolysin, favoring the maintenance of necrotic tissue and reduction of oxygen levels. Subsequently, TeTN is produced and is the predominantly responsible for the clinical signs (Popoff 2020). The disease is clinically characterized limb spasticity, mandibular trismus, hyperesthesia, third eyelid prolapse, and dysphagia (Reichamann et al. 2008).

The first description of horses in Brazil with clinical signs suggestive of tetanus was made by Lutz in 1908 (BRASIL 1988). Later, Aragão (1913) published a manuscript illustrated with a photo of a donkey showing clinical signs of tetanus and described the disease in several species (BRASIL 1988). Most of the published data on tetanus from Brazil are sporadic case reports (Silva et al. 2010; Chabí et al. 2022) and proceedings abstracts. Reports usually describe wounds (mainly on limbs) and/or a history of surgical procedures, such as castration. The main reported treatment is the administration of tetanus antitoxin (TAT), doses ranging from 5,000 - 250,000

IU by the intramuscular or intravenous routes. However, the use of antimicrobials, wound dressings, sedatives, enteral nutrition, fluid therapy and nursing measures are fundamental to reduce mortality (Reichamann et al. 2008; Ribeiro et al. 2018). Vaccination with tetanus toxoid is the main prophylactic measure, as well as the correct management of accidental or surgical wounds, associated with the administration of TAT (Dennis et al. 2022).

In a retrospective study involving 78 horses with tetanus carried out by Reichmann et al. (2008) in the state of Paraná, Southern Brazil, the main clinical signs observed were limb spasticity, hyperesthesia, third eyelid prolapse, dysphagia, and recumbency. The therapeutical protocol consisted of the administration of antibiotics (penicillin), wound treatment, TAT, and fluid therapy. Most of the animals evaluated died or were euthanized (n=58; 76.32%), and the inability to maintain in a quadrupedal position was the main reason for choosing euthanasia.

Costa (2010) described 18 cases of equine tetanus in the state of Paraíba, Northeastern Brazil, with 88.8% (16/18) survival. The treatment performed in these cases consisted of administration of TAT, penicillin, acepromazine and fluid therapy.

Di Filippo et al. (2016) described 25 cases of tetanus in horses in the state of Rio de Janeiro, Southeastern Brazil. The main clinical findings were muscle stiffness, hyperexcitability, mandibular trismus, drooling, bruxism and third eyelid protrusion. The absence of preventive vaccination was observed in all cases, and the survival rate was 20% (5/25). The administration of 50,000 IU of TAT by the intrathecal route in the atlanto-occipital space was performed in three horses (two survived).

The description of 70 cases of horses with tetanus sent to a reference Veterinary Hospital in the state of São Paulo, Southeastern Brazil, was carried out by Ribeiro et al. (2018). The presence of umbilical infections, limb wounds and castration were the main predisposing factors. Hyperesthesia, spasticity and limbs, neck stiffness, tetanic spasms, dysphagia, restriction of jaw movements and lateral recumbency were the main findings during the physical examination. The treatment performed in these cases was based on the administration of antibiotics, TAT, and muscle relaxant. Among the animals studied, 51 (72.9%) died.

A retrospective study involving 17 cases of tetanus in horses in the state of Rio Grande do Norte in the northeast region described a mortality rate of 23% (Melo and Ferreira 2022). The main clinical findings were hyperesthesia, limb spasticity, hyperexcitation, third eyelid protrusion and muscle spasms.

The treatment consisted of the administration of 50,000 IU of TAT, procaine penicillin, muscle relaxant, fluid therapy, feeding via nasogastric tube and maintenance of the quadrupedal position.

In retrospective studies of neurological diseases affecting horses carried out in various regions of Brazil, the occurrence of tetanus is described in Table 1.

Table 1. Occurrence of tetanus in retrospective studies of neurological diseases affecting horses carried out in various regions of Brazil

Author	Year	State	Geographical Region	Affected Horses
Pimentel et al.	2009	Pernambuco	Northeastern	13/159 – (8.18%)
Pierezan et al.	2009	Rio Grande do Sul	Southern	4/355 – (1.1%)
Rissi et al.	2010	Rio Grande do Sul	Southern	4/19 – (21.05%)
Sousa	2013	Federal District and Goiás	Midwestern	3/76 (3.94%)
Marcolongo-Pereira	2014	Rio Grande do Sul	Southern	9/73 (6.62%)

Leukoencephalomalacia

Leukoencephalomalacia is degeneration/necrosis of the white matter of the brain caused by the ingestion of fumonisin B1, a thermostable mycotoxin produced by two species of *Fusarium* (*F. proliferatum and F. verticillioides*) (Meireles et al. 1994; Riet-Correa et al. 2013). The disease affects equines and has seasonal occurrence, and in Brazil, cases are concentrated between June and September, the winter period (dry) in the southern hemisphere (Riet-Correa et al. 2013; Reis Gomes et al. 2018).

Different clinical signs have been described depending on the affected brain region; however, abnormalities in the level of consciousness and ataxia and later recumbency are frequently observed (Riet-Correa et al. 2009; Albertino et al. 2021). In general, clinical signs may appear between 7-10 days after eating contaminated food. These evolve within the first 72 hours, and the animals die within a maximum of 12 days (Riet-Correa et al. 1982, Riet-Correa et al. 2009; Del Fava et al. 2010; Echenique et al. 2019). It is important to emphasize that even after ceasing the supply of feed contaminated by fumonisin, new cases of leukoencephalomalacia may occur within the next 18 days (Borges et al., 1995). At necropsy of affected horses, the presence of congestion of meningeal vessels and diffuse encephalic white matter malacia are observed. In addition, the presence of cavitations in the nervous system facilitates their macroscopic identification. Liquefactive necrosis is the main histopathological finding (Riet-Correa et al. 2009; Del Fava et al. 2010). The diagnosis is made by associating the macroscopic and microscopic findings with the detection of the mycotoxin.

Since the appearance of the first cases of leukoencephalomalacia described in the beginning of the 20th century in the USA (MacCallum and Buckley 1901), the association of the disease with the consumption of moldy corn has been suspected. In the following years, this finding was confirmed with the effective participation of corn in cases where this disease occurred (Graham, 1936; Schwarte et al. 1937), and later, it was found to be an important substrate for toxin-producing fungi. The association between the presence of fungi of the genus *Fusarium* (*Fusarium moniliforme*, renamed *Fusarium vertilicoides*) and leukoencephalomalacia was established from outbreaks that occurred in South Africa in 1970 (Wilson and Maronpot, 1970; Kellerman et al. 1972). The role of fumonisin B1 mycotoxin, produced by *Fusarium verticillioides* as the cause of the disease, was elucidated 80 years after the first descriptions of leukoencephalomalacia (Bezeidenhount et al. 1988; Thiel et al. 1991). This association was confirmed by the intravenous administration of fumonisin, with replication of neurological symptoms and necropsy findings (Marasas et al. 1988).

In Brazil, the first report of leukoencephalomalacia with an association between the consumption of moldy corn and the appearance of neurological signs in equines was described by Chaves in 1950 in the city of Pirassununga, São Paulo, Southeastern Brazil. During this investigation, ten animals were affected, six horses and four mules, of which only one mule survived. The affected animals showed muscle tremors, ataxia, pelvic limb paralysis, decreased levels of consciousness, and recumbency. On average, death occurred 10 hours after the onset of clinical signs. A correlation was observed between the supply of moldy corn and the development of the disease. At necropsy, areas of liquefaction and necrosis were observed in the cerebral hemispheres (Chaves 1950).

Riet-Correa et al. (1982) described leukoencephalomalacia in three outbreaks affecting horses from Rio Grande do Sul, Southern Brazil. During this study, 5 horses died with acute evolution (2 to 24 hours), with clinical signs of a cerebral syndrome. In all outbreaks, the horses were fed moldy corn, with the surface fungal growth. The affected horses developed inappetence, limb ataxia, lateral recumbency, and blindness. At necropsy, necrosis was observed with the formation of cavitations at the white matter of the brain.

Histopathology of the CNS, revealed areas of myelin and vascular degeneration, hemorrhages and edema. Three genera of fungi were isolated in the feed: *Aspergillus sp.*, *Rhizophus sp.*, and *Fusarium sp* (Riet-Correa et al. 1982). Although the toxin was not investigated in the feed samples, the clinical, epidemiological, and histopathological findings were able to determine the diagnosis.

In the same year, an isolated case was described in, Minas Gerais, Southern Brazil (Brito et al. 1982). Decreased levels of consciousness, ataxia, hyperexcitation, and lateral recumbency were observed during neurological examination. At necropsy, cavitations were observed at the left cerebral hemisphere, perivascular infiltration and leptomeningeal edema were present. The postmortem findings supported the diagnosis of leukoence-phalomalacia. No samples for fumonisin detection or mycological culture were submitted on this occasion.

Subsequently, an outbreak was described in the state of Minas Gerais, affecting 10 horses from 4 different farms (Barros et al. 1984). The clinical signs observed were anorexia, circling, ataxia, and recumbency. Necropsy revealed white matter malacia with the presence of cavitations. Histopathology detected degenerative changes in the vascular endothelium, perivascular hemorrhages, and edema. The occurrence of cases in the months of June and July was consistent with what was observed by Riet-Correa et al. (1982), demonstrating the relative seasonality of the disease in the coldest and driest months (southern hemisphere), where a greater amount of concentrate is usually offered. No samples for fumonisin detection or mycological culture were submitted on this occasion.

In 1991, Xavier et al. reported five cases of leukoencephalomalacia in different cities from the state of São Paulo in Southeastern Brazil. In all outbreaks *F. verticilioides* was isolated from moldy corn (Xavier et al. 1991). The clinical signs described were ataxia, blindness, dysphagia, circling, and seizures. Analysis of the cerebrospinal fluid (CSF) revealed pleocytosis with a predominance of lymphocytes in more severe cases, while areas of liquefactive necrosis with cavitary formations were in the white matter (Xavier et al. 1991).

In 1995, Borges et al. described an outbreak of leukoencephalomalacia affecting 10 horses from the same farm in the state of São Paulo, Southeastern Brazil. This outbreak occurred for 40 days, affecting 36 horses, aged between 18 months and 12 years. The affected animals presented several neurological signs, with visual deficit, motor incoordination and marked decrease in mental status being the most frequent. Facial, glossopharyngeal, and hypoglossal nerve deficits and head tilt were observed in two cases. The evolution of the disease, from the beginning of the signs to death, ranged from 6 hours to four days, and all affected animals died. Two of the animals were found dead, with no previous clinical sings reported (sudden death). The diet consisted of pasture (coast-cross grass) and supplementation with corn (corn cobs crushed with straw and cob) stored in bags. This corn supply was suspended soon after the first clinical visit, but even with the suspension of the corn roll, new cases (seven) continued to appear within an interval of 18 days. The fungus *F. verticillioides* was isolated from the feed, and the presence of fumonisin toxin was confirmed. Necropsy revealed extensive areas of cerebral softening, indicative of liquefaction white matter necrosis, in one or both cerebral hemispheres. Marginal regions of necrotic foci showed hemorrhage. Central nervous system microscopy revealed edema, perivascular hemorrhage, mono- and polymorphonuclear infiltrates in the vessel wall and perivascular spaces, bordering areas of necrosis.

Although less frequent when compared to horses, the description of this disease in mules was reported by Riet-Correa et al. (2007) in Pará, Northern Brazil, Câmara et al. (2008) in Pernambuco, Northeast, and Santos et al. (2013) in Mato Grosso, Midwestern Brazil. It was described in donkeys by Del Fava et al. (2010) in the state of São Paulo, Southeastern Brazil. Clinical, epidemiological and necropsy findings were similar to those previously described.

Recently, Albertino et al. (2021) described the findings of the analysis of the cerebrospinal fluid (CSF) of seven horses with leukoencephalomalacia presenting xanthochromia, hyperproteinorrachia and mixed pleocytosis in approximately 50% of the cases, with the remaining CSF being normal. However, the definitive diagnosis depends on postmortem macroscopic and microscopic findings (Albertino et al., 2021).

When observed within the context of neurological diseases in Brazil, leukoencephalomalacia is of great importance. The retrospective studies in horses that observed the occurrence of this disease are listed below (leukoencephalomalacia cases/total neurological cases included in the study): Pimentel et al. (2008) (1/159 – 0.63%) in Pernambuco, Northeastern Brazil; Pierezan et al. (2009) (8/37 – 21.62%) in Rio Grande do Sul, Southern Brazil. Sousa (2013) (5/76 – 6.58%) in Goiás and the Federal District, Midwest; Cunha et al. (2016) (20/218 -9.20%) in São Paulo, Southeastern Brazil.

The presence of fumonisin B1 in the feed was detected initially in Brazil by Sydenham et al. (1992) in the state of Paraná in the Southern Brazil. Mycotoxin was observed in samples of corn and corn residue obtained from seven outbreaks that occurred in the state, which resulted in the death of 16 horses. The detected values ranged from 0.2 to 38.5 ppm. The observation of mycotoxin in feed and/or corn fed to horses with leukoencephalomalacia was described years later by Mallmann et al. (1999). On that occasion, Mallmann et al. (1999) reported 46 and 53 ppm in moldy corn samples from leukoencephalomalacia cases that occurred in the Rio Grande do Sul-south region. Subsequently, the identification of fumonisin B1 in cases of leukoencephalomalacia in horses was described in 2003 in the Federal District, Midwestern Brazil (Salles-Gomes et al. 2003). On this occasion, mycotoxin values ranged from 5-10 ppm and were observed in commercial feed. These levels were responsible for causing the death of forty horses between April and November. Values of 6.6 ppm were observed by Santos et al. (2013), resulting in outbreaks of the disease affecting six horses and a mule, all of which died.

Corn that causes LEM and contains toxic amounts of fumonisin B1 may not be visibly moldy. Some outbreaks are caused by corn that is visually normal but contains high concentrations of Fumonisin B1 (Riet-Corrêa et al. 2013).

Usually, all outbreaks or isolated cases diagnosed and confirmed by the postmortem examination as leukoencephalomalacia in equines in Brazil were associated with the consumption of corn or feed; however, Vendruscolo et al. (2016) described cases of the disease associated with hay consumption, resulting in the death of 13 horses. In this report samples of feed and hay were subjected to fumonisin screening and only the presence of fumonisin B1 (0.02 to 0.12 ppm) in hay was observed.

The presence of fumonisin in green (immature) corn with 2 ppm was associated with disease in horses. Signs were observed seven days after supply and progressed over the next 24 hours, with animals dying at the end of that time (Echenique et al. 2019).

Table 2 lists the main studies that carried out the detection of fumonisin B1 in an outbreak of leukoencephalomalacia in Brazil, and Table 3 presents reports that carried out the investigation of fumonisin in products used in animal feed. It is observed that potentially toxic levels are present even in foods considered suitable by visual inspection, which may pose a risk to horses that are fed corn, which is the main substrate for the growth of *F. verticilioides*.

Table 2. Detection of fumonisin B1 associated with outbreaks of equine leukoencephalomalacia from different geographical regions of Brazil

Author	Year	State	Geographical Region	Concentration (ppm)	Sample
Hirooka et al.	1988	Paraná	Southern	Not detected	Mixed feed
Hirooka et al.	1990	Paraná	Southern	Not detected	Corn Residue
Sydenham et al.	1992	Paraná	Southern	0.2-38.5	Corn Residue
Mallmann et al.	1999	Rio Grande do Sul	Southern	46-53	Corn
Sales-Gomes et al.	2003	São Paulo	Southeastern	>10	Corn
Pimentel et al.	2008	Paraíba	Northeastern	47	Corn bran
Santos et al.	2013	Mato Grosso	Northeastern	5-10	Commercial feed
Vendruscolo	2016	São Paulo	Southeastern	0.02-0.2	Hay
Machado et al.	2018	Federal District	Midwestern	0.87-4.09	Commercial feed
Echenique et al.	2019	Rio Grande do Sul	Southern	2.0	Immature corn
Albertino et al.	2021	São Paulo	Southeastern	0.8–27.0	Commercial feed

Table 3. Investigations of fumonisin B1 in products frequently used in equine rations (without association with outbreaks of leukoencephalomalacia) in Brazil

Author	Year	State	Geographical Region	Concentration (ppm)	Sample
Hirooka et al.	1996	Paraná, Goiás and Mato Grosso	Southern and Midwestern	5.45 - 5.04	Stocked corn
Orsi et al.	2000	Paraná	Southern	3.0 - 24	Stocked corn
Vargas et al.	2001	-	Southern, Midwestern and Southeastern	0.2 - 6.1	Stocked corn
Ono et al.	2001	-	Midwestern, Southeastern, Southern and Northeastern	1.14 - 9.85	Freshly harvested corn
Gonçalvez et al.	2001	São Paulo	Southeastern	0.97->5.0	Corn cob
				>5.0	Corn germ
				2.38 - 78.5	Corn grits
				0.31 - 157.9	Corn residue
				>5.0 - 6.93	Corn roll
Ono et al.	2002	Paraná	Southern	3.6 - 15.0	Stocked corn
Ono et al.	2004	Paraná	Southern	2-89 - 14.54	Stocked corn

Author	Year	State	Geographical Region	Concentration (ppm)	Sample
Hassegawa et al.	2006	São Paulo	Southeastern	0.3 - 11.2	Immature corn
Neves et al.	2013	Minas Gerais	Southeastern	5 - 6.1	Corn grain
Gabriel et al.	2017	Paraná	Southern	2.1 - 5.46	Corn cob
German et al.	2022	Rio Grande do Sul	Southern	0.88 - 0.90	Stocked corn

Eastern Equine Encephalomyelitis (EEEv), Western Encephalomyelitis (WEEv) and Venezuelan Encephalomyelitis (VEEv)

Eastern equine encephalomyelitis virus (EEEv), Western encephalomyelitis virus (WEEv) and Venezuelan encephalitis virus (VEEv) belong to the family *Togaviridae*, genus Alphavirus (Chen et al. 2018). These are enveloped positive, single-stranded RNA virus of zoonotic character, that are transmitted by hematophagous arthropods, mainly those belonging to the genus *Cullex* sp, that affect several species of mammals (Iversson 1980). Migratory birds act as reservoirs (Ceballos and Setien, 2015).

Although there are no classical signs, the most frequent clinical manifestations described in horses affected by these viruses include ataxia, decreased consciousness, circling, head pressing, dysphagia, pelvic limb paresis or paralysis, and seizures. In the most severe cases the affected horse dies within a week (Taylor and Paessler 2013). Diagnosis of this disease can be accomplished by identifying high concentrations of IgM in serum or CSF (comparative serology), RT-PCR in CSF and CNS, immunohistochemistry, and viral isolation in affected horses (Long 2014).

The first descriptions of EEEv and WEEv, with viral detection, occurred in the United States (Haring and Howitt 1931; Tenbroeck et al. 1935; Meyer et al.1931) and VEEv in Venezuela in the 1930s (Kubes and Rios 1939).

In Brazil, in 1937, at least 60 horses presented a disease considered unknown (state of São Paulo, Southeastern Brazil). Initially, the animals presented ataxia, followed by an inability to walk and seizures (Carneiro 1937). In this study, the isolation of a viral agent was performed, and it was possible to reproduce the disease in horses, obtaining similar clinical signs (Carneiro 1937). Associated with the detection of the viral agent and epidemiological findings of the disease, researchers associated the cases with encephalomyelitis observed in North America (Carneiro 1939). Years later, keeping the virus initially isolated, in monthly passages in guinea pigs, it was possible to prove, through biological tests, that the virus isolated by Carneiro (1937) was the EEEv (Carneiro and Cunha 1943; Carneiro 1944). After this first study, several epidemiological studies were performed to verify the presence of antibodies against EEEv, WEEv and VEEv in Brazil (Table 4).

Years later, viral isolation of the agent in outbreaks of neurological diseases in Brazil. EEEv was isolated in Bahia, Northeast Brazil (Alice 1951); São Paulo, Southeastern Brazil (Nilsson and Sugay 1962; Pereira et al. 1962) and Pará, Northern Brazil (Causey et al. 1962). After this series of isolations, EEEv was isolated again only after 30 years, according to Kotait et al. (1992), in the state of São Paulo. This later study suggested that there was no antigenic variation comparing this isolate and the first isolated virus in Brazil and those used as a standard vaccine production strain.

Another possible EEE case was reported in 1993. Although there was no viral isolation, a horse located in the state of Mato Grosso do Sul, Midwestern Brazil, with ataxia and walking in circles, was considered a case of EEEv because there was a fourfold increase in the titer of antibodies to EEEv compared to the acute and convalescent phases. Postmortem examination showed congestion of the leptomeninges, neuronal necrosis in the gray matter, areas of hemorrhage and perivascular inflammation (Iversson et al. 1993).

In 2000, Fernández et al. suggested a correlation of cases of encephalitis in horses from different regions of Paraná (Southern Brazil) with EEEv due to the presence of neutralizing antibodies to the virus, but it was not possible to isolate the agent.

The clinical observation of encephalomyelitis caused by EEEv and the identification of the etiologic agent were described in 2008 in the state of Pernambuco in Northeastern Brazil (Pimentel et al. 2009). An outbreak affecting 60 horses presenting neurological signs (compulsive walking, ataxia, blindness, salivation, head pressure and lateral recumbency) and acute evolution (3-5 days) was reported. At necropsy, diffuse encephalitis was detected, mainly in gray matter. The identification of EEEv was performed by the nested RT–PCR technique.

In 2008 and 2009, the presence of outbreaks with neurological manifestations were observed in horses in the states of Pernambuco, Ceará and Paraíba, Northeastern Brazil (Silva et al. 2011). The main clinical signs observed were ataxia, blindness, head pressing, decreased level of consciousness, hyperexcitability, paralysis, muscle fasciculation, lip tremors, and recumbency. Fever, facial paralysis, nasal and eye secretions were also observed, but less frequently. The time from onset of clinical signs to death was 3 to 15 days (Silva et al. 2011). Histology revealed diffused nonsuppurative lymphoplasmacytic encephalomyelitis with lymphocytic perivascular infiltrates, with similar lesions, but of less intensity, at the spinal cord. The participation of EEEv was confirmed by seminested RT–PCR (Silva et al. 2011).

EEEv was also isolated in horses in Pará, Northern Brazil (Campos et al. 2013). This region has a large amount of temporary flooded areas, favoring the proliferation of vectors. Ataxia, decreased level of consciousness, circling, muscle tremors and decreased tongue tone were the main findings during neurological examination. Nine animals were evaluated, four died, and the others recovered. Diffuse meningitis and encephalitis were the main histopathological findings. Virus identification was performed by seminested RT–PCR in three of the four animals tested (Campos et al. 2013).

A retrospective study with 670 CNS samples from equids with neurological abnormalities from different regions of Brazil and negative for rabies was submitted the identification of EEEv using the seminested RT–PCR technique (Oliveira et al. 2014). Eighteen samples were positive from the states of Mato Grosso (mildwest), São Paulo (southeastern), Pará (northern), Paraíba, Ceará and Pernambuco (northeastern).

Madariaga virus (MAVD), which belongs to the EEEv complex and has genetic differences from the North American strain, was isolated for the first time in Brazil in 2015 in the Paraíba, Northeast Brazil (Silva et al. 2015). A horse showing decreased level of consciousness, blindness, ataxia, head pressing against objects, circling, and lip ptosis. Frontal cortex histopathology showed diffuse multifocal nonsuppurative lymphoplasmocytic encephalomyelitis with perivascular infiltration by lymphocytes, plasma cells, macrophages and some neutrophils and vasculitis with endothelial swelling cells. Phylogenetic analysis of EEEv determined it to belong to lineage III (South American), genetically associated with isolates in South America.

Subsequently, the identification of MAVD was also reported; and was isolated from two horses from samples of different outbreaks that occurred in the state of Ceará, Northeastern Brazil (Gil et al. 2021). Clinical signs were ataxia, paresis, and circling, progressing to lateral recumbency and death within five days. Lymphoplasmocytic encephalitis mainly in the cerebral cortex (gray matter), swollen vascular endothelium with lymphocyte and plasma cell infiltrate, and nonsuppurative perivascular inflammation in leptomeninges were present on histopathology. The presence of EEEv was confirmed by seminested RT–PCR (Gil et al. 2021).

Table 4. Epidemiological studies of equine eastern encephalitis (EEEv), western encephalomyelitis (WEEv), and Venezuelan encephalitis (VEEv) in Brazil, in chronological order of publication

Author	Year	State(s)	Geographical Region	Technique	Total Animals	Reagent or Positive		
						EEEV	WEEv	VEEv
Lennette and Fox	1943	Minas Gerais and Rio de Janeiro	Southeastern	Seroneutralization	38	15 (39.47%)	NR	NR
Cunha	1943	Pernambuco, Ceará and Rio Grande do Norte	Northeastern	Seroneutralization	8	8 (100%)	0 (0%)	NR
Bruno-Lobo et al.	1961	Rio de Janeiro	Southeastern	Seroneutralization	500	50 (10%)	113 (22.6%)	NR
Pereira et al.	1962	São Paulo	Southeastern	Hemoagglutination	47	9 (19.15%)	0 (0%)	0 (0%)
Pereira et al.	1964	São Paulo	Southeastern	Hemoagglutination	8	2 (25%)	0 (0%)	0 (0%)
Iversson et al.	1993	Mato Grosso	Midwestern	Seroneutralization	432	29 (6.78%)	5 (1.2%)	NR
Fernadez et al	2000	Paraná	Southern	Seroneutralization	22	12 (55%)	0 (%)	0 (%)
Heinemann et al.	2006	Pará	Northern	Seroneutralization	95	26 (27.37%)	1 (1.05%)	NR
Aguiar et al.	2008	Rondônia	Northern	Seroneutralization	176	37 (21%)	0 (0%)	20 (11.36%)
Cunha et al.	2009	São Paulo	Southeastern	Hemoagglutination	50	1 (2%)	0 (%)	5 (10%)
Pauvolid-Corrêa et al.	2010	Mato Grosso	Midwestern	RT–PCR	135	0 (0%)	0 (0%)	0 (0%)
				Seroneutralization		64 (47.7%)	49 (36.4%)	0 (0%)
Araújo et al.	2012	Paraíba	Northeastern	Seroneutralization	182	23 (12.9%)	NR	NR
Melo et al.	2012	Mato Grosso	Midwestern	Immunodiffusion	437	168 (35.5%)	31 (6.5%)	0 (0%)
Pauvolid-Côrrea	2015	Mato Grosso	Midwestern	Seroneutralization	484	48 (9.8%)	1 (0.4%)	3 (1.3%)
Cunha et al.	2016	São Paulo	Southeastern	RT–PCR	218	0 (0%)	0 (0%)	0 (0%)
Lara et al.	2014	Minas Gerais	Southeastern	Seroneutralization	826	250 (30.2%)	0 (0%)	16 (1.9%)
Costa et al.	2015	Minas Gerais	Southeastern	PCR	217	0 (0%)	0 (0%)	0 (0%)
Ferreira et al.	2018	Rio Grande do Norte	Northeastern	Seroneutralization	118	13 (11.1%)	22 (19.3%)	NR
Nunes et al.	2021	Pará	Northern	Hemagglutination	89	7 (7.95)	1 (1.1%)	NR

WEEv was detected in horses in Brazil only once in the state of Rio de Janeiro in the southeastern Brazil in 1961 (Bruno-Lobo et al. 1961). During this occasion, the identification of the viral particle related to the WEEv/Sindbis group took place from a horse with neurological abnormalities at the Jockey Club in the city of Rio de Janeiro. The horse presented ataxia and a decreased level of consciousness and died within 3 days. The agent was isolated from CNS tissue, CSF, and serum. Subsequently, a sequence of studies was published on viral isolation, genetic classification and studies in animals and humans in contact. (Bruno-Lobo et al. 1961; Góes and Bruno-Lobo 1961; Rosa et al. 1961). WEEv in Brazil has already been isolated from mosquitoes (Wigg 1977), wild birds (Shope et al.1966; Vasconcelos et al. 1991) and rodents (Shope et al. 1996).

Several serological studies in horses have revealed the presence of antibodies to WEEv in Brazil (Table 4). However, when molecular biology techniques were applied, it was not possible to isolate the virus from horses (Pauvolid-Corrêa et al. 2010; Costa et al. 2015; Cunha et al. 2016).

VEEv was not isolated from horses with neurological abnormalities in Brazil. However, it was already isolated from mosquitoes in Brazilian territory (Calisher et al. 1982; Vasconcelos et al. 1991) and wild rodent (Souza-Lopes and Sacchetta 1978) monkeys (Causey et al. 1961). From a VEEv isolate obtained from samples of monkeys from the Amazon region (Causey et al. 1961), inoculation was performed in two healthy horses. Only one of these patients had fever and remained in the lateral position. However, he continued to eat normally, and 48 hours later, he returned to the quadrupedal position (Shope et al. 1964).

Epidemiological studies to identify the presence of antibodies in horses against VEEv were less frequently performed when compared to EEEv and WEEv (Table 1). The presence of VEEV antibodies was detected in five studies (Bruno-Lobo et al. 1961; Aguiar et al. 2008; Cunha et al. 2009; Lara et al. 2014).

West Nile Encephalitis (WNV)

The virus was first identified in Uganda in humans (Smithburn et al. 1940). Subsequently, outbreaks of fever occurred in the region of Egypt, mainly in children between 1937 and 1950 (Taylor et al. 1956). West Nile virus (WNV) is an arthropod-borne, single-stranded positive-sense RNA virus that belongs to the Japanese encephalitis virus (JEV) serocomplex within the Flaviviridae family (Campbell et al. 2002). Its genetic material is organized in the form of positive-sense single-stranded RNA. Within their epidemiological chain, birds present viral replication and are the reservoirs. Horses and humans are highly sensitive and are considered dead-end hosts (Petersen et al. 2013).

The first descriptions of this virus affecting horses and donkeys occurred in 1963 in Egypt, causing intermittent fever (Schimidt and Mansoury 1963). The development of cases with neurological manifestations (ataxia) was described in an outbreak in France in 1968 (Joubert et al. 1970).

This disease gained notoriety after the emergence of cases of encephalitis in humans and horses in the United States in 1999 (Nash et al. 2001). For many years, it has become one of the most important neurological diseases of horses in North America (Trock et al. 2001; Ostlund et al. 2001; Porter et al. 2003).

Infected horses usually present fever, but neurological signs occur in only some of these animals (Bunning et al. 2002). Muscle fasciculations (including the facial region) as well as ataxia are frequently described neurological signs (Furr and Reed 2015; Lindsey et al. 2015; Martins et al. 2019; Silva et al. 2019; Siconelli et al. 2021). Alterations in the level of consciousness, hyperesthesia, and cranial nerve deficits have also been described (Bernadette et al. 2001; Trock et al. 2001; Lindsey et al. 2015). The diagnosis of this disease can be performed with viral isolation or by molecular biology techniques (RT–PCR) (Castilo-Olivares and Wood, 2004; Silva et al. 2019).

Serological monitoring was carried out in different countries of South America, and evidence of positivity in horses was found in Colombia (Mattar et al. 2005) and Argentina (Hérbert et al. 2021) and in equids and wild birds in Venezuela (Bosch et al. 2007). The first isolation of the virus in horses with encephalitis in South America occurred in Argentina (Morales et al. 2006).

In the last 20 years, great concern has occurred in Brazil regarding the occurrence of a similar situation as occurred in the United States, since high temperatures and the presence of transmitting mosquitoes are present in different regions (Figueiredo et al. 2019). In Brazil, this virus has already been detected in mosquitoes (Pauvoloid-Corrêa et al. 2011), birds (Ometto et al. 2013, Chalhoub et al. 2021), humans (Ometto et al. 2013; Vieira et al. 2015), and monkeys (Oliveira-Filho et al. 2018; Almeida et al. 2019). The situation in horses will be described below.

The pioneering studies that sought to demonstrate the circulation of West Nile virus (WNV) in horses in Brazil were carried out by researchers from the Instituto Oswaldo Cruz-Fiocruz, and 55.4% of the horses located in the Pantanal region were seropositive (Pauvolid-Corrêa et al. 2011).

In summary, serological studies were carried out in different regions of Brazil, demonstrating the circulation of WNV. The number of serologically positive animals ranged from 0.3% to 60.5%. The studies performed, the diagnostic technique applied, the number of positive horses/number of analyzed horses, as well as the percentage of seropositive are listed in Table 5.

Table 5. Epidemiological studies of West Nile encephalitis (WNV) in Brazil, in chronological order of publication

Author	Year	State	Region	Technique	Reagent
Pauvolid-Corrêa et al.	2011	Mato Grosso	Midwestern	ELISA	93/168 -(55.4%)
Melandri et al.	2012	Mato Grosso	Midwestern	ELISA	3/38 -(60.5%)
Ommeto et al.	2013	São Paulo, Rondônia, Mato Grosso and Mato Grosso do Sul	Southeastern, Northeastern and Midwestern	ELISA	13/678 - (1.9%)
Silva et al.	2013	São Paulo, Minais Gerais, Rio de Janeiro, Paraíba and Mato Grosso	Southeastern, Northeastern and Midwestern	ELISA	79/753 – (10.5%)
Pauvolid-Corrêa et al.	2014	Mato Grosso	Midwestern	ELISA	2/78 -(0.3%)
Chalhoub et al.	2021	Ceará	Northeastern	Seroneutralization	11/24 – (44%)
Oliveira-Filho et al.	2021	Bahia	Northeastern	ELISA	32/713 - (4.5%)
Weber et al.	2021	Rio Grande do Sul	Southern	ELISA	86/465 - (18.5%)

RT–PCR or RT–qPCR results in healthy horses were negative in two studies that analyzed approximately two thousand horses. Even in individuals in regions where the circulation of the virus had already been confirmed and in seropositive or seronegative animals (Ometo et al. 2013; Weber et al. 2021).

The first report confirming the detection of WNV in horses in Brazil occurred in the state of Espírito Santo in 2018 (Southeast) in 12 animals (nine horses and three mules) that died (Silva et al. 2019). The animals showed acute neurological signs characterized by muscle tremors, dysphagia, and ataxia. Subsequently, paraparesis and permanent lateral recumbency were observed, evolving to death within 72 hours or being submitted to euthanasia (Silva et al. 2019). The histopathological examination revealed lesions compatible with viral encephalitis, characterized by the moderate presence of multifocal perivascular cuffs. The WNV genetic material was identified by nested PCR for the coding regions of the NS5 protein (Silva et al. 2019).

The following year, also in the state of Espírito Santo, a horse initially presented abdominal pain, evolving to neurological abnormalities. Dysphagia, ataxia, muscle tremors, opisthotonos, and lateral recumbency were observed. There was the presence of inflammatory infiltrate around the vessels with the presence of mononuclear and polymorphonuclear cells, neuronophagia, gliosis and neuronal necrosis. In immunohistochemistry, the presence of WNV antigen was observed by positive labeling (Martins et al. 2019). WNV was isolated from CNS samples.

Three horses with neurological abnormalities (Espírito Santo and Ceará - Southeastern and Northeastern) had CNS samples positive for WNV. Horses presented tremors/muscle stiffness, hyperesthesia, ataxia, and lateral recumbency. Isolation of WNV in cell culture was confirmed by RT–qPCR. Genetic sequencing confirmed WNV as the NY 99 strain, reinforcing the hypothesis that WNV has been circulating in Brazil for many years (Siconelli et al. 2021).

In 2021, the virus was also detected (RT–PCR) in red blood cells from two neurologic horses and one horse presenting chorioretinitis (Minas Gerais, São Paulo and Piauí) (Costa et al. 2021). The virus was also detected in two horses in the city of São Paulo (seizures and flaccid paralysis of the hind limbs) (Siqueira et al. 2022).

Due to positive case reports in horses and evidence of WNV circulation in Brazil (Silva et al. 2019; Martins et al. 2019; Siconelli et al. 2021), this disease should be considered among the differential diagnoses in horses with neurological signs. Health professionals should be alert to the emerging zoonotic potential of this disease (Chalhoub et al. 2021; Oliveira Filho et al. 2021; Siqueira et al. 2022; Weber et al. 2021.

Rabies

Rabies is the most important neurological disease in herbivores in Brazil (Babboni e Modolo 2011). The virus that causes rabies is *Lyssavirus*, belonging to the Rhabdoviride family. These are bullet-shaped with negative-sense RNA. It is able to transcribe five main proteins used structurally or for their replication (Pereira 2003; Scott and Nel, 2021). Among these, the G1 glycoprotein has the highest antigenicity (Banmansour et al. 1991).

Rabies has two main transmission cycles that occasionally intertwine. The urban cycle related to the spread by dogs and cats, and the rural one by the infection of herbivores, mainly cattle and horses, with hematophagous bats being the main responsible for transmitting the virus to herbivores (Batista et al. 2007). The presence of the virus in the saliva of horses has already been detected in Brazil (Carrieri et al. 2006). As well as cases of human rabies in which horses were responsible for the transmission (Araújo 2002).

In general, in horses, the clinical form associated with progressive paralysis is the most frequently described, but signs associated with brain abnormalities have also been reported (Lima et al. 2005; Achkar et al. 2013). The histopathology of rabies is characterised by nonsuppurative encephalomyelitis. The presence of perivascular lymphoplasmocytic inflammatory infiltrate, which can be observed in some neurological diseases of viral origin, is also remarkable in this disease. The observation of intracytoplasmic inclusion (Negri's body) is present in some cases (Hamir, Moser, Ruppercht, 1992; Pedroso et al. 2010; Merini et al. 2010; Achkar et al. 2013).

For the diagnosis of rabies in equids, it is necessary to collect different regions of the brain (hippocampus, cerebellum, cortex, and brainstem) and spinal cord. The samples must be sent to the reference laboratories for the performance of the biological test (cerebral inoculation) and direct fluorescent antibody test (dFAT) (Peixoto et al. 2000; Brasil, 2008).

The first official description of this disease in horses in Brazil occurred in the Itajaí Valley, in the state of Santa Catarina, Southern Brazil, in 1911, resulting in the death of more than 4000 cattle and 1000 horses (Horta 1911; BRASIL 1988). Subsequent studies conducted on the outbreak were able to determine the participation of the rabies virus (Carini 1911ab). Despite the identification of the Negri corpuscle in the brain of some animals, the diagnosis of rabies was discussed by international scientific members (Peixoto et al. 2000).

At that time, it was believed that for the development of rabies cases, it was necessary the bite of a rabid dog. The director of the Pasteur Institute in São Paulo, bacteriologist Antonio Carini, observed that the outbreaks occurred in places that were difficult to access. Associating the large presence of hematophagous bats in the region and strong evidence of the attack on the affected animals, the researcher assumed the participation of bats in the epidemiology of this disease (Carini 1911ab). The hypothesis raised was refuted by several researchers, who, even with the verification of the Negri corpuscle in some portions of the spinal cord, continued to deny the thesis (Carini, 1911). Only after verification and isolation of the virus in bats was this idea accepted years later (Hurst and Pawan, 1931; Lima 1934, Torres and Lima, 1934). The outbreak and the verifications carried out at the Pasteur Institute in São Paulo were fundamental for determining the participation of bats in the epidemiological chain.

As in herbivores, rabies is the neurological disease of greatest epidemiological importance in horses. Several studies have demonstrated that rabies is the main cause of encephalomyelitis in equids in Brazil (Silva et al. 1974, Lima et al. 2005; Achkar et al. 2010; Rissi et al. 2010; Pedroso et al. 2010; Marcolongo-Pereira et al. 2014; Torquato et al. 2020).

Several equine epidemiological studies have been published in the national territory (Silva e Menezes 1974; Lima et al. 2005; Santos et al., 2006; Pedroso et al. 2010; Achkar et al. 2010; Torquato et al. 2020). In general, these studies aimed to identify epidemiological patterns of the disease or improve detection techniques. Table 6 lists epidemiological studies on the occurrence of rabies in herbivores.

Table 6. Main published studies on the occurrence of rabies in horses in Brazil

Author	Year	State	Geographical Region	Technique	Affected
Silva et al.	1974	Rio de Janeiro	Southeastern	PB	2/2 (100%)
Peixoto et al.	2000	São Paulo	Southeastern	dFAT/PB	111/703 (15.78%)
Favoretto et al	2002	São Paulo	Southeastern	dFAT/IHQ	21/21 (100%)
Santos et al.	2006	Goiás	Midwestern	dFAT/PB	43 (100%)
Santos et al.	2007	Goiás	Midwestern	dFAT/PB	17/20 (85%)
Teixeira et al.	2008	Rio Grande do Sul	Southern	dFAT/PB	21/724 (2.91%)
Teixeira et al.	2008	Rio Grande do Sul	Southern	dFAT/PB/PCR	21/150 (14%)
Andrade et al.	2014	Paraíba	Northeastern	dFAT/PB	2/2 – (100%)
Dognani et al.	2016	Paraná	Southern	dFAT/PB	303/1411 – (21.5%)
Santos et al.	2016	Paraíba	Northeastern	dFAT/PB	1/2 (50%)
Rodrigues et al.	2018	Pará	Northern	dFAT/PB	8/23 (34.78%)
Silva et al.	2019	Maranhão	Northern	dFAT/PB	3/409 – (0.73%)
Silva et al.	2020	Amazonas	Northern	dFAT/PB	9/4 (44.44%)
Andrade et al.	2020	Ceará	Northeastern	dFAT/PB	44 (100%)

PB: biological test; dFAT: direct fluorescent antibody test. IQH: Immunohistochemistry.

In 1974, Silva et al. reported the observation of the virus in the spinal cord and medulla of two horses in the state of Rio de Janeiro, Southeastern Brazil.

During the neurological examination, paralysis of the pelvic limbs was observed, with death within 48 hours (Silva et al. 1974).

The evaluation of 703 samples of equine brains sent to the reference laboratory for the diagnosis of rabies in the state of São Paulo, Southeastern Brazil, 111 (15.78%) were positive using direct immunofluorescence and biological inoculation (Peixoto et al. 2000).

The description of four outbreaks of rabies in horses in the states of Paraíba and Rio Grande do Norte, Northeastern Brazil, represented 23.53% of neurological cases (Lima et al. 2005). The clinical course in these cases ranged from 2 to 8 days, with a decrease in the level of consciousness, ataxia, absence of pupillary reflex, and paralysis of the pelvic and thoracic limbs being observed. Inclusion bodies were observed in 40% of the cases, and areas of hemorrhage, neuronophagia and axonal spheroids were also described in the cerebral cortex, thalamus and brainstem.

The observation of 159 cases and/or disease outbreaks in horses in the semiarid region of Paraíba, Northeastern Brazil, revealed that 49 (30.8%) affected the CNS (Pimentel et al. 2009). On this occasion specifically, rabies was the third leading cause of mortality, affecting 10 horses and 1 donkey, corresponding to 22.4%. All were positive in immunohistochemistry, with higher immunostaining in the thalamus, cortex and cerebellum fragments. The main clinical findings were decreased tail and anus sensitivity, paresis and ataxia, followed by permanent lateral recumbency. Histopathologically, the presence of mononuclear inflammatory infiltrate with a predominance of lymphocytes was observed in all cases.

The comparison between the techniques of direct immunofluorescence, biological testing and immunohistochemistry of ten CNS samples from horses with neurological alterations sent to a reference center for the diagnosis of rabies in the state of São Paulo, Southeastern Brazil, showed similar results among them, suggesting that immunohistochemistry can also be used in rabies surveillance programs in large animals (Achkar et al. 2010). Samples from the hippocampus, cerebellum, brainstem, and cerebral cortex were used, the latter presenting a higher concentration of antigenic inclusions for the rabies virus.

Samples from 14 horses from the states of Mato Grosso, Midwestern Brazil, Rio Grande do Sul, Southern, Pará, Northern and Minas Gerais, Southeastern Brazil, all were positive for immunohistochemistry, and 55.5% were positive for dFAT (Pedroso et al. 2010). The main clinical signs were ataxia and pelvic limb paralysis. The histopathology of these cases revealed nonsuppurative meningoencephalitis and meningomyelitis with perivascular lymphoplasmacytic infiltrate.

A study involving samples of biological material from horses (tissues from necropsies, cytology, and histopathology) in the state of Rio Grande do Sul in Southern Brazil showed that rabies was the main viral disease (Marcologo-Pereira et al. 2014). Of the 31 samples in which a viral agent was diagnosed, 19 (61.29%) were positive for rabies.

The search for viral agents in 217 horses with neurological alterations in the state of Minas Gerais, Southeastern Brazil, found 47 (21.7%) positive for rabies in the direct immunofluorescence test (Costa et al. 2015). Non-suppurative meningoencephalitis was recorded in 55.5% of these samples. In addition, the presence of perivascular cuffs with lymphohistioplasmic infiltrate in the cerebral cortex, midbrain and brainstem regions was observed.

A retrospective study with 217 horses with neurological alterations was carried out in the state of São Paulo in Southeastern Brazil (Cunha et al. 2016). Of these, 37 (17%) were positive for rabies by indirect immune-fluorescence test (IFAT) and/or biological test.

The description of a case of rabies in a horse in the state of Piauí in Northern Brazil was carried out by Schawarz et al. (2020). The main clinical signs observed were decreased anus tone, dysphagia and progressive spasticity of the limbs. Samples of the cerebellum, cortex, hippocampus and spinal cord were sent, which were negative in the dFAT test, and the diagnosis was confirmed in the biological inoculation test.

Torquato et al. (2020) analyzed 174 CNS samples from horses with neurological abnormalities in the state of São Paulo, Southeastern Brazil. The techniques of direct immunofluorescence, isolation in cell culture, biological testing and RT–PCR were compared, observing the highest proportion of positive cases in the latter technique. The brainstem and hippocampus were the sections with the highest positivity.

Encephalitis Virus Saint Louis (SLEV)

SLEV was initially described to be associated with neurological abnormalities in humans in the city of Saint Louis, Missouri, USA approximately 100 years ago (U.S. Treasury Department 1935; Webster and Fite 1933). SLEV is a positive-stranded RNA virus belonging to the family Flaviviridae (arthropod-borne viruses), genus *Flavivirus*. Birds and mosquitoes of the genus *Culex sp.* gender are the main participants in this cycle (Ortiz-Martínez et al. 2017). In Brazil, it has already been isolated from vectors (Heinen et al. 2015), humans (Rocco et al. 2005; Vedovello et al. 2015), and nonhuman primates (Almeida et al. 2019; Costa et al. 2019). Humans and horses are considered terminal hosts due to low viremia (Vedovello et al. 2015). Saint Louis encephalitis virus is a problem of greater concern in humans than in horses, since only sporadic cases of encephalitis have been associated with this virus in horses, one of which is in Brazil (Rosa et al. 2013).

The first detection of SLEV by RT–PCR in the CNS of horses with neurological alterations was performed in the southwest region of Brazil (Costa et al., 2011), which was part of a retrospective study in horses with neurological abnormalities in which the CNS had been referred for evaluation. From this material, the isolation and characterization of this sample occurred (Rosa et al. 2013). It was a horse that presented with pelvic limb ataxia and depression. Death occurred 72 hours after the onset of clinical signs. In addition to the molecular biology techniques used to identify the agent, E protein gene sequencing was also performed. Phylogenetic analysis of a 903 bp amplified sequence of the partial envelope (E) gene region indicated that the horse isolate was within the genotype cluster (Rosa et al. 2013).

Due to its importance in humans, the search for Saint Louis encephalitis virus (SLEV) in animals, that can be considered circulating sentinels, is carried out within surveillance programs (Monat et al. 1985). Considering also that this virus was associated with a case of equine encephalitis in Brazil, serological studies on this species bring interesting details of the exposure of this species to this viral agent.

Table 7. Encephalitis Virus Saint Louis (SLEV) serological survey in horses in Brazil

Author	Year	State	Geographical Region	Technique	Reagent
Pauvolid-Corrêa et al.	2010	Mato Grosso	Midwestern	Seroneutralization	59/135 (43.7%)
Rodrigues et al.	2010	Acre, Amapá and Macapá	Northern	Seroneutralization	713/1401 (50.9%)
Silva et al.	2014	Paraíba	Northeastern	ELISA	93/753 – (12.35%)
Svoboda et al.	2014	Paraná	Southern	Hemagglutination inhibition	23/9 (39.13%)
Pauvolid-Corrêa et al.	2014	Mato Grosso and Mato Grosso do Sul	Midwestern	ELISA	24/760 – (3.16%)
Silva et al.	2014	São Paulo and Rio de Janeiro	Southeastern	ELISA	93/750 – (13.2%)
Gomes et al.	2019	Roraima	Northern	RIFI and ELISA	6/14 – (42.86%)
Costa et al.	2019	Minas Gerais	Southeastern	Seroneutralization	60/279 (21.5%)

Serological studies in horses were carried out in different regions of Brazil and found seropositivity between 3.16 and 50.91%. The studies are presented in chronological order, with the diagnostic technique used, the number of horses reactive to SLEV and total numbers sampled can be seen in Table 7.

It is interesting to note that three of the fomer studies also performed RT–PCR but did not obtain any positive animals (Costa et al. 2010; Pauvolid-Corrêa et al. 2010; Weber et al. 2021).

Considering the wide presence of antibodies to SLEV in horses in Brazil and a confirmed positive horse, we can consider this disease as a differential diagnosis when other viruses of more common occurrence have been ruled out.

Equine Herpesvirus Type 1 (EHV-1)

Equine herpesvirus type 1 (EHV-1) can cause respiratory and neurological problems, abortions, and neonatal mortality in horses. The neurological form causes great concern, as it usually occurs in outbreaks that affect several animals in a short period of time, and the most affected present recumbency and often need to be euthanized (Khusro et al. 2020). In recent years, it has caused outbreaks in different parts of the world (Pusterla et al. 2020; Gomez et al. 2021; Vereecke et al. 2021). This agent belongs to the *Alphaherpesvirinae* family presenting linear double-stranded DNA. The neurological presentation form has already been associated with a polymorphism at nucleotide 2254 in the DNA Polymerase gene (ORF 30), suggesting greater neuroinvasiveness, but it is known that the wild-type form can also cause neurological cases (Nugent et al. 2006). The spread of this disease occurs through direct contact with nasal secretions and/or environmental contamination, and closed places with higher population density and low air circulation can contribute to the emergence of cases (Khusro et al. 2020).

Neurological signs usually appear 7 to 10 days after infection and usually a few days after the initial respiratory signs observed (Mori 2000; Mori et al. 2003). Acute ataxia is usually seen, and many cases present with cauda equina syndrome. Urinary incontinence decreased sensation of the tail and anus, hemiparesis, and unilateral ataxia are commonly observed (Wilson 1997). The cerebral form of EHV-1 infection is less frequent but also described (Maanen, 2002; Pustrela and Hussey 2014).

The diagnosis can be made by isolation and/or identification in nasal swab, tissues or secretions and blood (Pustrela and Hussey 2014). Some horses present xanthochromic CSF and hyperproteinorraquia (100-500 mg/dL). Histopathologically, it is possible to verify necrosis and vasculitis of the meningeal vessels in the brain and spinal cord (Holz et al. 2019).

Table 8. EHV-1 serological surveys in horses in Brazil

Author	Year	State	Geographical Region	Technique	Reagents
Vargas and Weiblen	1991	Rio Grande do Sul	Southern	Seroneutralization	3/384 (0.9)
Carvalho et al	2000	Minas Gerais	Southeastern	ELISA	12/183 (6.56)
Cunha et al.	2002	São Paulo	Southeastern	ELISA	365/1341 (27.2)
Heinemann et al.	2002	Pará	Northern	Seroneutralization	17/96 (17.71)
Lara et al.	2003	Paraná	Southern	ELISA	10/70 (14.3)
Lara et al.	2003	São Paulo	Southeastern	ELISA	220/659 (33.4)
Diel et al.	2006	Rio Grande do Sul	Southern	Hemagglutination	67/1506 (4.5)
Pena et al.	2006	Pará	Northern	Seroneutralization	230/672 (45.45)
Lara et al.	2006	Paraná	Southern	ELISA	5/97 (4.1)
Cunha et al.	2009	São Paulo	Southeastern	ELISA	34/163 (21.0)
Lara et al.	2010	Minas Gerais	Southeastern	Seroneutralization	145/826 (17.6)
Alencar-Aratipe et al.	2014	Ceará	Northeastern	Seroneutralization	28/68 (41.2)
Diaz et al.	2015	Rio de Janeiro	Southeastern	Seroneutralization	172/581 (29.6)
Lara et al.	2017	São Paulo	Southeastern	ELISA	36/66 (55.4)
Pena et al.	2020	Bahia	Northeastern	Seroneutralization	225/622 (36.33)

The oldest description of the presence of EHV-1 in Brazil is from the 1960s, observed to be associated with abortion or neonatal mortality of foals in the state of São Paulo, southeast region (Corrêa e Nilson 1964), characterized by viral inclusion in tissues. The first isolation was performed by Nilsson and Corrêa in 1966 in the state of São Paulo, southeastern region, from liver samples from an aborted fetus with approximately six months of gestation. Clinical signs and histopathological findings were replicated (Nilsson e Corrêa 1966). At that time, the agent was called equine abortion virus. Later, virus was isolated again from aborted foals in the state of Rio Grande do Sul in the South region (Weiblen et al. 1994). Later studies showed that EVH circulates in different regions of Brazil. Being widely associated with cases of abortion and stillbirth in horses (Modolo et al. 1989; Vargas and

Weiblen 1991; Carvalho et al. 2000ab; Cunha et al. 2002; Lara et al. 2003). Table 8 lists the main serological surveys in equines in Brazil, and Table 9 lists studies that detected the presence of EHV-1.

Table 9. Studies that detected EHV-1 in horses in Brazil

Author	Year	State	Geographical Region	Technique	Positives	Tissue
Moreira et al.	1998	Paraná	Southern	Isolation	4/21 (19%)	Aborted fetuses
Carvalho et al	2000	Minas Gerais	Southeastern	PCR	2 (100%)	Semen
Lara et al.	2008	São Paulo	Southeastern	PCR	1/1(100%)	CSF and CSN
Costa et al.	2008	Minas Gerais	Southeastern	PCR	1/1 (100%)	CSF and CSN
Costa et al.	2009	Minas Gerais	Southeastern	PCR	39/52 (52%)	CSN
Mori et al.	2011	São Paulo e Minais Gerais	Southeastern	PCR	2/2 (100%)	CSN
Costa et al.	2015	Minas Gerais	Southeastern	PCR	20/170 (11.8%)	CSN
Silva et al.	2018	São Paulo	Southeastern	Nested PCR	0/105 (0%)	Aborted fetuses
Estima-Silva et al.	2019	Rio Grande do Sul	Southern	Nested PCR	2/2 (100%)	Aborted fetuses
Silva et al.	2020	São Paulo	Southeastern	PCR	2/2 (100%)	Aborted fetuses and stillbirths
Tomio	2020	Rio Grande do Sul	Southern	PCR	38/313 (12.14%)	Blood and Nasal Swab

The first report of EHV-1 causing neurological alterations occurred in the state of São Paulo, southeastern region of Brazil (Mori et al. 2007ab). A progressive evolution was described, initially reporting depression and reluctance to move, progressing to ataxia, paraparesis and lateral recumbency (Lara et al. 2008). The participation of EHV-1 was determined by PCR of CNS and CSF samples, viral isolation and serum neutralization. EHV-1 was detected again (PCR) by Costa et al. (2008) in the Minas Gerais-Southeast region in horses with neurological abnormalities. Ataxia, pelvic limb paresis, spontaneous falls, hyperexcitability (in pelvic limbs and lower back) and bladder distention were observed. Hours after admission, the clinical signs deteriorated. As a result, the animal was euthanized. In the leptomeninges, several areas of hemorrhage were found.

A retrospective study observed the presence of EHV-1 in 52% of CNS samples from horses presenting neurologic signs with negative test for rabies in the state of Minas Gerais, southeast region, by the seminested PCR technique (Costa et al. 2009). Ataxia, muscle spasms, pelvic limb paresis and recumbency were the main findings in affected horses. In most cases, the histopathological examination of the CNS revealed mild vasculitis with perivascular mononuclear cuffing, congestion, arterial thrombosis, and degeneration of nervous tissue.

Mori et al. (2011) described two horses with neurological signs in the states of Minas Gerais and São Paulo, southeastern region. One of the animals presented ataxia and paresis of limbs and signs of cauda equina injury (urinary incontinence, decreased tail and anal reflex and tone). CSF analysis revealed hyperproteinorraquia (109 mg/dL) and xanthochromia. At necropsy, congestion and foci of hemorrhage in the brain and spinal cord were observed. The main histological findings were demyelination, foci of hemorrhage in the cerebellum and brain, and neuronal necrosis. In the other animal, mental depression, dysphagia, nystagmus and ataxia were observed. During the histopathology evaluation, vasculitis, presence of thrombi in the meninges and neuronal ischemia were observed. In both cases, it was possible to confirm the participation of EHV-1 containing the ORF30 variant using PCR (Mori et al. 2011).

A retrospective study carried out with the CNS of 170 horses with neurological alterations and negative for rabies revealed positivity of 20 (11.8%) of EHV-1 with using PCR technique in the state of Minas Gerais in the southeast region (Costa et al. 2015). The main findings of the neurological examination were flaccid paralysis of the pelvic limbs and ataxia, with an evolution period ranging from one to nine days. Histopathologically, hyperemia and multifocal hemorrhages in the cerebellum and multifocal and diffuse nonsuppurative meningoencephalitis with the presence of perivascular cuffs were observed.

Aujeszky's Disease (SVH-1)

Porcine herpesvirus type 1 (SVH-1), a DNA virus, is the causative agent of Aujeszky's disease. It belongs to the genus Varicellovirus and the family Herpesviridade (subfamily Alphaherpesvirinae). The virus circulates in domestic and wild pigs, causing neurological sings. Being able to infect all mammals (Rziha et al. 1986; Zimmerman et al. 2019). In horses, this agent has already been detected associated with neurological alterations in the USA. Affected horses present excessive sweating, muscle tremors, behavioral changes, limb spasticity, seizures and lateral recumbency (Ingh et al. 1990; Kimman et al. 1990). Histopathology reveals nonsuppurative meningoencephalitis in these cases.

The first description of this disease in horses was made by Ingh et al. (1990) in Ultrecht, Netherlands. A horse showing behavioral changes, excessive sweating and seizures was confirmed for Aujesky's virus. Its detection in the brain by immunohistochemistry and in situ hybridization confirmed the diagnosis. On this occasion, soil fertilization with swine manure was recently reported. Subsequently, the virus of this former case was isolated (Ingh et al. 1990) and inoculated into healthy animals that showed the same clinical signs (Kimman et al. 1990).

In Brazil, this agent was identified (PCR technique with amplification of the gene encoding glycoprotein E in the state of Minas Gerais) in a horse with neurological signs. Microscopically, nonsuppurative meningoencephalitis was observed (Costa et al. 2015).

Malignant Catarrhal Fever

Sheep-associated malignant catarrhal fever (SA-MCF) is a widely studied disease in cattle. This disease is caused mainly by two agents, alcelaphine gammaherpesvirus (AlGHV1) and ovine gammaherpesvirus-2 (OvGHV2). Sheep and wildebeest are reservoirs for these viruses, respectively, with cattle, deer, buffalo, bison, and swine being susceptible or dead-end hosts (Russel et al. 2009; Headley et al. 2020). The only case reported in Brazil in horses and related to OvHGV2 was described in 2006 in a foal in the state of Minas Gerais in the southeastern region. The animal lived with other adult horses and goats. Presented muscle spasms, neck stiffness, spasticity followed by paralysis of the pelvic limbs, difficulty in maintaining a quadrupedal position. The animal died one day after the appearance of clinical signs. Moderate congestion and perivascular hemorrhage were observed in the brain.

Histopathological findings included lympho-histiocytic fibrinoid necrotizing vasculitis, primarily in small vessels of the kidney and liver, associated with interstitial lymphocytic nephritis and mild multifocal granulomatous mild hepatitis l. The histopathological pattern of vasculitis was similar to that observed in MCF caused by OvGHV2 and AlGHV-1. PCR of tissues and blood from this animal and from three other adult horses and eight contact goats was positive for OvGHV2 (Costa et al. 2009).

Equine Protozoal Myeloencephalitis (EPM)

Equine protozoal myeloencephalitis (EPM) is a neurological disease that affects horses and is caused by protozoa (Dubey et al. 2015). EPM is a very important disease in Brazil. *Sarcocystis neurona* is the main causative agent of EPM, and *Neospora hughesi* is occasionally reported (Lindsay et al. 1996; Johnson et al. 2013). The participation of *Toxoplasma gondii* in these cases has not yet been confirmed; however, there are studies seeking to associate seropositivity and clinical cases of motor incoordination, still without definitive proof (James et al. 2017; Schale et al. 2018).

The life cycle of *S. neurona* involves the participation of definitive and intermediate hosts. In North America, *Didelphis virginiana* and in Brazil and in South America, *Didelphis albiventris* are the definitive hosts. (Dubey et al. 2001; Dubey et al. 2015). In the study of Dubey et al., 2001, together with Dra. Claudia Kerber, the first isolation of *Sarcocystis neurona* from feces in South America was confirmed. Armadillos and raccoons are considered intermediate hosts. Equids are considered accidental or aberrant hosts and generally do not continue the cycle (Gondim et al. 2021). Contamination of water and feed with sporocyst-contaminated feces is the main form of equine infection. In horses, neurological signs result from the presence of the parasite in the central nervous system (Dubey 2022). The cycle of *Neospora hughesi* in horses has not been adequately established to date.

In general, EPM is considered a problem restricted to the American continent due to the presence of the definitive host. The disease in equids is generally progressive with signs of asymmetrical ataxia. Eventually, some horses may show acute signs. The spinal cord and brain stem are usually the affected areas that result in clinical signs, but other brain regions may also be affected. The clinical signs observed are directly associated with the location of merozoites in the CNS causing damage and local inflammation (Reed et al. 2016). Usually, animals initially show slight changes in their locomotion pattern that can be confused with musculoskeletal abnormalities. As the disease progresses, muscle weakness (paresis) and asymmetrical ataxia are the signs usually observed, with some cranial nerves being compromised (usually facial or trigeminal) (Dubey et al. 2001; Henker et al. 2020). The diagnosis in live animals is considered a process of exclusion of other diseases and confirmed with the comparison of the concentration of antibodies in the CSF in relation to the serum (Stelmann and Amorim 2010; Dubey 2022). The presence of the agent in the CSF of affected animals using molecular techniques has recently received attention (Bernardino et al. 2021). Visualization of the parasite in the postmortem CNS confirms the process.

The first reference to the presence of parasites in the CNS of equines with ataxia occurred in the USA in a description made by Rooney et al. (1970). At the time, the presence of focal lesions in the spinal cord of horses with chronic conditions of ataxia was observed. The disease was called focal myeloencephalitis. The same condition was observed by other research groups, which called it equine protozoal encephalomyelitis (Beech 1974) and equine protozoal myeloencephalitis (EPM) (Mayhew et al. 1976); the latter came to be used by most authors (Dubey 2022). The detection of Sarcocystis in CNS fragments of horses with EPM was performed in 1980 by Simpson and Mayhew in the United States. On this occasion, merozoites were observed concomitantly with necrotic lesions on histopathology. In electron microscopy, it was possible to visualize schizonts in the gray matter of the spinal cord. Later, this parasite was classified as *S. neurona* (Simpson and Mayhew 1980).

EPM in Brazil is an important and common neurological disease, and the first reference to parasites causing neurological alterations in horses in Brazil was made by Macruz et al. (1975) in the state of São Paulo in the southeastern Brazil. Despite the initial correlation between the case and *T. gondii*, this work became known as the first association of motor incoordination and protozoa in the country. In this study, serological evaluation for *T. gondii* was performed in horses with motor incoordination, mares that had a previous abortion and control animals. All animals with abnormalities were reactive for the presence of antibodies *to T. gondii* (Macruz et al. 1975). Later, the same author (Macruz) commented on his findings on the presence of cysts in the central nervous system of horses with neurological abnormalities, and despite initially being considered *T. gondii*, this may have been the first observation of *S. neurona* in the national territory. (Mayhew and Greiner 1986 and personal communication to the last author ASB). It is interesting to note that the relationship of *T. gondii* with neurological abnormalities in horses has received attention in the last 5 years (Bernardino et al. 2021).

Clinical cases compatible with EPM and the observation of lesions in the CNS were well characterized in 1986 in the Rio Grande do Sul, Southern Brazil (Barros et al. 1986ab). On this occasion, two horses presented progressive ataxia and spontaneous falls. The clinical signs had an evolution of fifteen days, until he adopted the permanent lateral decubitus, being submitted to the euthanasia. Focal areas with malacia and reddish coloration with a granular appearance in the thoracolumbar segment of the spinal cord have been described. Microscopically, a marked inflammatory reaction was observed, and oval structures measuring 2 μm were identified in neurons and endothelial cells of the medulla. Using silver impregnation and PAS, pseudocysts were observed around the parasite. Based on the neurological signs, epidemiological data and histopathological findings, it was concluded that it was EPM (Barros et al. 1986ab).

S. neurona was identified morphologically in the spinal cord of horses in the state of Paraná, Southern Brazil (Masri et al. 1992). They presented a history of falls during training, pelvic limb proprioceptive deficits and prolonged recumbency. The signs evolved gradually over a month until they present with permanent recumbency, and both were euthanized. Histopathology showed the presence of perivascular cuffs and mononuclear infiltrate. *S. neurona* (merozoites and schizonts) were associated with areas of gray matter necrosis. Immunohistochemistry confirmed the presence of parasites in the CNS (Masri et al.1992).

In a retrospective study of 35 EPM cases in the state of São Paulo in Southeastern Brazil (Baccarin et al. 2001), the main clinical signs observed were ataxia, muscle atrophy, decreased level of consciousness and sternal recumbency. The diagnosis was confirmed using the CSF western blot technique. After treatment with sulfametaxozole-trimethoprim and supportive therapy, 24 horses had complete improvement, and 11 horses did not respond to treatment.

A study was carried out by Teixeira et al. (2006) with 15 horses with EPM in the state of São Paulo, southeast region. The diagnosis was made with the detection of antibodies in the CSF using the Western blot technique. The main clinical signs were asymmetrical ataxia and paresis.

A retrospective study using CNS tissue samples from 54 horses with neurological abnormalities submitted to immunohistochemistry for anti-antibodies *S. neurona* detected only one positive result. It was a mare with a history of lip ptosis and tongue protrusion for two weeks. The condition progressed to ataxia, paralysis of the pelvic limbs and permanent lateral recumbency. Histopathological examination revealed nonsuppurative multifocal encephalitis predominantly in the gray matter of the brain, hypothalamus and brainstem. Numerous extracellular organisms were detected by immunohistochemistry, indicative of *S. neurona* (Paixão et al. 2007).

A study carried out by Lins et al. (2008) with 61 horses with ataxia in the state of Rio Grande do Sul, Southern Brazil, detected the presence of *S. neurona* antibodies in the CSF in 23 (37.7%). The main clinical signs observed were ataxia, muscle asymmetry and paresis. On this occasion, 61% of the animals improved their signs after treatment with toltrazuril or sulfa/trimethoprim combined with pyrimethamine.

Pierezan et al. (2009), in the Rio Grande do Sul, Southern Brazil, observed a low occurrence of this disease. In 355 horses submitted to necropsy, EPM was the cause of death in only one of the cases (0.28%), and in another study in the same state, it corresponded to 2.38% of the cases (Marcolongo-Pereira et al. 2014).

Sousa 2013 clinically diagnosed EPM in 4/76 (5.25%) horses with neurological alterations. The main clinical signs observed were ataxia, alteration in the pairs of cranial nerves, with evolution to the lateral recumbency. Confirmation of the diagnosis was performed using PCR technique in paraffin blocks and by the presence of antibodies comparing serum and CSF concentrations (Sousa 2013).

In a postmortem retrospective study with 218 equines presenting neurological diseases in the state of São Paulo, Southeastern Brazil, a case of EPM (*S. neurona*) was confirmed (Cunha et al. 2016). On this occasion, the identification of the agent in the brain was performed using the nested PCR-ITS1 technique. Interestingly, in this study, 12 horses were PCR positive for *T. gondii*. The participation of this agent in cases of protozoan myeloencephalopathy is still widely questioned, but these findings emphasize that further studies need to be carried out to verify whether *T. gondii* can actually cause neurological abnormalities in equids.

In a case reported by Faria et al. (2017), acute symptoms were observed in a horse with EPM in the state of Minas Gerais, Southeastern Brazil (acute permanent lateral recumbency). Subsequently, the patient presented convulsions, nystagmus and decreased level of consciousness, and euthanasia was performed. The CSF did not reveal any abnormalities. Histopathology showed areas of hemorrhage in the spinal cord, mainly in the thoracolumbar region. The diagnosis was based on the observation of *S. neurona* schizonts associated with multifocal lymphoplasmacytic myelitis in the lumbar spinal cord.

Postmortem retrospective studies involving 13 CNS samples from horses with neurological abnormalities and negative for rabies in the state of Rio Grande do Sul, Southern Brazil, of these 11 (85%) were positive for *S. neurona* by immunohistochemistry and PCR techniques of the ITS-1 gene

(Henker et al. 2020). The presentation of clinical signs ranged from 5 to 50 days. The main clinical findings were ataxia, circling, compulsive gait and permanent lateral recumbency.

Fantini et al. (2021) described a case of EPM (history of ataxia and muscle atrophy for more than two months) in Minas Gerais, Southeastern Brazil region. Clinically, ataxia (more accentuated in pelvic limbs) was observed. The presence of antibodies in the serum and CSF samples confirmed the diagnosis of EPM. After the initiation of treatment, the animal showed clinical improvement. Table 10 lists the studies that investigated the presence of antibodies to the causative agents of EPM and *T. gondii* in Brazil.

Serum antibodies against *S. neurona* and *T. gondii* were verified in horses without neurological alterations of different ages in the state of São Paulo, Southeastern Brazil (Dubey et al. 1999). Of the 101 PSI horses analyzed, 36 (35.64%) and 16 (15.84%) were positive for *S. neurona and T. gondii*, respectively.

An epidemiological study was carried out with serum samples from 961 horses from the states of São Paulo and Minas Gerais, Southeastern Brazil; Paraná, Santa Catarina and Rio Grande do Sul, southern; Bahia, northeastern; Rondônia, northern, Mato Grosso, Mato Grosso do Sul and Goiás, mildwest. Of these, 669 (69.6%) and 24 (2.4%) were positive for *S. neurona and Neospora* spp., respectively (Hoane et al. 2006). This study revealed the great exposure to protozoa to which horses are submitted, mainly *S. neurona*, confirming that the presence of antibodies in the serum alone is not enough to confirm the diagnosis.

A study published by Antonello et al. (2016) with samples collected from 195 mares and their foals immediately after birth (before colostrum ingestion). The mares presented 84.1% and the neonates 7.4% positivity for *S. neurona*. The results on the products show that this agent is possibly able to come into contact with horses during intrauterine life.

It was found that the *Sarcocystis falcatula-like* circulation between horses in Rio Grande do Sul and Bahia, Southern and Northeastern Brazil, respectively. Of the 409 horses submitted to immunofluorescence testing for both agents, 17.1% were positive for *S. neurona,* and 10.5% were positive for *S. falcatula-like*; coinfection was observed in 6.1% of horses (Borges-Silva et al. 2020).

Table 10. Epidemiological studies that investigated the circulation of EPM-causing agents in Brazil and *T. gondii*

Author	Year	State	Geographical Region	Technique	Total Animals	Agents		
						S. neurona	*T. gondi*	*Neospora spp*
Ishizuka et al.	1975	São Paulo	Southeastern	IFA	327	NR	228/327 - 70%	NR
Laranjeira et al.	1985	Mato Grosso do Sul	Midwestern	IFA	750	NR	246/750 - 32.8%	NR
Vidotto et al.	1997	São Paulo, Paraná, Mato Grosso e Mato Grosso do Sul	Southeastern, Southern and Midwestern	IFA	561	NR	177/561 - 31.55%	NR
Dubey et al.	1999	São Paulo	Southeastern	IFA	101	36/101 - 35.64%	16/101 -15.84%	NR
Mendonça et al.	2001	Bahia	Northeastern	IFA	343	NR	5/343 - 1.46%	NR
Hoane et al.	2006	São Paulo, Minas Gerais, Santa Catarina, Paraná, Mato Grosso, Mato Grosso do Sul, Bahia e Rondônia	Southern, Southeastern, Midwestern, Northern and Northeastern	IFA	961	669/961 – 69.6%	NR	24/961 – 2.4%
Locatelli-Dittrich et al.	2006	Paraná	Southern	IFA	45	NR	20/45 -44.4%	19/45 - 42.2%
Camossi et al.	2010	São Paulo	Southeastern	IFA	253	NR	15/253 - 5.9%	NR
Sangoni et al.	2011	Rio Grande do Sul	Southern	IFA	91	NR	NR	14/91 - 15.4%
Stelmam et al.	2011	São Paulo	Southeastern	Agglutination	23	NR	8/23 - 34.78%	NR
Stelmam et al.	2011	São Paulo	Southeastern	Agglutination	26	NR	NR	15/26 57.6
Villalobos et al.	2012	Paraná	Southern	IFA	97	NR	NR	14/97 - 14.4%

Author	Year	State	Geographical Region	Technique	Total Animals	Agents		
						S. neurona	*T. gondi*	*Neospora spp*
Evers et al.	2013	Paraná, Rio Grande do Sul, Rio de Janeior, Goiás, Mato Grosso do Sul e Minas Gerais	Southern, Midwestern and Southeastern	IFA	398	NR	60/398 – (15.0%)	NR
				PCR	398	NR	14/398 (3.52%)	NR
				Biological Test	398	NR	14/398 (3.52%)	NR
Finger et al.	2013	Paraná	Southern	IFA	10		17/100 (17%)	
Moura et al.	2013	Santa Catarina	Southern	IFA	615	NR	NR	25/615 (4.1%)
Abreu et al.	2014	Paraná and Santa Catarina	Southern	IFA	112	NR	14/112 (12.5%)	2/112 (1.78%)
Pivoto et al.	2014	Rio Grande do Sul	Southern	ELISA	181	12/547 (6.6%)	12/547 (6.6%)	15/181 (8.3%)
Laskoski et al	2015	Mato Grosso	Midwestern	IFA	200	NR	5/200 –(2.5%)	30/200 (15%)
Gennari et al.	2015	Minas Gerais	Southeastern	ELISA	453	NR	129/453 (28.47%)	NR
Borges et al.	2017	Mato Grosso	Midwestern	IFA	547	112/547 (20.4%)	138/547 (25.2%)	65/547 (11.8%)
Spohr et al.	2018	Roraima	Northern	IFA	303	131/303 (43.2%)	56/303 (18.5%)	91/303 (26.7%)
Valença et al.	2019	Alagoas	Northern	IFA	427	12/427 (1.67%)	NR	NR
Borges et al.	2017	Mato Grosso	Midwestern	IFA	547	112/547 (20.4%)	138/547 (25.2%)	65/547 (11.8%)

NR: not realized; IFA: indirect immunofluorescence assay.

It should be noted that although *T. gondii* antibodies are widely observed in horses (Levy et al. 2020), the association between this protozoan and the clinical signs of EPM is still unclear (James et al. 2017; Dubey 2022). In a previous study in Brazil, evaluating antibodies in the CSF of horses with ataxia, all horses presented no positive titles (Stelmann et al. 2011). Thus, several studies are directed to the investigation of *T. gondii* antibodies; however, most of these are epidemiological studies mainly related to abortion in mares.

Trypanosoma evansi

Trypanosoma evansi is the cause of an important neurological disease in horses in Brazil. This protozoan has a biological cycle with transmission by blood-sucking flies (inoculation of trypomastigotes that reach the bloodstream) and eventually in an iatrogenic way or vampire bats (Silva et al. 2002; Rodrigues et al. 2015; Buscher et al. 2019). Capybaras are the main reservoirs (Morales et al. 1976; Herrera et al. 2004). In Brazil, the parasite has already been identified in cattle (Silva et al. 2007), dogs (Colpo et al. 2005; Santalucia et al. 2012), and horses (Conrado et al. 2005; Rodrigues et al. 2005).

Infection in horses by *T. evansi* can result in two presentations. The first is more frequent, with progressive weight loss (muscle atrophy), weakness, anorexia, inappetence, ventral and limb edema, anemia and fever with a chronic course (Seiler, et al. 1981; Silva et al. 1995; Silva et al. 1996; Conrado et al. 2005). Another less frequent presentation causing neurological alterations is usually preceded by the first. Among the neurological signs, ataxia is often described (Conrado et al. 2005), as well as brain disorders such as decreased level of consciousness, amaurosis, circling and hyperexcitability (Rodrigues et al. 2005). Diagnosis can be performed by direct detection of the parasite (blood smear and buffy coat screening) and by molecular techniques such as PCR and qPCR in blood and tissues (Conrado et al. 2005; Rodrigues et al. 2005; Moraes et al. 2007; Buscher et al. 2019).

T. evansi was first observed in India in horses and camelids by Griffth Evans (1881) describing the parasite in blood. Later Steel (1885) classified the same agent as *Trypanosoma evansi*. This was the first *Trypanosoma* described as pathogenic in mammals. It is known as surra and was first reported in 1907 in Malaysia (Fraser 1907). At the beginning of the 20th century, T. evansi was called *T. hippiccum* e *T. equinum* (Hoare 1972, Desquesnes et al. 2013).

Table 11. Main case reports of horses infected by *T. evansi* with neurological alterations

Author	Year	State	Geographical Region	Technique	Affected/Dead	Capybaras (*Hidrochoerus hidrochaeris)*	Treatment	Results
Conrado et al.	2005	Rio Grande do Sul	Southern	Blood smear	8/0 (0)	ND	ND	ND
Rodrigues et al.	2005	Rio Grande do Sul	Southern	ELISA/IHQ/Blood smear	225/108 (46.78%)	Presence*	ND	ND
Zanette et al. Zanette and Silva	2008 2009	Rio Grande do Sul	Southern	Blood smear	8/0 (0)	Presence*	Diminazeno 7 mg/kg 7 days	Remission of Clinical Signs
Rodrigues et al.	2009	Rio Grande do Sul	Southern	ELISA/IHQ/Blood smear	09/09 (100%)	Presence*	ND	
Silva et al.	2010	Rio Grande do Sul	Southern	Blood smear/PCR	01/00 (0)	Presence*	3.5 mg/kg Single dose	Remission of Clinical Signs
Nunes et al.	2012	Minas Gerais	Southeastern	PCR	03/00 (0)	ND	Diminazeno 7 mg/kg 7days	Remission of Clinical Signs
Silva et al.	2016	Pará	Northern	IHQ/PCR	47/40 (85.1)	Presence*	ND	ND

ND: not described. *Presence of capybaras in the properties where the cases were described.

In Brazil, reports of horses with similar clinical disease are present in the nonspecialized literature since the 1830 but scientific observations about the disease were initially performed by Lacerda (1885) and later Lutz (1907) and Jansen (1941) described the presence of *T. equi*num in Marajo Island (North region). Later in 1994 Franke et al. carry out serological investigation and parasitological detection in horses in the Pantanal region, state of Mato Grosso, Midwestern Brazil, although (Table 11). Similar cases were observed in Brazil with outbreaks in the state of Pará, Northern Brazil and Pantanal Mato Grosso, Midwestern Brazil (Hoare 1972; Desquesnes et al. 2013).

In this study, Franke et al. (1994) detected *T. evansi* using blood smears in 0.3% of the horses and the presence of antibodies in 9.6% of the animals studied. All animals in which the presence of the parasite was confirmed were clinically healthy and came from the same farm, with reports of death of animals previously with the development of neurological signs.

In the same year, an outbreak of trypanosomiasis was reported in horses in the Pantanal region of the state of Mato Grosso, Midwestern Brazil (Silva et al. 1994ab). The caquetizing form was observed, characterized by the weight loss, atrophy of large muscle groups of the pelvic limbs, and generalysed weakness.

The experimental reproduction of the disease in horses with the inoculation of trypomastigones by the intravenous route in horses was described by Marques et al. (2000) in the state of São Paulo in Southeastern Brazil. After inoculation, the animals presented lymphadenomegaly, jaundice, apathy, progressive weight loss and edema. Pelvic limb ataxia and lateral recumbency were observed in two of the six animals. The immune response against *T. evansi* was observed by IFAT and ELISA techniques, occurring eight days after inoculation, reaching maximum levels in four weeks, remaining high for 145 days (Marques et al. 2001).

Research in horses, capybaras, dogs, marsupials, buffaloes and small rodents in the state of Mato Grosso, Midwestern Brazil, compared detection techniques using microhaematocrit, indirect immunofluorescence and PCR (Herrera et al. 2004). Low parasitemia was observed in horses (9.6%), and a high prevalence of *T. evansi* was observed in the PCR technique (73%). However, the horses studied did not present neurological alterations.

Description of horses with neurological alterations naturally associated with *T. evansi* in Brazil was performed by Conrado et al. (2005) in the state of Rio Grande do Sul, Southern Brazil. An epidemiological investigation was carried out after an episode of mortality in horses. The main clinical findings on this occasion, in addition to progressive weight loss and ventral edema, were pelvic limb ataxia and atrophy of muscle groups. The parasite was observed in the blood smear and in the investigation of the buffy coat (Conrado et al. 2005).

In the same year, an outbreak of trypanosomiasis was described in the same state, and 108 horses from two farms died, representing a mortality of 46.8%. In addition to the chronic clinical signs of the disease, neurological alterations were observed in eight horses. The clinical signs presented were consistent with cerebral syndrome. At necropsy, the presence of panencephalitis, demyelination, necrosis and perivascular lymphoplasmacytic infiltrate, affecting white and gray matter, were identified. The diagnosis was confirmed by the presence of flagellated protozoa observed in the blood, high antibody titers and direct (immunohistochemistry) observation of *T. evansi* in the CNS (Rodrigues et al. 2005).

The experimental infection in donkeys was carried out by Cadioli et al. (2006) in São Paulo, Southeastern Brazil, with intravenous inoculation of the pathogen. Parasites were observed on the blood smear five days after inoculation. Subsequently, anemia and hypoproteinemia were observed in the animals. At necropsy of these animals 145 days after inoculation, the presence of mononuclear infiltrate in the brain, spinal cord, meninges and choroid plexus was observed.

Experimental studies inoculating *T. evansi* into healthy horses resulted in changes in the CNS (Lemos et al. 2007; Lemos et al. 2008). On this occasion, all six animals developed ataxia, which was more pronounced in the pelvic limbs. Inflammatory infiltrate in the meninges and the presence of perivascular cuffs in the cortical and cerebellar regions were observed (Lemos et al. 2008). Immunohistochemistry detected the presence of *T. evansi* antigen in the CNS of infected horses. Nonsuppurative encephalomyelitis was observed, and the intensity of vascular lesions varied according to the different regions of the CNS (Lemos et al. 2007; Lemos et al. 2008).

Rodrigues et al. (2009) detailed the epidemiological, clinical and necropsy findings of eight horses with neurological abnormalities. The evolution ranged from two to twenty days, with the death of all affected animals. The main clinical findings were ataxia, decreased level of consciousness, atrophy of the pelvic limbs, blindness, circling, proprioceptive deficits and head tilt. It was possible to observe the presence of protozoa in the blood and high levels of antibodies. Perivascular lymphoplasmocytic meningoencephalitis, necrosis, edema and hemorrhage in the CNS were observed. The presence of the protozoan was confirmed by the immunohistochemical technique.

T. evansi was observed in the state of Rio Grande do Sul in Southern Brazil. Clinical examination revealed ataxia, with the presence of paresis and increased muscle tone. The property was located near a region in which capybaras (Hydrochaeris hydrochaeris) were present. In the blood smear of three of these horses, it was possible to observe the presence of the trypomastigote form of *T. evansi* (Zanette et al. 2008). Treatment with diminazene acetate resulted in gradual clinical improvement (Zanette and Silva 2009).

In the following year, another case of natural infection by *T. evansi* was described in horses in the state of Rio Grande do Sul in Southern Brazil (Silva et al. 2010). Clinically, the presence of fever and ataxia was observed. Trypomastigotes were observed in the blood smear, and the inoculation of blood from this animal in rats and subsequent PCR confirmed the diagnosis.

The presence of *T. evansi* in horses in the state of Minais Gerais in Southeastern Brazil was described by Nunes et al. (2012). On this occasion, on a farm with 16 horses, three had anemia, edema of the limbs, progressive weight loss, lameness, muscle atrophy and ataxia in the pelvic limbs. The diagnosis was confirmed by PCR.

Two outbreaks in the state of Pará, Northern Brazil, were described by Silva et al. (2016). From a population of 679 horses, 209 developed some type of abnormalities related to *T. evansi*, 183 (27%) died. Clinically, weight loss, subcutaneous edema, pale and icteric mucous membranes were observed. Specifically, the neurological examination revealed the presence of ataxia (mainly of the pelvic limbs) and atrophy of the muscle groups of the pelvic limbs. Lymphoplasmacytic encephalomyelitis was observed to affect the gray and white matter of the brain and spinal cord. Immunohistochemistry and PCR were able to detect the presence of *T. evansi* in CNS tissues.

Treatment with diminazene acetate has already been described as efficient by authors in Brazil (Zanette and Silva 2009; Silva et al. 2010; Nunes et al. 2012). It should be noted that in chronic and moderate cases, different from outbreaks (Rodrigues et al. 2005; Rodrigues et al. 2009; Silva et al. 2016). When there is neurological involvement, the response to treatment is less effective when compared to animals that only present weight loss and anemia (Moraes et al. 2007; Ranjithkumar et al. 2014; Buscher et al. 2019).

Halicephalobus gingivalis

Descriptions of neurological diseases caused by parasites are not common in Brazil, and only four descriptions of meningoencephalitis caused by

Halicephalobus gingivalis (or *H. gingivalis*) are present in the literature in this country. *H. gingivalis* is a free-living saprophytic nematode, and infecting horses can cause abnormalities in the central nervous system or even in other organs (eyes, kidneys, skin lesions, etc.) causing granulomatous lesions (Pearce et al. 2001). Neurological signs associated with this parasite in horses have been reported in Asia, North America and Europe. Neurological signs depend on the main site of the lesion, but the literature generally describes brain and spinal cord associated abnormalities, and there may be concomitant injuries in other organs (Henneke et al. 2014; Furr and Reed 2015).

The first published description of *H. gingivalis* in Brazil occurred in the Southeast region in a 10-year-old horse that presented acute neurological signs. Clinically, walking in circles and facial nerve paralysis were observed, rapidly progressing to lateral recumbency. In several regions of the cortex, diffusely distributed edema and gliosis and the presence of lymphocyte infiltrate were identified. In the meninges located close to the parasite, an intense lymphoplasmacytic infiltrate was observed. The nematode was found in several histological sections, identifying its rhabditiform esophagus (Vasconcelos et al. 2007).

A 6-year-old horse from the Midwest Brazil presented blindness, ataxia, nystagmus, depression and mydriasis and was euthanized five days after the onset of neurological signs. In the midbrain, thalamus, pons and more intensely in the cerebellum, the presence of perivascular infiltrate of lymphocytes, plasma cells and macrophages and nematode larvae characteristic of *H. gingivalis* was detected (Sant'ana et al. 2012).

Subsequently, three horses with neurological disease from different farms in the Midwest region were identified in a retrospective study. Ataxia, weakness, and head pressing were the clinical signs observed. No macroscopic changes were observed in the CNS. Histopathological examination revealed multifocal necrotizing granulomatous meningoencephalitis with the presence of adult and larval nematodes (Sousa et al. 2018).

The most recent case report describes a 9-year-old horse in the Southeastern Brazil with ataxia, bilateral strabismus, reduced menace response, depression and recumbency. CSF presented an increase in the number of nucleated cells (20 cells/μL). The presence of lymphoplasmacytic infiltrate was observed in the frontal cortex, brainstem, cerebellum, and neurohypophysis. Visualization of the parasite under microscopy confirmed the diagnosis (Santana et al. 2019).

Cryptococcal Meningoencephalomyelitis (*Cryptococcus neoformans*)

Cryptococcus neoformans is a fungal agent that causes several clinical manifestations in mammals, especially in immunosuppressed individuals. It has a polysaccharide capsule that favors its environmental resistance (Rathore et al. 2022). Soil contaminated by feces of pigeons and/or other birds and subsequent inhalation is the main form of infection (Carmo et al. 2022).

Cases of cryptococcosis in horses usually present with respiratory disorders (Riley et al. 1982; Kommers et al. 2005) and meningitis (Barton and Knight 1972; Barclay and DeLahunta, 1979). Ataxia, muscle tremors, decreased levels of consciousness and seizures are the main findings of the physical examination of animals that develop neurological sings (Barton and Knight 1972; Barclay and DeLahunta, 1979; Fava et al. 2011). In horses in Brazil, in addition to pneumonia in adults, this agent has been described as causing respiratory clinical signs (Kommers et al. 2005) and nasal obstruction by granulomas (Zoppa et al. 2008).

The first report of meningitis caused by *Cryptococcus neoformans* in Brazil occurred in the state of São Paulo (Fava et al. 2011). An adult horse initially presented with respiratory abnormalities (abdominal breathing, cough and intermittent fever). The condition progressed to chronic pneumonia and neurological abnormalities with ataxia, reduced level of consciousness, muscle and seizures. The animal was euthanized, and at necropsy, thickening of the meninges was observed. *C. neoformans* was observed in the histopathology of the meninges. Confirmation of the presence of mucoid capsules with numerous organisms.

A retrospective study of horses with neurological abnormalities performed by a referral center in the state of Minas Gerais identified a second case in Brazil. The identification of *C. neoformans* in the CNS occurred in a horse with seizures. The presence of unicellular microorganisms surrounded by a thick capsule was verified, which in the mucicarmine stain confirmed the diagnosis of cryptococcosis (Cunha et al. 2016). In other retrospective studies on the occurrence of neurological diseases in equids, cryptococcal meningoencephalomyelitis was not reported (Pimentel et al. 2009; Rissi et al. 2010; Sousa 2013; Costa et al. 2015).

Conclusion

Infectious or parasitic neurological diseases in equids in Brazil are frequent and economically import. This fact is demonstrated by the large number of scientific publications on the subject. In this context, the need for the proper elaboration of lists of differential diagnoses is highlighted, seeking with the aid of complementary exams to obtain the definitive diagnosis, and thus adopt preventive measures.

References

Abreu, R. A., Weiss, R. R., Thomaz-Soccol, V., Locatelli-Dittrich, R., Laskoski, L. M., Bertol, M. A. F., Koch, M. O., Alban, S. and Green, K. T. 2014. "Association of antibodies against *Neospora caninum* in mares with reproductive problems and presence of seropositive dogs as a risk factor." *Veterinary Parasitology* 202, no. 3-4 (May): 128-131.

Achkar, S. M., E. R. Fernandes, M. L. Carrieri, A. B. M. Castro, A. M. Batista, M. L. Duarte, and I. Kotati. 2010. "Sensitivity of the Immunohistochemistry technique in central nervous system fragments of cattle and horses naturally infected by rabies vírus." *Pesquisa Veterinária Brasileira* 3, no. 30 (March): 211-218.

Achkar, S. M., Fernandes, E. R., Guedes, F., Mori, E., Del Fava, C., Duarte, M. I. 2013. "Indissociabilidade da presença de corpúsculos de Negri e da inflamação parenquimatosa em amostras de sistema nervoso central de herbívoros acometidos pela raiva [*Inseparability of the presence of Negri bodies and parenchymal inflammation in central nervous system samples from herbivores affected by rabies*]." R*evista de Educação Continuada em Medicina Veterinária e Zootecnia do CRMV-SP* 11, no. 3: 41-41.

Aguiar, D. M., Cavalcante, G. T., Lara, M. C. C. S. H., Villalobos, E. C., Cunha, E. M. S., Okudam L. H., Stéfano, E., Nassar, A. F. G., Souza, G. O., Vasconcellos, S. A., Labruna, M. A. and gennari, S. M. 2008. "Prevalência de anticorpos contra agentes virais e bacterianos em eqüídeos do município de Monte Negro, Rondônia, Amazônia Ocidental Brasileira [*Prevalence of antibodies against viral and bacterial agents in horses from Monte Negro, Rondônia. Brazilian Western Amazon*]." *Brazilian Journal of Veterinary Research and Animal Science* 45, no. 4: 269-276.

Aguilar, P. V., Estrada-Franco, J. G., Navarro-Lopez, R., Ferro, C., Haddow, A. D. and Weaver, S. C. 2011. "Endemic Venezuelan equine encephalitis in the Americas: hidden under the dengue umbrella." *Future Virology* 6, no. 6: 1-31.

Albas, A., Zoccolaro, P. T., Rosa, T. Z. and Cunha, E. M. S. 2005. "Diagnóstico laboratorial da raiva na região oeste do Estado de São Paulo [*Laboratory diagnosis of rabies in the west region of São Paulo State*]." *Revista Brasileira da Sociedade Brasileira de Medicina Tropical* 38, no. 6 (December): 493-495.

Albertino, L. G., Dias, N. M., Moreira, J. J., Oliveira-Filho, J. P., Takahira, R. K., Laufer-Amorim, R., Borges, A. S. and Amorim, R. M. 2021. "Clinical findings of equine leukoencephalomalacia." *Pesquisa Veterinária Brasileira*, no. 1 (November), 1 -4.

Alencar-Araripe, M. G., Maia, D. C. B. S. C., Campelo, C. C., Silva Júnior, A., Silva, M. C., Dias, A. V., Medeiros, C. M. O. and Pinheiro, D. C. S. 2014. "Evidências sorológicas de EHV-1/EHV-2 em cavalos de vaquejadas no estado de Ceará, Brasil [*Serological evidence of EHV-1/EHV-2 in vaquejada horses in the state of Ceará, Brazil*]." *Revista Brasileira de Higiene e Sanidade Anima*l 8, no. 4(April): 203-217.

Alice, F. J. 1951. "Encefalomielite equina na Bahia: estudo de três amostras isolada [*Equine encephalomyelitis in Bahia: study of three isolated samples*]." *Revista Brasileira de Biologia* 11, no. 2 (June): 127-144.

Almeida, G. L. G., D'Almeida and J. M., Horn, S. C. 1988. *Doenças Animais no Brasil. História das primeiras observações* [*Animal Diseases in Brazil. History of the first observations*]. 1ª ed. Brasília: SNAP/SDSA.

Almeida, M. A. B., Santos, E., Cardoso, J. C., Noll, C. A., Lima, M. M. Silva, F. A., Ferreira, M. S., Vasconcelos, P. C. and Bicca-Marques, J. C. 2019. "Detection of antibodies against Icoaraci, Ilhéus, and Saint Louis Encephalitis arboviruses during yellow fever monitoring surveillance in non-human primates (*Alouatta caraya*) in southern Brazil." *Journal of Medical Primatology* 48, no. 4 (August): 211-217.

Anderson, R. C., Linder, K. E. and Peregrine, A. S. 1998. "*Halicephalobus gingivalis* (Stefanski, 1954) from a fatal infection in a horse in Ontario, Canada with comments on the validity of *H. deletrix* and a review of the genus." *Parasite* 5:255-261.

Andrade, E. A., Monteiro, F. D. O., Solório, M. R., Raia, V. A., Xavier, D. A., Colino, E., Guimarães, R. J. P. and Abel, I. 2020. "Livestock rabies in Pará state, Brazil: a descriptive study (2004 to 2013)." *Pesquisa Veterinária Brasileira* 40, no. 4 (April): 234-241.

Andrade, J. S. L., Azevedo, S. S., Peconick, A. P., Pereira, S. M., Barçante, J. M., Vilar, A. L. T., Silva, M. L. C. 2014. "Estudo retrospectivo da raiva no Estado da Paraíba, Brasil, 2004 a 2011 [*Retrospective survey of rabies in Paraíba State, Brazil, from 2004 to 2011*]." *Brazilian Journal of Veterinary Research and Animal* Science 51, no. 3 (March): 12-16.

Antonello, A. M., Pivot, F. L., Camilo, G., Brauning, P. Sangioni, O. E., Pompermayer, M. C. Godim, L. F. P. and Vogel, F. S. F. 2016. "Intra-uterine exposure of horses to *Sarcocystis spp.* Antigens." *Arquivo Brasileiro de Medicina Veterinária e Zootecnia* 68, no.42 (March): 271-275.

Aragão, J. M. 1911. "Um caso de tétano [*A case of tetanus*]." *Revista de Veterinária e Zootchenia* 1, no. 2: 83-89.

Araújo, F. A. A., Andrade, M. A., Jayme, V. S., Santos, A. L., Romano, A. P. M., Ramos, D. G., Cunha, E. M. S., Lara, M. C. C. S. H., Villalobos, E. M. C. and Martins, L. C. 2012. "Anticorpos antialfavírus detectados em equinos durante diferentes epizootias de encefalite equina, Paraíba, 2009 [*Antibodies to alphavirus detected in horses during different epizootics of equine encephalitis, Paraiba state, Brazil, 2009*]." *Revista Brasileira de Ciências Veterinárias* 19, no. 1 (May): 80-85.

Argenta, F. F., Konradt, G., Bassuino, D. M., Caprioli, R. A., Laisse, C. J., Borsanelli, A. C., Dutra, I. V., and Driemeier, D. 2017. "Surto de botulismo tipo C em equinos no

Rio Grande do Sul [*Outbreak of type C. botulism in horses in Rio Grande do Sul*]." *Pesquisa Veterinária Brasileira* 37, no. 12 (December): 1369-1372.

Babboni, S. D., and J. R. Modolo. 2011. "Raiva: Origem, Importância e Aspectos Históricos [*Rabies: Origin, importance and historical aspects*]." *Científica Ciências Biológicas e Saúde* 13, no. 1: 349-356.

Baccarin, R. Y. A., Fernandes, W. R., Vicenzi, R. C., Rêgo, E. B. and Silva, L. C. L. C. 2001. "Estudo da evolução clínica e tratamento da mieloencefalite protozoária equina [*Study of clinical evolution and treatment of the equine protozoal myeloencephalitis*]." *Veterinária Notícias* 7, no. 2:79-85.

Barclay, W. P. and DeLahunta, A. 1979. Cryptococcal meningitis in a horse." *Journal of The American Veterinary Medical Association* 174, no. 11 (June): 1236-1238.

Barros, C. S. L., Barros, C. C. and Santos, M. N. 1986. "Equine protozoal myelo-encefaphalitis in southern Brazil." *Veterinary Records* 119, no.1 (September): 283-284.

Barros, C. S. L., Barros, S. S., Santos, M. N., Souza, M. A. 1984. "Leucoencafalomalácia em equinos no Rio Grande do Sul [*Leukoencephalomalacia in horses in Rio Grande Sul*]." *Pesquisa Veterinária Brasileira* 4, no. 3: 101-107.

Barros, C. S. L., S. S. Barros, M. N. Santos, C. A. M. Silva, and F. Waihrich.1986. "Mieloencefalite eqüina por protozoário [*Equine protozoan myeloencephalitis*]." *Pesquisa Veterinária Brasileira* 6, no. 2: 45-49.

Barton M. D. and Knight, I. 1972. "Cryptococcal meningitis of a horse." *Australian Veterinary Journal* 48, no. 1 (September): 523-525.

Batista, H. B. C., Franco, A. C. and Roehe, P. M. 2007. " Raiva uma breve revisão [*Rabies: a brief review*]." *Acta Scientiae Veterinariae* 35, no. 2: 125-144.

Bedenice, D. and Johnson, A. L. 2018. "Neurologic conditions affecting the Equine Athlete." *Veterinary Clinics of North America: Equine practice* 34, no. 2 (August): 277-297.

Beech, J. 1974. "Equine protozoan encephalomyelitis." *Veterinary Medicine Small Animal Clinician* 69, no. 4: 1562–1566.

Benmansour, A.; Leblois, H., Coulon, P., Gaudin, Y., Flamand, A. and Lafat, F. 1991. "Antigenicity of rabies virus glycoprotein." *Journal of Virology* 65, no. 8: 4198-4203. 10.1128/jvi.65.8.4198-4203.1991.

Benzuidenhount, S. C., Gelderblom, W. C. A., Gorst-Allman, C. P., Horak, R. M., Marasas, W. F. O., Spieteller, G., Vieggar, R. 1988. "Structure elucidation of the fumunisins mycotoxins from *Fusarium moniliforme*." *Journal of the Chermical Society, Chemical Communications* 11, no. 1: 743-745.

Bernadette, M., Murri, S., Zientara, S., Durand, B., Durand, J. P. and Zeller, H. 2001. "West Nile Outbreak in Horses in Southern France, 2000: The Return after 35 Years." *Emerging Infectious Diseases* 7, no. 4 (August): 692-698.

Bernadino, P. D. Smith, W. A., Conrad, P. A., Packham, A. E. Tamez, E. A. Barnum, S. and Pusterla, N. 2021. "Molecular detection of *Sarcocystis neurona* in cerebrospinal fluid from 210 horses with suspected neurologic disease." *Veterinary Parasitology* 291, no. 3 (March): 1-6.

Borges, A. M. C. M., Yearg, M. R., Silva, L. G., Taques, I. G. G., Howe, D. and Aguiar, D. M. 2017. "Antibodies Against *Sarcocystis neurona*, *Neospora* spp., and

Toxoplasma gondii in Horses and Mules from the Northern Pantanal Wetland of Brazil." *Journal of Equine Veterinary Science* 56, no. 2: 19-25.

Borges, A. S., Luvizotto, M. C. R., Alves, A. L. G. and Garcia, S. D. 1995 "Leucoencefalomalacia – relato de 10 casos" [Leukoencephalomalacia - Report of 10 cases]. In: *Encontro Nacional de Patologia Veterinária – ENAPAVE* 7, Belo Horizonte. Belo Horizonte, 1995. p.98.

Borges-Silva, W., Jesus, R. F., Ferreira, R. and Godim, L. F. P. 2020. "Reactivity of horse sera to antigens derived from *Sarcocystis falcatula-like* and *Sarcocystis neurona.*" *Frontiers in Veterinary Science* 2, no. 7 (November): 1-8.

Bosch, I., Herrera, F., Navarro, J. C., Lentino, M., Dupuis, A., Maffei, J. and Kremer, L. 2007. "West Nile Virus, Venezuela." *Emerging Infectious Diseases* 13, no. 4 (September): 651-653.

Brito, L. A. B., Nogueira, R. H. G., Pereira, J. J. and Chquiloff, M. A. G. 1982. "Leucoencefalomalácia em equinos associada à alimentação com milho mofado [*Leucoenchepalomalacia of horses associated with the feeding with mouldy corn*]." *Arquivos da Escola de Medicina Veterinária* UFMG 34, no. 1(April).

Broeck, B. T., Hurst, W. and Traub, E. 1935. "Epidemiology of equine encephalomyelitis in the Eastern United States." *Journal of Experimental Medicine* 62, no. 5 (January): 677-685.

Bruno-Lobo, G., Bruno-Lobo, M. Travasso, J., Pinheiros, F. F. and Pazin, I. P. 1961. "Estudos sôbre os arbovírus III. Isolamento de um vírus sorològicamente relacionado ao sub-grupo Western-Sindbis, de um caso de encefalomielite eqüina, ocorrido no Rio de Janeiro [*Studies on arboviruses III. Isolation of a virus serologically related to the Western-Sindbis subgroup, from a case of equine encephalomyelitis, which occurred in Rio de Janeiro*]." *Anais de Microbiologia* 9, no. 1: 183-195.

Bunning, M. L., Bowen, R. A., Croop, C. B., Sullivan, K. G., Davis, B. S., Komar, N., Godsey, M. S., Baker, D., Hettler, D. L., Holmes, D. A., Biggerstaff, B. J., Mitchell, C. J. 2002. "Experimental infection of horses with West Nile vírus." *Emerging Infectious Diseases* 8, no. 4 (April): 380-386.

Buscher, P., Gonzatti, M. I., Herbert, L., Inoue, N., Pascucci, I., Schnaufer, Suganuma, K., Touratier, L. and Reet, N. V. 2019. "Equine Trypanosomosis: enigmas and diagnostic challenges." *Parasites & Vectors* 12, no. 234: 1-8.

Cadioli, F. A., marques, L. C., Machado, R. Z., Alessi, A. C., Aquino, L. P. C. T., and Barnabé, P. A. 2006. "Experimental Trypanosoma evansi infection in donkeys: hematological, biochemical and histopathological changes." *Arquivo Brasileiro de Medicina Veterinária* 58, no. 5 (October): 749-756.

Cai, S., Singh, B. R. and Sharma, S. 2007. "Botulism diagnostics: from clinical symptoms to in vitro assays." *Critical Reviews in Microbiology* 33, no. 2 (April-June): 109-125.

Calisher, C. H., Kinney, R. M., Lopes, O. S., Trent, D. W., Monath, T. P. and Francy, D. B. 1982. "Identification of a New Venezuelan Equine Encephalitis Virus from Brazil." *The American Journal of Tropical Medicine and Hygiene* 31, no. 6: 1260-1272.

Câmara, A. C. L., Afonso, J. A. B., Riet-Correa, F., Dantas, A. F. M., Mendonça, C. L., Costa, N. A., Dantas, A. C., Costa Neto, H. A., Campos, A. G. S. S. and Souza, M. I. 2008. "Leucoencefalomalácia em equideos no estado do Pernambuco

[*Leukoencephalomalacia in equids in the state of Pernambuco*]." *Ciência Animal Brasileira* 9, no. 2: 470-479.

Campbell, G. L., Marfin, A., Lanciotti, R. S., and Gubler, D. J. 2002. "West Nile Virus." *The Lancet* 2, no. 9 (September): 519-529.

Campos, K. F., Oliveira, C. H. S., Reis, A. B., Yamasaki, E. M., Brito, M. F., Andrade, S. J., Duarte, S. J. T. and Barbosa, J. D. 2013. "Surto de encefalomielite equina Leste na Ilha de Marajó, Pará [*Eastern equine encephalitis on Marajó Island, Pará state, Brazil*]." *Pesquisa Veterinária Brasileira* 33, no. 4 (April):443-448.

Carini, A. 1911. "Sur une grand epizootie de rage [*On a great epizootic of rabies*]." *Annales de L'Institut Pasteur* 25, no. 8 (November): 843-846.

Carmo, F. N., Fenley, J. C., Garcia, M. T., Rossoni, R. D., Junqueira, J. C., Barros, P. P. and Scorzoni, L. 2022. "*Cryptococcus* spp and Cryptococcosis: focosing on the infection in Brazil." *Clinical Microbiology* 10, no. 1 (March):1-17.

Carneiro, V. 1937. "Encephalomyelite infecciosa dos equinos no Brasil [*Infectious encephalomyelitis of horses in Brazil*]." *Arquivos do Instituto Biológico 2*:115-134.

Carneiro, V. 1939. "A encephalomyelites in Brazil." *Proceedings of the Sixth Pacific Science Congress of the Pacific Science Association* 5, no. 1 (July): 251-258.

Carneiro, V. 1944. "Estudos sobre uma amostra de vírus da encefalomielite infecciosa do cavalo e os vírus americanos – pelas provas de soroneutralização [*Studies on a sample of horse infectious encephalomyelitis virus and American viruses – by serum neutralization tests*]. " *Arquivos do Instituto Biológico* 15, no. 6: 209-238.

Carneiro, V. and Cunha, R. 1943. "Estudos sobre a encefalomielite infecciosa dos equídeos no Brasil [*Studies on equine infectious encephalomyelitis in Brazil*]." *Arquivos do Instituto Biológico* 14, no. 10 (December): 157-194.

Carrieri, M. L., Peixoto, Z. M., Paciencia, M. L. B., and Germano, P. M. L. 2006. "Laboratory diagnosis of equine rabies and its implications for human postexposure prophylaxis." *Journal of Virological Methodos* 138, no. 1-2 (December): 1-9. doi.org/10.1016/j.jviromet.2006.07.005.

Carvalho, F. S. R., Coelho, H. E. and Ribeiro, S. M. 1995. " Micotoxicose em equino associada a ingestão de milho mofado [*Equine mycotoxicosis associated with moldy corn ingestion*]." *Veterinária Notícias* 1, no. 1: 37-43.

Carvalho, R. F., Spiki, F. R., Cunha, E. M. and Arns, C. W. 2012. "Molecular data og UL24 homolog gene (ORF37) from Brazilian isolates of equine herpesvirus type 1." *Research in Veterinary Science* 93, no.1: 494-497.

Carvalho, R., Oliveira, A. M., Souza, A. M., Passos, L. M. F. and Martins, A. S. 2000. "Prevalence of equine herpesvirus type 1 latency detected by polymerase chain reaction." *Archives of Virology* 145: 1773-1787.

Carvalho, R., Passos, L. M. F. and Martins, A. S. 2000. "Development of a Differential Multiplex PCR Assay for Equine Herpesvirus 1 and 4 as a Diagnostic Tool." *Zoonoses and Public Health* 47, no. 5 (June):351-359.

Carvalho, R., Passos, L. F. M. Oliveira, A. M., Henry, M. and A. S. Martins. 2000. "Detection of equine herpesvirus 1 DNA in single embryo and in horse sêmen by polymerase chain reaction." *Arquivo Brasileiro de Medicina Veterinária e Zootecnia* 52, no. 4 (August): 1-10.

Carvalho, R., Passos, L. F. M., Gouvea, A. M. G., Resende, M., Martins, A. S. and Franco, G. C. 2000. "Use of an ELISA system for detection of equine herpesvirus 1 (EHV-1) antibodies in non-symptomatic pregnant mares and neonatal foals." *Arquivo Brasileiro de Medicina Veterinária e Zootecnia* 53, no. 2 (June): 1-6.

Castilo-Olivares, J. and Wood, J. 2004. "West Nile vírus infection of horses." *Veterinary Research* 35, no. 4 (July-August): 467-483.

Causey, O. R., Causey, C. E., Maroja, O. M. and Macedo, D. G. 1961. "The isolation of arthropod-borne viruses, including members of two hitherto undescribed serological groups, in the Amazon region of Brazil." *Journal of Tropical Medicne and Hygiene* 10, no. 2 (March): 227-249.

Causey, O. R., Shope, R. E., Sutmoller, P. and Laemmert, H. 1962. "Epizootic eastern equine encephalitis in the Bragança region of Pará, Brazil." *Revista do Serviço Especial de Saúde Pública* 12, no. 1: 39-45.

Ceballos, N. A. and Setien, A. A. 2015. "Les encephalomyelitis équines (de I' Est, de I' Ouest et vénézuélienne) dues à de alphavirus [*Equine encephalomyelitis (Eastern, Western and Venezuelan) due to alphaviruses*]." *Revues Scientifique et Technique* 34, no. 2(august): 491-501. doi.org/10.20506/rst.34.2.2374.

Chabí, E. S., Peixoto, A. P. C., Miranda, C. A., Pinheiro, D. N. S., Souza, L. Q., Abareu, T. S. and Pereira, T. O. 2022. "Tétano em um equino: Relato de caso [*Responsive treatment of a horse with tetanus: A case report*]." *PubVet* 16, no. 07: 186-190.

Chalhoub, F. L. L., Queiroz-Júnior, E. M., Durte, B. H., Sá, M. E. P., Lima, P. C., Oliveira, A. C. and Pauvolid-Corrêa, A. 2021. "West Nile vírus in the State of Ceará, Northeast Brazil." *Microorganisms* 9, no. 8 (August): 1-31.

Chaves, L. R. 1950. "Doença de sintomatologia nervosa causada pela intoxicação pelo milho [*Nervous symptomatology disease caused by corn intoxication*]." *Revista Milenar Remédios e Veterinária* 10: no. 4:199-217.

Chen, R., Mukoádhyay, S., Merits, A., Bolling, B., Nasar, F., Coffey, L. L., Powers, A. and Weaver, S. C. 2018. "ICTV Virus Taxonomy Profile: Togaviridae." *Journal of General Virology* 99, no. 1 (June): 761-762, 2018.

Clark, E. G., Towsend, H. G. G., and McKenzie, N. T. 1981. "Equine Protozoal myeloencephalitis: a report of two cases from Western Canada." *The Canadian Veterinary Journal* 22, no. 5 (May): 140-140.

Coelho, H. E., Carvalho, F. S. R., Mineo, J. R., Silva, D. A. O., Manzan, R. M. and Francisco Júnior, A. 2000. "Surto de botulismo tipo C em equinos [*Outbreak of type C botulism in horses*]." *Veterinária Notícias* 6, no. 2: 99-103.

Colpo, C. B., Monteiro, S. G., Stainki, D. R., Colpo, E. T. B. and Henriques, G. B. 2005. "Infecção natural por Trypanosoma evansi em cães [*Natural infection by Trypanosoma evansi in dogs*]." *Ciência Rural* 35, no. 3 (June): 717-719.

Conrado, A. C., Lopes, S. T. A., Oliveira, L. S. S., Monteiro, S. G., Vargas, D. L. B. and Bueno, A. 2005. "Infecção natural por Trypanosoma evansi em cavalos na região Central do Estado do Rio Grande do Sul [*Natural infection by Trypanosoma evansi in horses in the central area of the state of Rio Grande do Sul, Brazil*]." *Ciência Rural* 35, no. 4 (July-August): 928-931.

Correa, W. M., and M. R. Nilsson. 1964. "Observações preliminares sobre aborto por vírus equino no Brasil [*Preliminary observations on equine virus abortion in Brazil*]." *Arquivos do Instituto Biológico* 31, no.3: 13-15.

Costa, E. A., Bomfim, M. R. Q., Fonseca, F. G., Drumond, B. A., Coelho, F. M., Vasconcelos, A. C., Furtini, R., Paixão, T. A., Tsolis. 2009. "Ovine Herpesvirus 2 Infection in foal, Brazil." *Emerging Infectiuos Diseases* 15, no. 5 (May): 844-845.

Costa, E. A., Five, G. B. L., Castro, R. T., Furtini, R., Portilho, R. V. and Resende, M. 2008. "Meningoencephalitis in a horse associated with equine herpesvirus 1." *Arquivo Brasileiro de Medicina Veterinária e Zootecnia* 60, no. 6 (December):1580-1583.

Costa, E. A., Giovanetti, M., Catenacci, L. S., Fonseca, V., Aburjaile, F. F., Chalhoub, F. L. L. and Alcantara, L. C. J. 2021. "West Nile Virus in Brazil." *Pathogens* 10, no. 7 (May): 1-12.

Costa, E. A., Rosa, R., Oliveira, T. S., Furtini, R. Fonseca Júnior, A. A., Paixão, T. A. and Santos, R. L. 2015. "Diagnóstico etiológico de enfermidades do sistema nervoso central de equinos no Estado de Minas Gerais, Brasil. [*Etiologic diagnosis of diseases of the central nervous system of horses in Minas Gerais State, Brazil*]." *Arquivo Brasileiro de Medicina Veterinária e Zootecnia* 62, no. 2 (April): 391-399. doi.org/10.1590/1678-6765.

Costa, E. A., Rosa, R., Oliveira, T. S., Furtini, R., Fonseca Júnior, A. A., Paixão, T. A. and Santos, R. L. 2011. " Encefalites equinas em Minas Gerais e o primeiro isolamento do vírus da encefalite de Saint Louis no Brasil [*Equine encephalitis in Minas Gerais and the first isolation of Saint Louis encephalitis virus in Brazil*]." *Revista de Educação Continuada em Medicina Veterinária e Zootecnia do CRMV-SP* 9, no. 3: 42-43.

Costa, E. A., Vasconcelos, A. C., Bomfim, M. R. Q., Silva, M. X., Haddad, J. P. A. Amorim, H. B., Lima, G. B. L., Furtini, R. and Resende, M. 2009. "Epidemiological and clinical aspects of equine Herpesvirus encephalitis infection in horses that died with neurological signs from Minas Gerais state, Brazil." *Brazilian Journal of Veterinary Research and Animal Science* 46, no. 4 (August): 262-272.

Costa, G. B., Marinho, P. E. S., Vilela, A. P. P. Saraiva-Silva, A. T., Crispim, A. P. C., Borges, I. A., Dutra, A. G. S., Lobato, Z. I. P., Reis, J. K. P., Oliveira, D. B., Drumoun, B. P. Kroon, E. G. and Trindade, G. S. 2019. "Silent Circulation of the Saint Louis Encephalitis Virus among Humans and Equids, Southeast Brazil." *Viruses* 5, no. 11 (November):1-10. 10.3390/v11111029.

Cunha, E. M. S., Ferraria, C. I., Lara, C. C. S. H. and Silva, L. H. Q. 2002. "Presença de anticorpos contra o herpesvirus eqüino 1 (HVE-1) em eqüinos do noroeste do estado de São Paulo [*Presence of antibodies against equine Herpesvirus 1 (HVE-1) in horses from the northwest of the state of São Paulo*]." *Arquivo do Instituto Biológico* 69, no. 1 (January): 1-5.

Cunha, E. M. S., Lara, M. C. C. S. H., Villalobos, E. M. C., Nassar, A. F. C., Fava, C. D., Scannapieco, E. M., Cunha, M. S. and Mori, E. 2016. "Causes of Encephalitis and Encephalopathy in Brazilian Equids." *Journal of Equine Veterinary Science* 38, no. 3 (March): 8-13. doi.org/10.1016/j.jevs.2016.01.002.

Cunha, E. M. S., Vilallobos, E. M. C., Nassar, A. F. C., Lara, M. C. C. S. H., Peres, N. F., Palazzo, J. C. P., Silva, A., Stéfano, E. D. and Pino, F. A. 2009. "Prevalence of antibodies against viral agents in equids in the south of the state of São Paulo." *Arquivos do Instituto Biológico* 76, no. 2 (April): 165-171.

Cunha, R. 1943. "Verificação de Anticorpos para o vírus "Este" da encefalomielite equina em sôro de cavalos no nordeste Brasileiro [*Antibodies to equine encephalomyelitis "Este" virus in horse serum in northeastern Brazil*]." *Revista Brasileira de Biologia* 3, no. 4 (December):425-430.

Dávila, A. M. R., Herrera, H. M., Schlebinger, T., Souza, S. S. and Y. M. Traub-Cseko. 2003. "Using PCR for unraveling the cryptic epizootiology of livestock trypanosomosis in the Pantanal" Brazil. *Veterinary Parasitologic* 117, no. 1-2 (November): 1-13.

Del Fava, C., Lara, M. C. C. S. H., Villalobos, E. M. C., Nassar, A. F. C., Cabral, A. D., Torelli, E. M. C., Cunha, M. S. and Cunha, E. M. S. 2010. "Occurrence of leukoencephalomalacia in equids in São Paulo state, Brazil: anatomopathological findings." *Brazilian Journal of Veterinary Research and Animal Science* 47, no. 6:488-497.

Dennis, S. T., Hage, C. M. E. and Brookes, V. J. 2022, "A survey of veterinarians' practices, recommendations and perceptions associated with the prevention of tetanus in horses in Australia." *Australian Veterinary Journal* 100, no. 4 (April): 181-186.

Desquesnes, M., Holzmuller, P., Lai, D. H., Dargantes, A., Lun, Z. R. and Jittaplapong, S. 2013. "*Trypanosoma evansi* and Surra: A Review and Perspectives on Origin, History, Distribution, Taxonomy, Morphology, Hosts, and Pathogenic Effects." *BioMed Research International* 3, no. 7 (August): 1-22.

Di Filippo, P. A., Graça, F. A. S., Costa, A. P. D., Coutinho, I. S. and Viana, I. S. 2016. "Clinical and epidemiological findings and response to treatment of 25 cases of tetanus in horses occurred in Norte Fluminense, Rio de Janeiro, Brazil." *Brazilian Journal Veterinary Medicine* 38, no. 1 (January-March):33-38.

Diaz, K. A. F., Rodrigues, P. R. C., Lilenbaum, W., and Lima, M. 2015. " Ocorrência de anticorpos contra o herpesvírus equino e virus da arterite equina em rebanhos equinos do estado do Rio de Janeiro [*Occurrence of Antibodies Against Equine Herpesvirus and Equine Arteritis Virus in Horse Herds of Rio De Janeiro State, Brazil*]." *Ciência Animal Brasileira* 16, no. 3:410-418.

Diel, D. G., Almeida, S. R., Weiblen, R., Frandoloso, R. Anziliero, Kreutz, L. C., Groof, F. H. S. and Flores, E. D. 2006. "Prevalência de anticorpos contra os vírus da influenza, da arterite viral e herpesvírus em eqüinos do Estado do Rio Grande do Sul, Brasil [*Prevalence of antibodies to influenza virus, viral arteritis and herpesvirus in horses of the Rio Grande do Sul state, Brazil*]." *Ciência Rural* 36, no. 5 (October): 1467-1673.

Dognani, R., Pierre, E. J., Silva, M. C. P., Patrício, M. A. C., Costa, S. C., Prado, J. R. and Lisbôa, J. A. N. 2016. "Epidemiologia descritiva da raiva dos herbívoros notificados no estado do Paraná entre 1977 e 2012 [*Epidemiology of rabies in large animals of Paraná, Brazil, from 1977 to 2012*]." *Pesquisa Veterinária Brasileira* 36, no. 12 (December): 1145-1154.

Doutre, M. P. 1969. "First observation of type D animal botulism in Senegal [*Premiere observation of type D animal botulism in Sénégal*]." *Revue d'Elevage et de Médecine Vétérinaire des Pays Tropicaux* 22, no. 1: 25-27.

Dubey, J. P. 2022. "*Sarcocystis neurona, Neospora spp. and Toxoplasma gondii* infections in horses and equine protozoal myeloencephalitis (EPM): five decades of personal experience, perspectives and update." *Parasitology* 179, no. 3 (March): 717-728.

Dubey, J. P., Howe, D. K., Furr, M., Saville, W. J., Marsh, A. E., Reed, S. M. and Grigg, M. E. 2015. "An update on *Sarcocystis neurona* infections in animals and Equine Protozoal Myeloencephalitis (EPM)." *Veterinary Parasitologic* 209, no. 1 (April): 1-14.

Dubey, J. P., Kerber, C. E. and Granstrom, D. E. 1999. "Serologic prevalence of *Sarcocystis neurona, Toxoplasma gondii, and Neospora caninum* in horses in Brazil." *Journal of the American Veterinary Medical Association* 1, no. 215 (October): 970-972.

Dubey, J. P., Lindsay, D. S., Kerber, C. E., Kasai, N., Pena, H. F. J., Gennari, S. M., Kwok, O. C., Shen, S. K. and Rosenthal, B. M. 2001. "First isolation of *Sarcocystis neurona* from the South American opossum, *Didelphis albiventris*, from Brazil." *Veterinary Parasitology* 95, n. 3 (Februray): 295-304.

Dubey, J. P., Lindsay, D. S., Saville, W. J. A., Reed, S. M., Granstrom, E. and Speer, C. A. 2001. "A review of *Sarcocystis neurona* and equine protozoal myeloencephalitis (EPM)." *Veterinary Parasitology* 95, no. 2-4 (February): 89-131.

Echenique, J. V. Z., Estima-Silva, P., Pereira, D. B., Marques, L. S., Ribeira, L. S. and Schild A. L. 2019. "Leukoencephalomalacia in horses associated with immature corn consumption." *Ciência Rural* 49, no. 3: 1-4.

Estima-Silva, P., Riet-Correa, F., Coelho, A. C. B., Echenique, J. V. Z., Marcolongo-Pereira, C., Lima, M., Diel, D. G. and Schild, A. L. 2019. "Identification of equine herpesvirus type 1 as cause of abortion in mares in Southern Brazil." *Arquivo Brasileiro de Medicina Veterinária e Zootecnia* 71, no. 4: 1421-1424.

Evans, G. 1881. "On a horse disease in India known as surra, probably due to a haematozoon." *Veterinary Journal* 13, no. 3 (July): 1-10.

Evers, F., Garcia, J. L., Navarro, I. T., Lipe, D. L., Nino, B. S. L., Carvalho, M. P., Pagliari, S., Almeida, J. C. and Freire, R. L. 2012. "Diagnosis and isolation of *Toxoplasma gondiiin* horses from Brazilian slaughterhouses." *Revista Brasileira de Parasitologia* 22, no. 1 (March): 58-63.

Fantini, P., Sampaio, I. S. and Silva, M. O. 2021. "Mieloencefalite protozoária equina: relato de caso [*Equine Protozoal Myeloencephalitis: Case Report*]." *ARS Veterinaria* 37, no. 4 (April) 242-246.

Faria, T. T. R., Pessoas, G. O., Biihrer, D. A., Lima, A. P., Varaschim, M. S. and Sousa, T. M. 2017. "Mieloencefalite p rotozoária e quina de evolução clínica aguda: Relato de caso [*Equine protozoal myeloencephalitis of acute clinical course: case report*]." *PubVet* 11, no. 1:40-45.

Farias, A. X., Rocha, E. S. and Costa, P. P. 2002. "Fumonisina em Milho: um risco a saúde humana e animal [*Fumonisin in Corn: a risk to human and animal health*]." Technical Communication 51, no. 1: 1-2.

Fava, C. D., Levy, F. L., Scannapieco, E. M., Lara, M. C. C. S. H., Villalobos, E. M. C. Nassar, A. F. C., Cunha, M. S., and Cunha E. M. S. 2011. "Cryptococcal pneumonia and meningitis in a horse." *Journal of Equine Veterinary Science* 31, no. 12 (December): 693-695.

Favoretto, S. R., Carrieri, M. L., Cunha, E. M. S., Aguiar, E. A. C., Silva, L. H. Q., Sodré, M. M., Souza, M. C. A. M. and Kotait, I. 2002. "Antigenic typing of brazilian rabies virus samples isolated from animals and humans, 1989-2000." *Revista do Instituto de Medicina Tropical de São Paulo* 2, no. 44 (March): 91-95.

Fernández, Z., Richartz, R., Travassos Da Rosa, A. P. A. and Soccol V. T. 2000. "Identificação do vírus causador de encefalomielite eqüina, Paraná, Brasil [*Identification of the virus causing equine encephalomyelitis, Paraná, Brazil*]." *Revista de Saúde Pública* 34, no. 3 (June): 232-235.

Ferreira, H. I. P., Calabulg, C., Borges, P. A. C. and Oliveira, I. V. P. M. 2018. "Seroepidemiology of viral agents in vaquejada horses." *Brazilian Journal of Veterinary Medicine* 40, no. 1: 210-218.

Figueiredo, L. T. M. 2019. "West Nile virus infection in Brazil." *Revista da Sociedade Brasileira de Medicina Tropical* 52, no. 1 (May): 1-2.

Finger, M. A., Villalobos, E. M. C., Lara, M. C. S. H., Cunnha, E. M. S., Barros Filho, I. R., Deconto, I., Dorbusch, P. T., Ullmann, L. S. and Biondo, A. W. 2013. "Detection of anti-*Toxoplasma gondii* antibodies in carthorses in the metropolitan region of Curitiba, Paraná, Brazil." *Revista Brasileira de Parasitologia Veterinaria* 22, no. 1 (March): 179-181.

Franke, C. R., Greiner, M. and Mehilitz D. 1994. "Investigations on naturally occurring *Trypanosoma evansi* infections in horses, cattle, dogs and capybaras (*Hydrochaeris hydrochaeris*) in Pantanal de Pocono (Mato Grosso, Brazil). *Acta Tropica* 58, no. 1 (november): 159-169.

Fraser, H. 1907. "Surra in the federated Malay states." *The Lancet* 170, no. 4381 (August): 466.

Furr, M. and Reed, S. 2015. *Equine Neurology*. 2° ed. Hoboken: Wiley Blackwell.

Gabriel, L. C., Pereira, C. B., Bavia, G. P., Coan, M., Donel, A. G., Tessmann, D. J. Scapim, C. A. 2017. "Evaluation of the resistance of popcorn genotypes to fumonisin accumulation and fusarium ear rot." *Summa Phytopathology* 44, no. 3: 286-288.

Galvão, C. M. M. Q., Gondim, M. M. R., Chaves, A. C. R., Schares, G., Ribas, J. R. L. and Gondim, L. F. P. 2015. "Brazilian donkeys (*Equus asinus*) have a low exposure to *Neospora spp.*" *Revista Brasileira de Parasitologia* 24, no. 3 (July): 340-344.

Gennari, S. M., Esmerini, P. O., Lopes, M. G., Soares, H. S., Vitaliano, S. N., Cabral, A. D., Pena, H. F. J., Horta, M. C., Cavalcante, P. H., Fortes, K. P. and Villalobos, E. M. C. 2015. "Occurrence of antibodies against *Toxoplasma gondii* and its isolation and genotyping in donkeys, mules, and horses in Brazil." *Veterinary Parasitology* 209, no. 1-2 (April): 129-132.

Gil, L. H. V. G., Magalhães, T., Santos, B. S. A. S., Oliveira, I. V.; Oliveira-Filho, E. F., Cunha, J. L. R., Fraiha, A. L. S., Rocha, B. M. M., Longo, B. C., Ecco, R., Faria, G. C. and Costa, E. A. 2021. "Active Circulation of Madariaga Virus, a Member of the Eastern Equine Encephalitis Virus Complex, in Northeast Brazil." *Pathogens* 10, no. 8: 1-13.

Góes, P. and Bruno-Lobo, M. 1961. "Estudos sobre o Arbovirus E – Resumo do problema e plano de trabalho inicial [*Studies on Arbovirus E – Summary of the problem and initial work plan*]." *Annais de Microbiologia* 9, no. 1: 164-182.

Gomes, F. A., Jansen, A. M., Machado, R. Z., Pena, H. F. J., Fumagalli, M. J., Silva, A. S. Alves, B. F., Roque A. L. R., and Figueiredo, L. T. M. 2019. "Serological evidence of arboviruses and coccidia infecting horses in the Amazonian region of Brazil." *Plos Ones* 14, no. 12 (December): 1-13.

Gomez, D. E., Arroyo, L. G., Brandon, L. and Scott, W. J. 2021. "Nasal bacterial microbiota during an outbreak of equine herpesvirus 1 at a farm in southern Ontario." *Canadian Journal of Veterinary Research* 85, no. 1 (January): 3-11.

Gonçalvez, E., Pinto, M. M., and Felicio, J. D. 2001. "Análise de Micotoxinas no Instituto Biológico de 1989 a 1999 [*Analysis of Mycotoxins at the Biological Institute from 1989 to 1999*]." *Biológico* 63, no. 1-2 15-19.

Gondim, L. F. P., Soares, R. M., Moré, G., Jesus, R. F. and Liano, H. A. B. 2021. "*Sarcocystis neurona* and related S*arcocystis* spp. shed by opossums (*Didelphis* spp.) in South America." *Brazilian Journal of Veterinary* Parasitology 30, no. 3 (March): 1-22.

Haagsma, J., Haesebrouck, F., Devriese, L. and Bertels, G. 1990. "An outbreak of botulism type B in Horses." *The Veterinary Record* 25, no. 127 (August): 206-208.

Hamir, A. N., Moser, G., Rupprecht, C. E. 1992. "A Five Year (1985-1989) Retrospective Study of Equine Neurological Diseases with Special Reference to Rabies." *Journal of Comparative Pathology* 106, no. 4 (May): 411-421.

Hassegawa, R., Zorzete, P., Reis, T. A., Fancelli, A. L., Fonseca, H., Almeida, A. P. and Corrêa, B. 2006. "Influência de nutrientes no crescimento fúngico e na produção de fumonisinas e aflatoxinas em grãos de milho [*The nutrients effect on mycoflora, and for fumonisins and aflatoxinsproduction in corn grain*]." *Revista do Instituto Adolfo Lutz* 65, no. 1: 21-26.

Headley, S. A., Oliveira, T. E. S. and Cunha, C. W. 2020. "A review of the epidemiological, clinical, and pathological aspects of malignant catarrhal fever in Brazil." *Veterinary Microbiology* 51, no. 1: 1405-1432.

Hébert, L., Polledo, G., Lecouturier, F., Giorgi, M., Beck, C., Lowenski, S., Loraucau, K., Buscher, P., Hans, A. and Bécu, T. 2021. "Serological evidence of equine infectious anaemia, West Nile fever, surra and equine piroplasmosis in a herd of horses in northern Argentina." *Veterinary Parasitology: Regional Studies and Reports* 24, no. 4: 1-10.

Heinemann, M. B., Cortez, A., Sousa, M. C. C., Gotti, T., Ferreira, F., Homem, V. S. F., Neto, J. S. F., Soares, R. M., Sakamoto, S. M., Cunha, E. M. S. and Richtzenhain, L. J. 2002. " Soroprevalência da anemia infecciosa eqüina, da arterite viral dos eqüinos e do aborto viral eqüino no município de Uruará, PA, Brasil [*Seroprevalence of equine infection anemia, equine viral arteritis and equine viral abortion in Uruará municipality, Pará state, Brazil*]." *Brazilian Journal Veterinary Research Animal Science* 39, no. 1: 50-53.

Heinemann, M. B.; Souza, M. C. C., Cortez, A., Ferreira, F., Homem, V. S. F., Ferreira Neto, J. S., Soares, R. M., Cunha, E. M. S. and Richtzenhain, L. J. 2006. "Soroprevalência da encefalomielite eqüina do Leste e do Oeste no Município de Uruará, PA, Brasil [*Seroprevalence of eastern and western equine encephalomyelitis in the municipality of Uruará, Referencias, PA, Brazil*]." *Brazilian Journal of Veterinary Research and Animal Science* 43:137-139.

Heinen, L. B. S.; Zuchi, N., Serra, O. P., Cardoso, B. F., Godin, B. H. F., Santos, M. A. M., Souto, F. J. D., Paula, D. A. J., Dutra, V. and Slhessarenko, R. D. 2015. "Vírus da encefalite de Saint Louis em Mato Grosso, Centro-Oeste, Brasil [*Saint Louis encephalitis virus in Mato Grosso, central-western Brazil*]." *Revista do Instituto de Medicina Tropical* 57, no. 3(May-June): 215-220.

Henker, L. C., Bandinelli, M. B., Andrade, C. P., Bianchi, M. V., Sonne, L. Driemeier, D., Soares, J. F. and Pavarini, S. P. 2020. "Pathological, immunohistochemical, and molecular findings of equine protozoal myeloencephalitis due to *Sarcoscystis neurona* infection in Brazilian horses." *Tropical Animal Health and Production* 52, no.1 (November): 3809-3818. doi: 10.1007/s11250-020-02419-y.

Henneke, C., A. Jespersen, S. Jacobsen, M. K. Nielsen, F. Mcevoy, and H. E. Jensen. 2014. "The distribution pattern of *Halicephalobus gingivalis* in a horse is suggestive of a haematogenous spread of the nematode." *Acta Veterinaria Scandinavica* 56, no. 1 (September): 1-4.

Herrera, H. M., Dávila, A. M. T., Norek, A., Souza, S. S., D'andrea, P. S. and Jansen, A. M. 2004. "Enzootiology of *Trypanosoma evansi* in Pantanal, Brazil." *Veterinary Parasitologic* 125, no. 3-4 (July): 263-275.

Hirooka, E. Y., Viotti, N. M. A., Marochi, M. A. and Ishii, K. 1990. "Leucoencefalomalácia em equinos do norte do Paraná [*Leukoencephalomalacia in horses from northern Paraná*]. " *Revista de Microbiologia* 21, no. 3 (September): 223-227.

Hirooka, E. Y., Viotti, N. M. A., Soares, L. M. V., and Alfieri, A. A. 1988. "Intoxicação em equinos por micotoxinas produzidas por *Fusarium moniliforme* no norte do Paraná [*Poisoning in horses by mycotoxins produced by Fusarium moniliforme in northern Paraná*]." *Semina* 9, no. 3: 135-141.

Hirooka, E. Y., Yamaguchi, M. M., Aoyama, S., and Sugiura, Y. 1996 "The natural ocurrence of fumonisins in Brazilian corn kernels." *Food Additives & Contaminants* 13, no. 2 (November): 173-183.

Hoane, J. S., Gennari, S. M., Dubey, J. P., Ribeiro, M. C., Borges, A. S., Yai, L. E., Cavalcante, T. C. Bonesi, G. L. and Howe, D. K. 2006. "Prevalence of *Sarcocystis neurona and Neospora spp*. infection in horses from Brazil based on presence of serum antibodies to parasite surface antigen." *Veterinary Parasitology* 136, no. 2 (March): 155-159.

Hoare, C. A. *The Trypanosomes of Mammals. A Zoological Monograph*. 1ª ed. Blackwell Scientific Publications, 5 Alfred Street, Oxford. 79p.

Holz, C. L., Sledge, D. G., Kiupel, M., Nelli, R. K., Goehring, L. S. and Hussey, G. S. 2019. "Histopathologic Findings Following Experimental Equine Herpesvirus 1 Infection of Horses." *Frontiers in Veterinary Science* 6, no. 59 (March): 1-10.

Horta, P. F. P. 1911. "Sobre a epizzotia de "Raiva" observada no Estado de Santa Catarina: morcegos propagadores da Moléstia? [*On the "Rava" epizzotia observed in the State of Santa Catarina: disease propagating bats?*]" *Chácaras e Quintais* 3, no. 6: 4-5.

Horta, P. F. 1911. " A epizootia de .Biguassú – Nota preliminar [*The epizootic of .Biguassú – Preliminary note*]." *O Brazil-Medico* 25, no. 5 :71-74.

Hurst, E. W. and Pawan, J. L. 1931. "An Outbreak of Rabies in Trinidad." *Lancet* 2, no. 2: 622-628.

Ingh, T. S. S. G. A., Binkhorst, G. J., Kimman, T. G., Vreeswijk, J., Pol, J. M. and Oirschot, J. T. 1990. "Aujeszky's disease in a horse." *Journal of Veterinary Medicine* 37, no. 7: 532-538.

Ishizuka, M. M., Miguel, O., and Brogliato, D. F. 1975. "Avaliação da Prevalência de Anticorpos Anti-Toxoplasma em Cavalos PSI Clinicamente Normais [*Evaluation of the Prevalence of Anti-Toxoplasma Antibodies in Clinically Normal PSI Horses*]." *Revista da Faculdade de Medicina Veterinária e Zootecnia da Universidade de São Paulo* 12, no. 3: 289-292.

Iversson, L. B. 1980. "Aspectos da epidemia de encefalite por arbovírus na região do Vale do Ribeira, S. Paulo, Brasil, no período de 1975 a 1978 [*Aspects of the encephalitis epidemic caused by arbovirus in the Ribeira Valley, S. Paulo, Brazil, during 1975-1978*]." *Revista de Saúde Pública* 14, no. 1 (March): 9-35.

Iversson, L. B., Silva, R. A. M. S., Rosa, A. P. A. and Barros, V. L. R. S. 1993. "Circulation of Eastern equine encephalitis, Western equine encephalitis, Ilhéus, Maguari and Tacaiuma viruses in equines of the Brazilian Pantanal, South America." *Revista do Instituto de Medicina Tropical de São Paulo* 35, no. 4 (August):1-2.

James, K. E., Smith, W. A., Packham, A. E., Conrad, P. A. and Pusterla, N. 2017. "*Toxoplasma gondii* seroprevalence and association with equine protozoal myeloencephalitis: A case–control study of Californian horses." *The Veterinary Journal* 224, no. 1: 38-43.

Jansen, K. 1941. " Contribuição ao estudo do mal de cadeiras na Ilha do Marajó [*Contribution to the study of chair disease on Marajó Island*]." *Memórias do Instituto Oswaldo Cruz* 36, no. 3 (November): 347-363

Johnson, A. L., McAdams, S. C. and Whitlock, R. H. 2010. "Type A botulism in horses in the United States: A review of the past ten years (1998–2008)." *Journal of Veterinary Diagnostic Investigation* 22, no. 2(March): 165-173.

Johnson, A. L., McAdams-Gallagher, S. C. and Aceto, H. 2015. "Outcome of adult horses with botulism treated at a veterinary hospital: 92 cases (1989–2013)." *Journal of Veterinary Internal Medicine* 29, no. 1 (November): 311-319.

Johson, A. L., Morrow, J. K. and Sweeney, R. W. 2013. "Indirect Fluorescent Antibody Test and Surface Antigen ELISAs for Ante mortem Diagnosis of Equine Protozoal Myeloencephalitis." *Journal of Veterinary Internal Medicine* 27, no. 3 (May-June): 596-599.

Joubert, L., Oudar, J., Hannoun, C., Beytout, D., Corniou, B. Guilion, J. C. and Panthier, R. 1970. "Epidemiology of the West Nile virus: study of a focus in Camargue. IV. Meningo-encephalomyelitis of the horse." *Annales de l'Institut Pasteur* 118, no. 2: 239-247.

Junco, S. M., Furr, M., Howe, D. K., Johnson, A. L., MacKay, R. J., Pusterla, N. and Witonsky, S. 2016. "Equine Protozoal Myeloencephalitis: An Updated Consensus Statement with a Focus on Parasite Biology, Diagnosis, Treatment, and Prevention." *Journal of Veterinary Internal Medicine* 20, no. 2 (March):491-502.

Kellerman, T. S., Marasas, W. F. O., Pienaar, J. G., Naude, T. W. 1972. "A mycotoxicosis of equidae by *Fusanium moniliforme* Sheldon." *The Onderstepoort Journal of Veterinary Research* 39, no. 1: 205-208.

Kelly, A. P. Jones, R. T., Gillick, J. C. and Sims, L. D. 1984. "Outbreak of botulism in horses." *Equine Veterinary Journal* 16, no. 6: 519-521.

Khusro, A., Aarti, C., Rivas-Caceres, R. R. and Barbosa-Pilego, A. 2020. Equine Herpesvirus-I Infection in Horses: Recent Updates on its Pathogenicity, Vaccination, and Preventive Management Strategies. *Journal of Equine Veterinary Science* 87, no.1: 1-8. doi.org/10.1016/j.jevs.2020.102923.

Kimman, T. G., Binkorst, G. J. Ingh, Ingh, T. S. S. G. A., Gielkens, A. L. and Roevink, M. E. 1991. "Aujeszky's disease in horses fulfils Koch's postulates." *The Veterinary Record* 185, no. 2 (February): 103-106. DOI: 10.1136/vr.128.5.103.

Kinde, H., Bettey, R. L., Ardans, A., Galey, F. D., Daft, B. M., Walker, R. L., and Byrd, J. W. 1991. "Clostridium botulinum Type-C intoxication associated with consumption of processed alfalfa hay cubes in horses." *Journal of the American Veterinary Medical Association* 199, no. 6:742-746.

Koch, M. O., Laskoski, L. M., Aguiar, D. M. Régio, R. R., Ishikura, J. I., Vaz, F. F. and Locatteli-Dittrich, R. 2019. "Detection of antibodies against *Sarcocystis neurona, Neospora caninum and Toxoplasma gondii* in horses, dogs and cat." *Brazilian Journal of Veterinary Research and Animal Science* 56, no. 2: 1-8.

Kommers, G. D., Souza, T. M., Souto, M. A. M., La Corte, F. D. and Barros, C. S. L. 2005 "Criptococose pulmonar granulomatosa em um eqüino [*Granulomatous cryptococcal pneumonia in a horse*]." *Ciência Rural* 34, no. 4 (August): 938-940.

Kotai, I., Peixoto, Z. M. P., Coimbra, T. L. M., Cunha, E. M. S., Cunha, L. H., Queiroz, R., Macruz, R. and Nagamori, A. H. 1992. "Isolamento e identificação do vírus da encefalomielite equina, tipo oriental, em equinos do estado de São Paulo, Brasil [*Isolation and identification of equine encephalomyelitis virus, eastern type, in horses from the state of São Paulo, Brazil*]." *Arquivos do Instituto Biológico* 59, no. ½ (January-December): 37-41.

Kubes, V. and Rios, F. A. 1939. "The Causative Agent of Infectious Equine Encephalomyelitis in Venezuela." *Science* 90, no. 2323: 20–21.

Lara, M. C. C. H., Barros-Filho, I., Viana, F., Gregory, L., Cunha, E. M. S. and Castro, M. 2003. "Pesquisa de anticorpos contra o vírus da arterite equina (EAV) e herpes eqüino tipo 1 (HVE-1) em equinos criados em Curitiba, PR [*Research of antibodies against equine arteritis virus (EAV) and equine herpes type 1 (HVE-1) in horses raised in Curitiba, PR*]." *A Hora de Veterinária* 23, no. 135 (September): 26-28.

Lara, M. C. C. S. H., Beghin, G., Cunha, E. M. S., Villalobos, E. M. C., Nassar, A. F. C. Bello, A. C. P. P., Cunha, A. P., Reis, J. K. P., Leite, R. C. and Mori, E. 2014. "Levantamento sorológico da infecção pelo vírus da encefalomielite equina no estado de Minas Gerais, Brasil [*Serological survey of equine encephalomyelitis virus infection in the state of Minas Gerais, Brazil*]." *Brazilian Journal of Veterinary Research and Animal Science* 51, no. 1:37-41.

Lara, M. C. C. S. H., Cunha, E. M. S., Nassar, A. F. C., Gregory, L., Birgel, E. H. and Fernandes. W. R. 2003. "Ocorrência do herpesvírus eqüino 1 (HVE-1) em cavalos criados no Estado de São Paulo, Brasil (2003) [*Occurrence of equine herpesvirus 1 (EVH-1) in horses bred in the state of São Paulo, Brazil*]." *ARS Veterinaria* 19, no. 3: 254-259.

Lara, M. C. C. S. H., Cunha, E. M. S., Villalobos, E. M. C., Nassar, A. F. C., Asano, K. M., Fernandes, W. R., Richtzenhain, L. J., Brandão, P. E and Mori, E. 2008. "First isolation of equine herpesvirus type 1 from a horse with neurological disease in Brazil." *Arquivo do Instituto Biológico* 75, no.2 (April): 221-224.

Lara, M. C. C. S. H., Torelli, C. S., Cunha, E. M. S., Villalobos, E. M. C., Cunha, M. S., Bello, A. C. P. P., Cunha, A. P., Reis, J. K. P., Leite, R. C. and Mori, E. 2010. "Inquérito sorológico da infecção por herpesvírus equino no Estado de Minas Gerais [*Serological survey of equine herpesvirus infection in Minas Gerais state*]." *Brazilian Journal of Veterinary Research Animal* 47, no. 5: 352-356.

Lara, M. C. C. S. H., Villalobos, E. M. C., Cunha, E. M. S., Oliveira, J. V., Castro, V., Nassar, A. F. C., Silva, L. M. P., Okuda, L. H., Romalndini, A. H. C. N., Cunha, M. S., Marques, E. C. and Mori, E. 2017. "Ocorrência de enfermidades virais em asininos (Equus asinus) no estado de São Paulo, Brasil [*Occurrence of viral diseases in donkeys (*Equus asinus*) in São Paulo State, Brazil*]." *Brazilian Journal of Research Animal Science* 54, no. 2: 154-158.

Lara, M. C. C. S., Furman, K. E., Barros-Filhos, I. V., Villalobos, E. M. C., Cunha, E. M. S., Deconto, I., Bonacim, J. and Biondo, A. W. 2006. "Detection of antibodies against equine viral arteritis virus (EVAV) and equine herpesvirus type 1 (EHV-1) in cart horses from Curitiba and surroundings, southern Brazil." *Archives of Veterinary Science* 6. No. 3: 11-14.

Larangeira, N. L. Ishizuka, M. M. and Hyakutake, S. 1985. "Prevalencia Da Toxoplasmose Equina Avaliada pela Técnica de Imunofluoresncia Indireta, Mato Grosso Do Sul, Brasil [*Prevalence of Equine Toxoplasmosis Assessed by Indirect Immuno-fluorescence Technique, Mato Grosso Do Sul, Brazil*]." *Boletin de La Oficina Sanitaria Panamericana* 99, no. 2: 158-162.

Laskoski, L. M., Muraro, L. S., Dittrich, R. L., Abreu, R. A., Koch, M. O. Silva, F. T. and Hagi, R. H. 2015. "Occurrence of anti-*Neospora caninum* and anti-*Toxoplasma gondii* antibodies in horses in the Pantanal of Mato Grosso, Brazil." *Semina Ciências Agrárias* 36, no. 2 (March): 895-900.

Lemos, K. R., and Alessi, A. C. 1999. "Astrócitos imunorreativos à proteína glial fibrilar ácida (GFAP) em sistema nervoso central de equinos normais e de equinos com leucoencefalomalácia [*Glial fibrillary acidic protein (GFAP) immunoreactive astrocytes in the Central Nervous System of normal horses and horses with leukoencephalomalacia*]." *Pesquisa Veterinária Brasileira* 19, no. ¾ (July-December): 104-108.

Lemos, K. R., Marques, L. C., Aquino, L. P. C. T., Alessi, A. C. and Zacarias, R. Z. 2008. "Astrocytic and microglial response and histopathological changes in the brain of horses with experimental chronic *Trypanosoma evansi* infection." *Revista do Instituto de Medicina Tropical de São Paulo* 50, no. 4 (August): 243-249.

Lemos, K. R., Marques, L., Deaquino, L. P. C. T., Alessia, A. C. and Machado, R. Z. 2007. "Immunohistochemical characterization of mononuclear cells and MHC II expression in the brain of horses with experimental chronic *Trypanosoma evansi* infection." *Revista Brasileira de Parasitologia Veterinária* 16, no. 4 (October):186 -191.

Lennette, E. H. and Fox, J. P. 1942. "Anticorpos neutralizantes para a amostra leste do vírus de encefalomielite equinos em equídeos no Brasil [*Neutralizing antibodies to the equine encephalomyelitis virus eastern sample in equids in Brazil*]." *Memórias do Instituto Oswaldo Cruz* 38, no. 1: 85-92.

Levy, S. Y., Steinman, A., Minderigiu, A., Arieli, O., Savitski, I., Flederovitz, L., edery, N., Schvartz, G. and Mazuz, M. L. 2020. "High Exposure to *Toxoplasma gondii* and *Neospora Spp.* in Donkeys in Israel: Serological Survey and Case Reports." *Animals* 10, no. 10 (March): 1-10.

Lima, E. F., F. Riet-Correa, R. S. Castro, A. A. B. Gomes, and F. S. Lima. 2005. "Sinais clínicos, distribuição das lesões no sistema nervoso e epidemiologia da raiva em herbívoros na região Nordeste do Brasil [*Clinical signs, distribution of the lesions in the central nervous system and epidemiology of rabies in northeastern Brazil*]." *Pesquisa Veterinária Brasileira* 25, no.4 (December): 250-264.

Lima, E. Q. 1934. "A transmissão da raiva dos herbívoros pelos morcegos hematófagos da família *Desmodontidae* [*The transmission of herbivore rabies by vampire bats of the Desmodontidae family*]." *Revista do Departamento Nacional de Produção Animal* 1, no. 1: 165-175.

Lindsay, D. S., Seteinberg, H., Dubielzig, R. R., Semrad, S. D., Konkle, D. M., Milller, P. E. and Biagburn, B. L. 1996. "Central nervous system neosporosis in a foal." *Journal of Veterinary Diagnostic Investigation* 8, no. 1 (October): 507-510.

Lindsey, N. P., Lehman, J. A., Erin, Staples, J. E. and Fischer, M. 2015. "West Nile Virus and Other Nationally Notifiable Arboviral Diseases — United States, 2014." *Morbidity and Mortality Weehly Report* 64, no. 34 (September): 929-934.

Lindströrm, M. and Korkeala, H. 2006. "Laboratory Diagnostics of Botulism." *Clinical Microbiology Reviews* 19, no. 2 (April): 298-314.

Lins, L. A., Feijó, L. S. and Nogueira, C. E. W. 2008. "Mieloencefalite protozoária equina nas regiões da Campanha e do Sul do Rio Grande do Sul no período de 1998-2006 [*Equine protozoal myeloencephalitis in the Campanha and Southern regions of Rio Grande do Sul in the period 1998-2006*]." *Revista de Ciências Agroveterinárias* 11, no.3: 248-250.

Lins, L. A., Frey Junior, F., Berne, M. E. A. and Nogueira, C. E. W. 2008 "Mieloencefalite protozoária equina em equinos de Bagé, Sul do Brasil [*Equine protozoal myeloencephalitis in horses from Bagé, Southern Brazil*]." *Revista Portuguesa de Ciências Veterinárias* 103, no. 1 (December): 177-180.

Locatelli-Dittrich, R., Dittrich, J. R., Richartz, R. R. T. B., Joineau, M. E. G., Antunes, J., Pinckney, R. D., Deconto, I., Hoffmann, D. C. S. and Thomaz-Soccol, V. 2006. "Investigation of *Neospora sp.* and *Toxoplasma gondii* antibodies in mares and in precolostral foals from Parana State, Southern Brazil." *Veterinary Parasitology* 135, no. 3-4 (February): 215-221.

Long, M. T. 2014. "West Nile virus and equine encephalitis viruses: new perspectives." *Veterinary Clinics of North America: Equine Pratice* 30, no. 3 (December): 523-542. doi.org/10.1016/j.cveq.2014.08.009.

Lutz, A. 1907. "Estudo r observações sobre o quebrabunda ou peste de cadeiras [*Study and observations about the cracker or chair pest*]." *Revista da Sociedade Scientifica de São Paulo* 3, no.1 (July):34-58.

Maanen, C. 2002. "Equine herpesvirus 1 and 4 infections: an update." *Veterinary Quarterly* 24, no. 2: 57-78.

MacCallum, W. G. and Buckley, S. S. 1901. Acute epizootic leucoencephalitis in horses. *Journal of Exeperimental Medicine* 6, no. 1: 65-74. 10.1084/jem.6.1.65.

Machado, M., Andrade, L. R., Moraes, D. D. A., Castro, M. B., Neto, A. R. T., Keller, K. M., Soto-Blanco, B. and Câmara, A. C. L. 2018. "Intoxicação por antibióticos ionóforos e leucoencefalomalácia concomitantes pelo consumo de ração comercial contaminada em equinos [*Concurrent Ionophore Poisoning and Leukoencephalomalacia by Consumption of Contaminated Commercial Ration in Horses*]." *Acta Scientiae Veterinarie* 46, no. 336: 1-6.

Macruz, R. 1980. Personal communication. Mayhew, I. G. and Greiner, E. C. 1986. "Doenças Protozoárias [*Protozoal Diseases*]." *Parasitology* 2, no. 2 (August): 439-459.

Macruz, R., Lenci, O., Ishizuka, M. M., Miguel, O. and Cunha, R. A. F. 1975. "Toxoplasmose em equinos psi. Estudo sorológico [*Toxoplasmosis in horses PSI serological study*]." *Revista da Faculdade de Medicina Veterinária e Zootecnia* 12, no. 1 (December): 277-282.

Mallmann, C. A., J. M. Santurio, and P. Dilkin. 1999. "Equine leukoencephalomalacia with ingestion of corn contaminated with fumonisin B_1." *Revista de Microbiologia* 30, no. 1 (July): 249-252.

Marasas W. F. O. 2001. "Discovery and ocorrence or the Fumoisins: a historical perspective." *Environmental Health Perspectives* 109, no. 2 (May): 239-243.

Marasas, W. F., Kellerman, T. S., Gelderblom, W. C., Coetzer, J. A., Thiel, P. G. and Lugt, J. J. V. 1988. "Leukoencephalomalacia in a horse induced by fumonisin B1 isolated from *Fusarium moniliforme*." *The Onderstepoort Journal of Veterinary Research* 55, no. 4: 197-203.

Marcologno-Pereira, C., Silva, P. E., Soares, M. P., Sallis, E. S. V. Greccom F. B., Raffi, M. B., Fernandes, C. G., and Schild, A. L. 2014. "Doenças de equinos na região Sul do Rio Grande do Sul [*Equine diseases in Southern Brazil*]." *Pesquisa Veterinária Brasileira* 34, no. 4 (March): 205-210.

Marques, L. C., Machado, R. Z., Alessi, A. C., Aquino, L. C. P. T., and Pereira, G. T. 2000. "Experimental infection with Trypanosoma evansi in horses: clinicla and haematological observations." *Revista Brasileira de Parasitologia Veterinária* 9, no. 1: 11-15.

Marques, L. C., Machado, R. Z., Alessia, A. C. and Aquino L. P. C. T. 2001. "Humoral immune response of horses experimentally infected with *Trypanosoma evansi*." *Semina Ciências Agrárias* 22, no. 2 (July): 131-133.

Martins, L. C., Silva, E. V. P., Casseb, L. M. N., Silva, S. P., Cruz A. C., Pantoja, J. A. S., Medeiros, D. B. A., Filho, A. J. M., Cruz, E. R. M., Araújo, M. T. F., Cardoso, J. F., Cunha, M. A. C. R., Almada, G. L., Romano, A. P. M., Santos, M. G. D. P., rodrigues, G. A. P. R., Chiang, J. O. Quaresma, J. A. S., Carvalho, V. L. and Vasconcelos, P. F. C. 2019. "First isolation of West Nile virus in Brazil." *Memórias do Instituto Oswaldo Cruz* 11, no.1: 1-7.

Masri, M. D., Alda, J. L., and Dubey. J. P. 1992. "Sarcocystis neurona-associated ataxia in horses in Brazil." *Veterinary Parasitology* 44, no. 3 (October): 311-314. doi.org/10.1016/0304-4017(92)90128-V.

Mattar, S., Edwards, E., Laguado, J., González, M., Alvares, J. and Komar, N. 2005. "West Nile Virus Antibodies in Colombian Horses." *Emerging Infectious Diseases* 11, no. 9 (September): 1497-1498. 10.3201/eid1109.050426.

Mayhew, I. G., De Lahunta A., Whitlock, R. H., and Pollock, R. V. H. 1976 "Equine protozoal myeloencephalitis." *Proceedings of the 22nd Annual Convention of the American Association of Equine Practitioners* 7, (December): 107–114.

Meireles, M. C. A., B. Corrêa, O., Fischman, W. Gambale, C. R. Paula, N. O., Chacon-Reche, and C. R. Pozzi.1994. "Mycoflora of the toxic feeds associated with equine leukoencephalomalacia (ELEM) outbreaks in Brazil." *Mycopathologia* 127, no. 1 (September): 183-188. doi.org/10.1007/BF01102919.

Melandri, V., Guimarães, A. E., Komar, N., Nogueira, M. N., Mondini, A., Sesma, A. F., Alencar, J. and Bosch, I. 2012. "Serological detection of West Nile virus in horses and chicken from Pantanal, Brazil." *Memórias do Instituto Oswaldo Cruz* 107, no. 8 (December): 1073-1075.

Melo, R. M., Cavalcanti, R. C., Villalobos, E. M. C., Cunha, E. M. S., Lara, M. C. C. S. H., and Agiiar, D. M. "Ocorrência de equídeos soropositivos para os vírus das encefalomielites e anemia infecciosa no Estado de Mato Grosso [*The occurrence of equids seropositive for encephalomyelitis and infectious anemia virus in Mato Grosso State, Brazil*]." *Arquivos do Instituto Biológico* 79, no. 2 (May-June): 169-175.

Melo, U. P. and Ferreira, C. 2022. "Clinical findings and response to treatment of 17 cases of tetanus in horses (2012–2021)." *Brazilian Journal of Veterinary Medicine* 44, no. 1 (April): 1-7.

Mendonça, A. O., Cerqueira, E. J. L., Araújo, W. N., Silva, E. M., Shimabukuru, F. H., Sarkis, D. T., Sherlock, I. Langoni, H. 2001. "Inquérito Sorológico para toxoplasmose em equídeos procedentes de duas regiões do estado da Bahia Brasil [*Serological survey toxoplasmosis in equids from two regions of Bahia State, Brazil*]." *Semina Ciências Agrárias* 22, no. 2 (July-December): 115-118.

Merini, L. P. Cormelato, T. C. B. T., Garbade, P., Bueno, F. U., Pedroso, P. M. O. and Carnesella, S. 2010. "Raiva em equino no município de Porto Alegre – RS, Brazil [*Equine rabies in the city of Porto Alegre - RS, Brazil*]." *Acta Scientiae Veterinariae* 38, no. 2: 213-216.

Meyer, K. F., Haring, C. M. and Howitt, B. F. 1931. "The epidemiologic of epizootic encephalomyelitis of horses in the San Joaquin Velley. *Science* 74, no. 1913: 227-228. Doi:10.1126/ science.74.1913.227.

Minami, L. P. G. Meirelles, E. Y. Hirooka, and E. Y. Ono. 2004. "Fumonisinas: efeitos toxicológicos, mecanismo de ação ebiomarcadores para avaliação da exposição [*Fumonisins: toxicological effects, mechanism of action and biomarkers for exposure assessment*]." *Semina* 25, no. 3 (July): 207-224.

Modolo, J. R., Petzoldt, K., Gotts-Chalk, A. F., Margatho, L. F. F., Forlin, W. and Carreira, E. L. C. 1989. "Investigação sorológica do Herpesvirus equi-1 em equinos pelo teste de fixação do complemento, considerações sobre seu uso na saúde do haras [*Serological investigation of Herpesvirus equi-1 in horses by the complement fixation test, considerations about its use in the health of the stud*]." *A Hora Veterinária* 8, no. 8 (March-April): 25-28.

Monath, T. P., Sabattini, M. S., Pauli, R., Daffner, J. F., Mitchell, C. S., Bowen, G. S. and Cropp, C. B. 1985. "Arbovirus investigations in Argentina, 1977-1980. IV. Serologic surveys and sentinel equine program." *The American Journal of Tropical Medicine and Hygiene* 34, no. 5(September): 966-975.

Moraes, C. M., Curcio, B. R., Frey Júnior, F., Ribas, L. M., Nizoli, L. Q. and Nogueira, C. E. W. 2007. "Iinfecção por *Trypanosoma evansi* em equinos no Brasil [*Infection by Trypanosoma evansi in horses from Brazil*]." *Revista Portuguesa de Ciências Veterinária* 102, no. 561: 159-163.

Morales, G. A., Wells, E. A. and Angel, D. 1976. "The capybara (*Hydrochoerus hydrochaeris*) as a reservoir host for *Trypanosoma evansi*." *Journal of Wildilfe Diseases* 12, no. 4 (October): 572-574.

Morales, M. A., Barraguay, M., Fabbri, C., Garcia, J. B., Vissani, A., Trono, K., Guitierrez, G., Pigretti, S., Menchaca, H., Garrido, N., Taylor, N., Fernandez, F. and Enría, D. 2006. "West Nile Virus Isolation from Equines in Argentina, 2006." *Emerging Infectious Diseases* 12, no. 10 (October): 1559-1561.

Moreira, N., Kruher, E. R., Warth, J. G. G., Biesdorf, S. M., Goularte, M. M. M. and Weiss, R. R. 1998. "Aspectos etiológicos e epidemiológicos do aborto equino [*Etiological and epidemiological aspects of equine abortion*]." *Archives Veterinary Science* 3, no. 1: 25-30.

Mori, E., Borges, A. S., Delfiol, D. J. Z., Oliveira-Filho, J. P., Gonçalves, R. C., Cagnini, D. Q., Lara, M. C. C. S. H., Cunha, E. M. S., Villalobos, E. M. C., Nassar, A. F. C., Castro, A. M. M. G., Brandão P. E. and Richtzenhain, L. J. 2011. "First detection of the equine herpesvirus 1 neuropathogenic variant in Brazil." *Revue Scientifque et Techinique* 30, no. 3: 949-954.

Mori, E., Lara, M. C. C. S. H., Cunha, E. M. S., Villalobos, E. M. C., Mori, C. M. C., Soares, R. M., Brandão, P. E., Fernades, W. R., Ritchzenhain, L. J. 2015. "Molecular characterization of Brazilian equid herpesvirus type 1 strains based on neuropathogenicity markers." *Brazilian Journal of Microbiology* 46, no. 1 (June): 565-570.

Mori, E., Mori, C. M. C., Libera, A. M. M. P. D., Lara, M. C. C. S. H. and Fernandes, W. R. 2003. "Evaluation of alveolar macrophage function after experimental infection with equine herpesvirus-1 in horses." *Arquivo Brasileiro de Medicina Veterinária e Zootecnia* 55, no. 3 (June): 1-5.

Moura, A. B., Silva, M. O., Farias, J. A., Neto, A. V., Souza, A. P., Sartor, A. M., Fonteque, J. H., and Bunn, S. 2013. "Antibodies against *Neospora spp.* in horses from two geographic regions of the State of Santa Catarina, Brazil." *Revista Brasileira de Parasitologia Veterinária* 22, no. 4: 597-601.

Nash, D., Mostashari, F., Fine, A., Miller, J., O'Leary, D., Murray, L., Hung, A. Rosenberg, M. D., Wong, S., Campbell, M. D. G. and Layton, M. 2001. "The Outbreak of West Nile Virus Infection in the New York City Area in 1999." *The New England Journal of Medicine* 344, no. 24 (June): 1807-1814.

Neiva, C. 1911"Adolfo Lutz e a Medicina Veterinária [*Adolfo Lutz and Veterinary Medicine*]." *Revista do Instituto Adolfo Lutz* 1, no. 1 :95-114.

Neves, J. F., Queiroz, V. A. V., Costa, R. V., Guimarães, L. J., Mendes, F. F. and Miguel, R. A. 2013. "Atraso na Colheita e Incidência de teores de Fumonisinas Totais em

Grãos de Milho [*Harvest Delay and Incidence of Total Fumonisin Contents in Corn Grains*]." *Seminário de Iniciação Científica* 5, no. 5: 1-4.

Nilson, M. R. and Corrêa, W. M. 1966. "Isolamento do virus do aborto equino no estado de São Paulo [*Isolation of equine abortion virus in the state of São Paulo*]." *Arquivos do Instituto Biológico* 33, no. 3:23-25.

Nilson, M. R. and Sugay, W. 1962. "Ocorrência da encefalomielite eqüina em Itaporanga, estado de São Paulo [*Occurrence of equine encephalomyelitis in Itaporanga, state of São Paulo*]." *Arquivos do Instituto Biológico* 29, no. 7 (April): 64-68.

Nugent, J., Birch-Machin, I., Mumford, J. A., Swann, Z., Newton, J. R., Bowden, R. J., Allen, G. P. and Davis-Poynter, N. 2006. "Analysis of Equid Herpesvirus 1 Strain Variation Reveals a Point Mutation of the DNA Polymerase Strongly Associated with Neuropathogenic versus Nonneuropathogenic Disease Outbreaks." *Journal of Virology* 80, no. 8 (April): 4047-4060.

Nunes, J. S. S. S., Casseb, L. M. N., Guimarães, R. J. P. S.; Reis, W. D. M., Ferreira, M. S., Chiang, J. O., Pinheiro, H. H. C., Vasconcelos, P. F. C. and Cruz, A. C. R. 2021. "Serological evidence of circulation of eastern equine encephalitis in equids in the state of Pará, Brazil." *Revista Brasileira de Medicina Veterinária* 43, no. 1 (March): 1-11.

Nunes, J. T. S., Silva, A. S., Dorneles, F. S., Tonin, A. A., Lazzarotto, C., Miletti, L. C. and Monteiro, S. G. 2012. "Occurrence of *Trypanosoma evansi* in Horses in the State of Minas Gerais, Brazil" *Journal of Equine Veterinary Science* 32, no. 4 (April): 205-207.

Oliveira, M. S., Frota, F. P., Carvalho, M. P., Bersano, P. R. O., Dias, F. E. F., Cavalcante, T. V., Santos, H. D. and Minharro, S. S. 2013. "Frequência de Raiva em herbívoros e humanos no Estado do Tocantins de 1999 a 2010: Relatório Técnico [*Survey of rabies in herbivores and humans in state of tocantins from 1999 to 2010: Technical report*]." *Acta Veterinária Brasilica* 7, no. 3: 180-183.

Oliveira, R. N., Iamamoto, K., Silva, M. L. C. R., Achkar, S. M., Castilho, J. G., Ono, E. D., Lobo, R. S. V., Brandão, P. E., Carnieli, P., Carrieri, M. L., Kotait, I. and Macedo, C. I. 2014. "Eastern equine encephalitis cases among horses in Brazil between 2005 and 2009." *Archives of Virology* 159, no. 5 (May): 2615-2620.

Oliveira-Filho, E. F., Fisher, C., Nerneck, B. S., Carneiro, I. O., Kuhne, A., Campos, A. C. A., Ribas, J. R. L., Netto, E. M., Franke, C. R., Ulbert, S. and Drexler, J. F. 2021. "Ecologic Determinants of West Nile Virus Seroprevalence among Equids, Brazil." *Emerging Infectious Diseases* 27, no. 9 (September): 2466-2470.

Oliveira-Filho, E. F., Oliveira, R. A. S., Ferreira, D. R. A., Laroque, P. O., Pena, L. J., Velença-Montenegro, M. M., Mota, R. A., Gil, L. H. V. G. 2018. "Seroprevalence of selected flaviviruses in free-living and captive capuchin monkeys in the state of Pernambuco, Brazil." *Transboundary and Emerging Diseases* 65, no. 4 (February): 1094-1097.

Ometto, T., Durigon, E. D., Araujo, A., Aprelon, J. R., Aguiar, D. M., Cavalcante, G. T. and Lefrançois T. 2013. "West Nile virus surveillance, Brazil, 2008–2010." *Transactions of The Royal Society of Tropical Medicine and Hygiene* 107, no.14 (September): 723-730.

Ono, E. Y. S., Ono, M. A., Funo, F. Y., Medina, A. E., Oliveira, T. C. R., Kawamura, O., Ueno, Y. and Hirooka, E. Y. 2001. "Evaluation of fumonisin-aflatoxin co-ocorrencie in Brazilian corn hybrids by ELISA." *Food Additives and Contaminants* 18, no. 8: 719-729.

Ono, E. Y. S., Sasaki, E. Y., Hashimoyo, E. H., Hara, L. N., Corrêa, B., Itano, E. N., Sugiura, T., Ueno, Y. and Hirooka, E. Y. 2002. "Post-haverst storage of corn: effext to beginning moisture contente on mycoflora and fumonisin contamination." *Food Additives and Contamination* 19, no. 11: 1081-1090.

Ono, E. Y., Fungaro, M. H. P., Sofia, S. H., Figueira, E. L. Z., Gerage, A. C., Ichinoe, M., Sugiura, Y., Ueno, Y. and Hirooka, E. Y. 2004. "Trends of fumonisin contamination and animal intoxication through monitoring 1991 to 1997 corn crop in the State of Paraná, Brazil." *Mycopathologia* 158, no. 6 (December): 451-455.

Orsi, R. B., Corrêa, B., Possi, C. R., Schammass, E. A., Nogueira, J. R., Dias, S. M. C. and Malozzi, M. A. B. 2000. "Mycoflora and occurence of fumonisins in freshly harvested and stored hybrid maize." *Journal of Stored Products Research* 36, no. 3: 75-87.

Ortiz-Martínez, Y., Vega-Useche, L., Villamil-Gómez, W. E. and Rodriguez-Morales, A. J. 2017. "Saint Louis Encephalitis Virus, another re-emerging arbovirus: a literature review of worldwide research." *Le Infezioni in Medicina*, no. 1: 77-79.

Ostlund, E. N., Crom, R. L., Pedersen, D. D., Johnson, D. J., Williams, W. O. and Schimitt, B. J. 2001. "Equine West Nile encephalitis, United States." *Emerging Infectious Diseases* 7, no. 4 (July-August): 665-669.

Ostrowski, S. R., Kubiski, S. V., Palmero, J., Reilly, C. M., Higgins, J. K., Cook-Cronin, S. and Uzal, F. A. 2012. "An outbreak of equine botulism types A associated with feeding grass clippings" *Journal of Veterinary Diagnostic Investigation* 24, no. 3 (April): 601-603.

Paixão. T. A., Rêgo, I. O. P. and Santos, R. L. 2007. "Anti-*Sarcocystis neurona* immunostaining associated with equine protozoal myeloencephalitis in Brazil." *Ciência Rural* 37, no. 6 (December): 1820-1823.

Pauvolid-Corrêa, A., Campos, Z., Juliano, Velez, R. J., Nogueira, R. M. R. and Komar, N. 2014. "Serological Evidence of Widespread Circulation of West Nile Virus and Other *Flaviviruses* in Equines of the Pantanal, Brazil." *Plos Neglected Tropical Diseases* 8, no. 2 (Februray): 1-11.

Pauvolid-Corrêa, A., Juliano, R. S., Campos, Z., Velez, J., Nogueira, R. M. R., and Komar, N. 2015. "Neutralising antibodies for Mayaro virus in Pantanal, Brazil." *Memórias do Instituto Oswaldo Cruz* 110, no. 1 (February):125-134.

Pauvoloid-Corrêa, A., Morales, M. A., Levis, S., Moraes, S. T., Figueiredo, L. T. M., Couto-Lima, D., Campos, D., Nogueira, M. F., Silva, E. E., Nogueira, R. M. R., Schatzmayr, H. G. 2011. "Neutralising antibodies for West Nile virus in horses from Brazilian Pantanal." *Memórias do Instituto Oswaldo Cruz* 106, no. 4 (June): 467-474.

Pauvolid-Corrêa, A., Tavares, F. N., Costa, E. V., Burlandy, F. M., Murta, M., Pellegrin, A. O., Nogueira, M. F. and. Silva, E. D. 2010. "Serologic evidence of the recent circulation of Saint Louis encephalitis virus and high prevalence of equine encephalitis viruses in horses in the Nhecolândia sub-region in South Pantanal, Central-West Brazil." *Memórias do Instituto Oswaldo Cruz* 103, no. 6 (September): 829-833.

Pearce, S. G., J. A. Bouré, J. A. Taylor, and A. S. Peregrine. 2001. "Treatment of a granuloma caused by *Halicephalobus gingivalis* in a horse." *Journal of the American Veterinary Medical Association* 219, no. 12 (December): 1735-1738.

Pedroso, P. M. O., Colodel, E. M., Gomes, D. C., Varaschin, M. S., Bezerra Júnior, P. S., Barbosa, J. T., Tokarnia, C. H. and Driemeier, D. 2010. "Aspectos clínico-patológicos e imuno-histoquímicos de equídeos infectados pelo vírus da raiva [*Clinic-pathological and immunohistochemical aspects of equids infected with rabies vírus*]." *Pesquisa Veterinária Brasileira* 30, no. 11 (November): 909-914.

Peinado, R. S., Eberle, R. J., Pacca, C. C., Arni, R. K. and Coronado, M. A. 2022. "Review of -omics studies on mosquito-borne viruses of the Flavivirus genus." *Virus Research* 307, no. 3 (Jnuary): 1-18.

Peixoto, Z. M. P., Cunha, E. M. S., Sacramento, D. V. R., Souza, M. C. A. M., Silva, L. H. S., Germano, P. L., Kroeff, S. S. and Kotait, I. 2000. "Rabies laboratory diagnosis: peculiar features of samples from equine origin." *Brazilian Journal of Microbiology* 31, no. 1: 71-75.

Pena, L. J., Pena, D. A., Dale, R., Lamêgo, M. R. A. and Moraes, M. P. 2006. "Levantamento soro-epidemiológico da infecção pelo vírus da Anemia Infecciosa Eqüina, da Influenza Eqüina-2 e do Herpesvírus Eqüino-1 em rebanhos do sul do Estado do Pará, Brasil [*Seroepidemiological survey of infection of equine infectious anemia, equine influenza type 2 and equine herpesvirus type 1 in herds of south Pará State, Brazil*]." *Brazilian Journal of Veterinary Research Animal Science* 43, no.4: 537-542.

Pereira, A. O., Moreira, L. P. and Rojas, E. 1962. "Encefalomielite equina em Conchas, São Paulo, Brasil: incidência de anticorpos inibidores da hemaglutinação no homem e em equídeos [*Equine encephalomyelitis in Conchas, São Paulo, Brazil: incidence of hemagglutination inhibitor antibodies in humans and horses*]." *Revista do Instituto de Medicina Tropical* 4, no. 3 (May-June): 149-151.

Pereira, O. A., Nilson, M. R., W. Sugay and Trapp, E. E. 1964. "Ocorrência da encefalomielite equina em Itaporanga, Estado de São Paulo. II Estudos sorológicos [*Occurrence of equine encephalomyelitis in Itaporanga, State of São Paulo. II Serological studies*]." *Arquivos do Instituto Biológico, São Paulo* 6, no. 1 (January-February):1-4 63-68.

Petersen, L. R., Brault, A. C. and Nasci, R. S. 2013. "West Nile Virus: Review of the literature." *Clinical Review & Education* 310, no. 3 (July): 308-315.

Pierezan, F., D. R. Rissi, R. R. Rech, R. A. Fighera, J. S. Brum, and C. S. L. Barros. 2009. "Achados de necropsia relacionados com a morte de 335 eqüinos: 1968-2007 [*Necropsy findings related to the cause of death in 335 horses: 1968-2007*]." *Pesquisa Veterinária Brasileira* 29, no. 3 (March): 275-280.

Pimentel, L. A., D. M. Oliveira, G. J. N. Galiza, R. O. Rego, A. F. M. Dantas, and F. Riet-Correa. 2009. "Doenças do sistema nervoso central de equídeos no semi-árido [*Diseases of the central nervous system in equidae in the Brazilian semiarid*]." *Pesquisa Veterinária Brasileira* 29, no. 7 (July): 589-597.

Pivoto, F. L., Macêdo-Junior, A. G., Silva, M. V., Ferreira, F. B., Silva, D. A. O., Pompermayer, E., Sangioni, L. A., Mineo, T. W. P. and Vogel, F. S. F. 2014. "Serological status of mares in parturition and the levels of antibodies (IgG) against protozoan family *Sarcocystidae* from their pre colostral foals." *Veterinary Parasitology* 199, no. 1-2 (January): 107-111.

Popoff, M. R. 2020. "Tetanus in animals." *Journal of Veterinary Diagnostic Investigation* 32, no. 2: 184-191.

Porter, M. B., Long, M. T., Getman, L. M., Giguérre, S., Mackay, R. J., Lester, S., Alleman, A. R., Wamsley, H. R., Franklin, R. P., Jacks, S., Buergelt, C. D. and Detrisac, C. 2003. "West Nile Virus encephalomyelitis in horses: 46 cases (2001)." *Journal of the American Veterinary Medical Association* 222, no. 9: 1241-1247.

Póvoas, D. R., Chaves, N. P., Bezerras, D. C., Almeida, V. M. and saraiva, L. Q. 2012. "Raiva em equinos no estado do Maranhão: um estudo retrospectivo [*Rabies in horses in the state of Maranhão: a retrospective study*]." *Revista Brasileira de Ciências Veterinárias* 19, no. 2 (May): 86-89.

Pozzi, C. R., Arcaro, J. R. P., Arcaro Júnior, I. and H. F. B. Corrêa. 2002. "Aspectos relacionados à ocorrência e mecanismo de ação de fumonisinas [*Occurrence and fumonisins pathophisiology-reviews*]." *Ciência Rural* 32, no. 5 (October): 901-907.

Pusterla, N., Hatch, K., Crossley, B., Wademan, C., Barnum, S. and Flynn, K. 2020. "Equine herpesvirus-1 genotype did not significantly affect clinical signs and disease outcome in 65 horses diagnosed with equine herpesvirus-1 myeloencephalopathy." *The Veterinary Journal* 255, no. 1: 1-3.

Pustrela, N. and Hussey, G. S. 2014. "Equine Herpesvirus 1 Myeloencephalopathy." *Veterinary Clinics of North America: Equine practice* 30, no. 3 (December): 489-506.

Queiroz, L. H., Carvalho, C., Buso, D. S., Ferrari, C. I. L. Pedro, W. A. 2009. "Perfil epidemiológico da raiva na região Noroeste do Estado de São Paulo no período de 1 3 a 2007 [*Epidemiological profile of rabies in the northwestern region of São Paulo State, from 1993 to 2007*]." *Revista da Sociedade Brasileira de Medicina Tropical* 42, no. 1:9-14.

Rademaker, V., Herrera, H. M., Raffael. T. R., D'Andrea, P. S., Freitas, T. P. T., Abreu, U. G. P., Hudson, P. J., Jansen, A. M. 2009. "What is the role of small rodents in the transmission cycle of *Trypanosoma cruzi* and *Trypanosoma evansi* (Kinetoplastida Trypanosomatidae)? A study case in the Brazilian Pantanal." *Acta Tropica* 111, no. 2 (August): 102-107.

Ranjithkumar, M., Saravanan, B. C., Yadav, S. C., Kumar, R., Singh, R. and Dey, S. 2014. "Neurological trypanosomiasis in quinapyramine sulfate-treated horses--a breach of the blood-brain barrier?." *Tropical Animal Health and Production* 46, no. 2 (February): 371-377.

Rathore, S. S., Sathiyamoorthy, J., Cheepurupalli, L. and Ramakrishnan, J. 2022. "A holistic review on *Cryptococcus neonformans*." *Microbial Pathogenesis* 166, no. 1(may): 1 -11. doi.org/10.1016/j.micpath.2022.105521.

Reichmann, P., J. A. N. Lisbôa, and R. G. Araújo. 2008. "Tetanus in Equids: A review of 76 cases." *Journal of Equine Veterinary Science* 28, no. 8 (September): 518-523.

Reis-Gomes, A., Marcolongo-Pereira, C., Sallis, E. S., Bruhn, F. R. P., Faria, R. O., Schild, A. L., and Meireles, C. A. 2018. "Epidemiologia de micoses, pitiose e micotoxicoses em equinos no sudeste do Rio Grande do Sul [*Epidemiology of mycoses, pitiosis and micotoxicosis in horses in southeastern Rio Grande do Sul, Brazil*]." *Pesquisa Veterinária Brasileira* 38, no. 6: 110- 116. 10.1590/1678-5150-PVB-5182.

Ribeiro, M. G., G. Nardi Júnior, J. Megid, M. M. J. Franco, S. T. Guerra, F. V. R. Portilho, F. V. R., Rodrigues, S. A. and A. C. Paes. 2018. "Tetanus in horses: an overview of 70 cases." *Pesquisa Veterinária Brasileira* 38, no. 2 (February): 285-293.

Ricketts, S. W., Greet, T. R., Glyn, P. J., Ginnett, C. D., McAllister, E. P., McCaig, J., Skinner, P. H., Webon, P. M., Frape, D. L. and Smith G. R. 1984. "Thirteen cases of botulism in horses fed big bale silage." *Equine Veterinary Journal* 16, no. 5 (November): 515-518.

Riet-Correa, F., Medeiros, R. M. T., Pfister, J., Schild, A. L., Dantas, A. F. M. *Intoxicações por plantas, micotoxinas e substâncias relacionadas na pecuária brasileira* [*Poisonings by plants, mycotoxins and related substances in Brazilian Livestock*]." 2009. 1ª ed. Sociedade Vicente Palloti: Patos. 246p.

Riet-Correa, F., Meirelles, M. C. A., Soares, J. M. and Zambrano, F. 1982. "Leucoencefalomalácia em cavalos associada à ingestão de milho mofado [*Leukoencephalomalacia in horses associated with moldy corn ingestion*]." *Pesquisa Veterinária Brasileira* 2, no. 2: (27-30).

Riet-Correa, F., Rivero, R., Odriozola, E., Adriano, M. L., Medeiros, R. M. T. and Schild, A. l. 2013. "Mycotoxicoses of ruminants and horses." *Journal of Veterinary Diagnostic Investigation* 25, no. 3: 692-708.

Riet-Correa, F., Soares, M. P. and Mendez, M. C. 1998. "Intoxicação em equinos no Brazil [*Intoxitacations in horses in Brazil*]." *Ciência Rural* 28, no. 4: 715-722.

Riley, C. B., Bolton, J. R., Mills, J. N. and Thomas, J. B. 1992. "Cryptococcosis in seven horses." *Australian Veterinary Journal* 69, no. 6 (June): 135–139.

Rissi, D. R., Pierezam, F., Oliveira-Filho, J. C., Lucena, R. B., Carmo, P. M. S. and Barros, C. S. L. 2010. "Abordagem diagnóstica das principais doenças do sistema nervoso de ruminantes e equinos no Brasil [*Diagnostic approaches for the main neurological diseases of ruminants and horses in Brazil*]." *Pesquisa Veterinária Brasileira* 30, no. 1 (November): 958-967.

Rocco, I. M., Santos, C. L. S., Bisordi, I., Petrella, S. M. C. N., Pereira, L. E., Coimbra, T. L. M., Bessa, T. A. F., Oshiro, F. M., Lima, L. B. Q., Cerroni, M. P., Marti, A. T., Barbosa, V. M., Katz, G. and Suzuki, A. 2005. "St. Louis encephalitis vírus: first isolation from a human in São Paulo state, Brazil." *Revista do Instituto de Medicina Tropical* 47, no. 5 (September): 281-285.

Rodrigues, A., Fighera, R. A., Souza, T. M., Schild, A. L. and Barros, C. S. L. 2009. "Neuropathology of Naturally Occurring *Trypanosoma evansi* Infection of Horse." *Veterinary Pathology* 46, no. 1: 251-258.

Rodrigues, A., Fighera, R. A., Souza, T. M., Schild, A. L., Soares, M. P., Milano, J. and Barros C. S. L. 2005. "Surtos de tripanossomíase por Trypanosoma evansi em eqüinos no Rio Grande do Sul: aspectos epidemiológicos, clínicos, hematológicos e patológicos [*Outbreaks of trypanosomiasis in horses by Trypanosoma evansi in the state of Rio Grande do Sul, Brazil: epidemiological, clinical, hematological, and pathological aspects*]." *Pesquisa Veterinária Brasileira* 25, no. 4 (December): 239-249.

Rodrigues, C. M. F., Batista, J. S., Lima, J. M., Freitas, F. J. C., Barros, I. O., Garcia, H. A., Rodrigues, A. C., Camargo, E. P. and Teixeira, M. M. G. 2015. "Field and experimental symptomless infections support wandering donkeys as healthy carriers of *Trypanosoma vivax* in the Brazilian Semiarid, a region of outbreaks of high mortality in cattle and sheep." *Parasites Vectors* 8, no. 564 (October): 1-11. doi: 10.11 86/s13071-015-1169-7.

Rodrigues, E. D. L., Freitas, T. A., Paiva, F. A. S., Pereira, A. S., Coelho, T. F. S. B., Rosa, E. S. T., Casseb, A. R. and Casseb, L. M. N. 2018. "Prevalência de raiva animal no estado do Pará, no período de 2004 a 2013 [*Prevalence of animal rabies in Pará State, Brazil, from 2004 to 2013*]." *Revista Pan-Amazônica de Saúde*, 9, no. 4 (December): 1-6.

Rodrigues, S. G., Otávio, P. O., Araújo, F. A. A., Martins, L. C., Jannifer, O. C., Henriques, D. F., Prazeres, A. S. C., Tavares-Neto, J. and Vasconcelos, P. F. C. 2010. "Epidemiologia do vírus da encefalite Saint Louis na Amazônia brasileira e no Estado do Mato Grosso do Sul, Brasil: elevada prevalência de anticorpos em equinos [*Epidemiology of Saint Louis encephalitis virus in the Brazilian Amazon region and in the State of Mato Grosso do Sul, Brazil: elevated prevalence of antibodies in horses*]." *Revista Pan-Amazônica de Saúde* 1, no.1: 81-86.

Rooney, J. R., Prickett, M. E., Delaney, F. M. and Crowe, M. W. 1970. "Focal myelites-encefalites in horses." *The Cornel Veterinarian* 60, no. 3 (July): 494-501.

Rosa, J. T., Bruno-Lobo, M. and G. Bruno-Lobo. 1961. "Estudos sobre os arbovirus. V. Inquérito sorológico e avaliação da imunidade pós vacinal em eqüinos no Rio de Janeiro [*Studies on arboviruses. V. Serological survey and evaluation of post-vaccination immunity in horses in Rio de Janeiro*]." *Annual Microbiol 9*: 213-228.

Rosa, R., Costa, E. A., Marques, R. E., Oliveira, T. S., Furtini, R., Bomfim, M. R. Q. Teixeira, M. M. A. P. Tatiane, and R. L. Santos. 2013. "Isolation of Saint Louis Encephalitis Virus from a Horse with Neurological Disease in Brazil." *Plos Neglected Trpical Diseases* 7, no. 11 (November): 1-8.

Russell, F. C., Stewart, J. P. and Haig, D. M. 2009. "Malignant catarrhal fever: A review." *The Veterinary Journal* 179, no. 3 (March): 324-335.

Rziha, H. J., Mettenleiter, T. C., Ohlinger, V., Wittmann, G. "Herpesvirus (pseudorabies virus) latency in swine: occurrence and physical state of viral DNA in neural tissues." *Virology* 155, no. 2 (December):600-613.

Salles-Gomes, T. L., Almeida, P. E., Moreira, M., Canola, J. C. and Souza, H. 2003. "Surto de leucoencefalomalácia equina causado por ração comercial com concentração de fumonisina inferior a 10 ppm [*Outbreak of equine leukoencephalomalacia caused by commercial feed with a fumonisin concentration lower than 10 ppm*]." *Ars Veterinária* 19, no. 3:267-271.

Sangoni, L. A., Botton, S. A., Cargnelutti, J. F., Cadore, G. C. Cezar, A. S., Weiblen, R., Lopes, S. T. A. and Vogel, F. S. F. 2011. "Pesquisa de anticorpos anti-Neospora spp. e anti-herpersvírus equino em cavalos de tração no município de Santa Maria, RS, Brasil [*Looking for antibodies anti-Neospora spp. and anti-equine herpersvirus in carter horses in Santa Maria, Brazil*]." *Ciência Rural* 41, no. 2: 321-323.

Sant'ana, F. J. F., Ferreira Júnior, J. A., Costa, Y. L., Resende, R. and Barros, C. S. L. 2012. "Granulomatous meningoencephalitis due to *Halicephalobus gingivalis* in a horse." *Brazilian Journal of Veterinary Pathology* 5, no. 1 (March): 12-15.

Santalucia, S., Castro, J. L. C., Raiser, A. G., Castro, V. S. P., Braseiro, C. R., and Corrêa, L. F. D. 2012. "Uveíte associada à infecção por Trypanosoma evansi em cães no município de Uruguaiana, RS, Brasil [*Uveitis associated with the infection by Trypanosoma evansi in dogs from Uruguaiana, RS, Brazil*]." *Ciência Rural* 42, no. 12 (December): 2225-2228.

Santana, C. H., Oliveira, L. B., Pimentel, S. P., Mendes, B. L. L., Silva, A. P. R. Maranhão, R. P. A., Teixeira, R. B. C. and Ecco, R. 2019. "Granulomatous lesions in multiple organs in a horse caused by *Halicephalobus gingivalis.*" *Brazilian Journal of Veterinary Pathology* 12, no. 3 (November): 111-116.

Santos, A. V. P., Caldas, M. L., Klein Júnior, M. H., Silva, A. L. D. and Cardoso Filho, F. C., 2016. "Raiva em herbívoros no estado do Piauí no período de 2007 a 2011 [*Rabies in herbivores in the state of Piauí during 2007 to 2011*]." *Acta Veterinaria Brasilica* 10, no.3: 224-228.

Santos, C. E. P., Souto, F. S. M., Santurio, J. M. and Marques, L. C. 2013. "Leucoencefalomalácia em equídeos da região Leste de Mato Grosso [*Leukoencephalomacia in Equidae of the Eastern Region of Mato Grosso, Brazil*]." *Acta Scientiae Veterinariae* 41, no. 1119: 1-6.

Santos, M. F. C., Resende, R. M., Sobrinho, R. N. and Vieira, S. 2006. "Diagnóstico laboratorial da raiva no estado de Goiás no período de 1976 a 2001 [*Laboratory Diagnosis of Rabies in the State of Goiás from 1976 to 2001*]." *Ciência Animal Brasileira* 7, no. 1 (March): 77-83.

Schale. S., Howe, D., Yeargan, M., Morrow, J. K. and Graves, A. 2018. "Protozoal coinfection in horses with equine protozoal myeloencephalitis in the eastern United States." *Journal Veterinary Internal Medicine* 32, no. 3 (May):1210-1214.

Schawarz, D. G. G., Barreto, F. M., Branco, M. A. C., Marinho, F. L. O., Farias, M. P. O., Monteiro, H. M. A., Castro, R. J. S. and Tolentino, M. L. D. L. 2020. "Raiva em equino na região Sul do estado do Piauí [*Equine rabies in the Southern region of Piauí State*]." *Acta Scientiae Veterinarie* 48, no. 538: 1-5.

Schimidt, J. R. and Mansoury, H. K. 1963. "Natural and experimental infection of Egyptian Equines with West Nile Virus." *Annals of Tropical Medicine & Parasitology* 57, 4: 415-427. doi.org/10.1080/00034983.1963.11686194.

Schoenbaum, M. A., Hall, S. M., Glock, R. D., Grant, K., Jenny, A. L., Schiefer, T. J. and Whitlock, R. H. 2000. "An outbreak of type C botulism in 12 horses and a mule." *Journal of the American Veterinary Medical Association* 217, no. 3: 365-368.

Scoot T. P. and Nel, L. H. 2021. "Lyssaviruses and the fatal encephalitic disease rabies." *Frontiers in Immunology* 12, no. 1 (December): 1-7.

Seidl, A. F., Moraes, A. S. and Silva, R. A. 2001. "*Trypanosoma evansi* control and horse mortality in the Brazilian Pantanal." *Memórias do Instituto Oswaldo Cruz* 96, no. 5 (July): 599-602.

Seidl, A., Moraes, A. S., R. Aguilar, and Silva M. S. S. 1995. "A financial analysis of treatment strategies for *Trypanosoma evansi* in the Brazilian Pantanal." *Preventive Veterinary Medicine* 33, no. 1 (January): 219-234. doi: 10.1016/s0167-5877(97)00 049-4.

Seiler, R. J., Omar, S. and Jackson, A. R. 1981. "Menigoencephalitis in naturally ocurring *Trypanosoma evansi* infection (surra) of horses." *Veterinary Pathological* 18, no. 1: 120-122.

Shnaiderman-Torban, A., Elad, D., Kelmer, G., Avni, G., Shalit, U. and Steinman, A. 2018. "An outbreak of equine botulism type D in Israel." *Equine Veterinary Education* 30, no. 11 (January): 594-597. doi.org/10.1111/eve.12725.

Shope, R. E., Andrade, A. H. P., Bensabath, G., Causey, O. R. and Humphrey, P. S. 1966. "The epidemiology of EEE, WEE, SLE and Turlock viruses, with special reference to birds, in a tropical rain forest near Belém, Brazil." *American Journal of Epidemiology* 84, no. 3 (November): 467 – 477.

Shope, R. E., Causey, O. R., Andrade, A. H. P., and Theiler, M. 1964. "The Venezuelan equine encephalomyelitis complex of group A arthropod-borne viruses including Mucambo and Pixina from the Amazon region of Brazil." *American Journal of Tropical Medicine and Hygiene* 13, no. 5 (September): 723-727.

Siconelli, M. J. L., Jorge, D. M. M., Castro-Jorge, L. A., Fonseca-Junior, A. A., Nascimento, M. L. Floriano, V. G., Souza, F. R., Querioz-Júnior, E. M., Camargos, M. F., Costa, E. D. L., Carvalho, A. A. B. and Fonseca, B. A. L. 2021. "Evidence for current circulation of an ancient West Nile virus strain (NY99) in Brazil." *Revista da Sociedade Brasileira de Medicina Tropical* 54, no. 2: 1-5.

Silva, A. A., Cunha, E. M. S., Lara, M. C. C. S. H., Villalobos, E. M. C., Nassar, A. F. C., Mori, E., Zanuzzi, C. N. Mônica, C. and Fava, C. D. 2018. "Low occurrence of equine herpesvirus 1 (EHV-1) as cause of abortion and perinatal mortality in Brazil." *Arquivos do Instituto Biológico* 85, no. 1: 1-7.

Silva, A. A., Stelmann, U. J. P., Papap, J. P., Fonseca, E. F., Ignácio, F. S., Ferreira, J. C., Farreira, J. C., Ribeiro Filho, J. D. 2010. "Administração intratecal e intravenosa de antitoxina tetânica para tratamento de tétano em equino: relato de caso [*Intrathecal and intravenous tetanus antitoxin administration for the treatment of tetano in a horse: case report*]." *Revista Científica Eletrônica de Medicina Veterinária* 8, no. 14 (January):1-11.

Silva, A. P., Villalobos, E. M. C., Cunha, E. M. S., Lara, M. C. C. S. H., Nassar, A. F. C., Piatti, R. M., Castro, V., Pinheiro, E. S., Carvalho, A. F. and Fava, C. D. 2020. "Causes of equine abortion, stillbirth, and perinatal mortality in Brazil." *Arquivos do Instituto Biológico* 87, no.1: 1-9.

Silva, A. S. G., Matos, A. C. D., Cunha, M. A. C. R., Vrehfeld, I. S., Galinari, G. C. F. Marcelino, S. A. C. L., Saraiva, L. H. G., Martins, N. R. S., Maranhão, R. P. A., Lobato, Z. I. P., Pierezan, F., Guedes, M. I. M. C. and Costa, E. A. 2018. "West Nile virus associated with equid encephalitis in Brazil, 2018." *Transboundary and Emerging Diseases* 66, no. 1 (January): 445-453. 10.1111/tbed.13043.

Silva, A. S., Neto, O. A. S. A., Costa, M. M., Wolkmer, P., Mazzantti, C. M., Santurio, J. M., Lopes, S. T. A. and Monteiro, S. G. 2010. "Tripanossomose em equinos na região sul do Brasil [*Trypanosomosis in equines in southern Brazil*]." *Acta Scientiae Veterinariae* 38, no. 2: 113-120.

Silva, A. S., Oliveira, C. B., Zanette, R. A., Soares, C. M. D., Polenz, G. H., Santurio, J. M., and Monteiro, G. S. 2007. "Ocorrência de Trypanosoma evansi em bovinos de uma propriedade leiteira no município de Videira - SC, Brasil [*Occurrence of Trypanosoma evansi in bovines from a dairy farm in the municipality of Videira - SC, Brazil*]." *Acta Scientiae Veterinarea* 35, no. 3: 373-379.

Silva, E. M. C., Pinto, C. S., Rosa, T. D. S., Braga, M. S. C., Martins, N. S. Oliveira, R. A., Santos, H. P., Carvalho Neta, A. V., Ribeiro, D. L. S. and Santos, L. S. 2019. "Estudo retrospectivo da raiva em herbívoros e animais silvestres no estado do Maranhão [*Retrospective Study of Rabies in Herbivores and Wild Animals in the State of Maranhão*]." *ARS Veterinária* 35, no. 2: 56-62.

Silva, J. A., Dominicano, T. O., Montão, D. P., Sousa, P. G. S., Ramos, L. L., Paredes, L. J. A., Monteiro, S. G., Rivero, G. R. C., Scofield, A., Bezerra Júnior, P., Bezerra, I. A. and Cerqueira, V. D. 2016. "Reemerging of natural infection by *Trypanosoma evansi* in horses in Arari, Marajó Island, Brazil." *Ciência Rural* 46, no. 12 (December): 2170-2176.

Silva, J. R., Medeiros, L. C., Reis, V. P., Chavez, J. H., Munhoz, T. D., Borges, G. P., Soares, O. A. B., Campos, C. H. C., Machado, R. Z., Baldani, C. D., Silva, M. L. C. R., Faria, J. L. M., Silva, E. E. and Figueiredo, L. T. M. 2013. "Serologic survey of West Nile virus in horses from Central-West, Northeast and Southeast Brazil." *Memórias do Instituto Oswaldo Cruz* 108, no. 7 (November): 921-923.

Silva, J. R., Romeiro, M. F., Souza, M. W., Munhoz, T. D. Borges, G. P. Soares, O. A. B., Campos, C. H. C., Machado, R. Z., Silva, M. L. C. R., Faria, J. L. M., Chávez, J. H. and Figueiredo, L. T. M. 2014. "A Saint Louis encephalitis and Rocio virus serosurvey in Brazilian horses." *Revista Brasileira de Medicina Tropical* 47, no. 4 (July): 414-417.

Silva, L. P., Pinto, A. P. V. B., Pontes, A. N. and Bichara, C. N. C. 2020. "Epidemiologia da raiva em herbívoros domésticos em uma localidade na Amazônia brasileira [*Epidemiology of rabies in domestic herbivores in a locality in the Brazilian Amazon*]." *Revista Ibero Americana de Ciências Ambientais* 11, no. 3: 105-112.

Silva, M. L. C. R., Auguste, A. J., Terzian, A. C. B., Vedovello, D., Riet-Corrêa, F., Marcário, V. M. K. 2015. "Isolation and Characterization of Madariaga Virus from a Horse in Paraíba State, Brazil." *Transboundary and Emerging Diseases* 64, no. 3 (June): 990-993. doi.org/10.1111/tbed.12441.

Silva, M. L. C. R., Galiza, G. J. N., Dantas, A. F. M., Oliveira, R. N., Iamamoto, K. Achkar, S. M. and F. Riet-Correa. 2011. "Outbreaks of Eastern equine encephalitis in northeastern Brazil." *Journal of Veterinary Diagnostic Investigation* 23, no. 3 (June): 570-575.

Silva, R. A. M. S., Arosemena, N. A. E., Herrera, H. M., Sahib C. A. and M. S. J. Ferreira. 1995. "Surto de tripanossomose por *Trypanosoma evansi* em cavalos do Pantanal Mato-grossense, Brasil [*Outbreak of trypanosomiasis by Trypanosoma evansi in horses from the Pantanal Mato Grosso, Brazil*]." *Veterinary Parasitologic* 60, no. 1 (November): 167-171. doi.org/10.1590/S0100-736X2005000400010.

Silva, R. A. M. S., Barros, A. T. M. and Herrera, H. M. 1995. "Surtos de tripanossomose por *Trypanosoma evansi* no Pantanal, Brasil. Uma abordagem preliminar dos fatores de risco [*Outbreaks of trypanosomiasis in horses by Trypanosoma evansi in the state of Rio Grande do Sul, Brazil: epidemiological, clinical, hematological, and pathological aspects*]." *Revue d'Élevage Médicine Vétrinarie Pays Tropicaux* 4, no. 1: 315-319.

Silva, R. A. M. S., Herreira, H. M., Domingos, L. B. S., Ximenes, F. A. and Dávila, A. M. 1995. "Pathogenesis of *Trypanosoma evansi* infection in dogs and horses: hematological and clinical aspects." *Ciência Rural* 25, no. 2: 233-238.

Silva, R. A. M. S., Seidl, A., Ramirez, L. and Dávila, A. M. R. 2002. *Trypanosoma evansi e Trypanosoma vivax: biologia, diagnóstico e controle* [*Trypanosoma evansi and Trypanosoma vivax: biology, diagnosis and control*]." Corumbá: Embrapa Pantanal, 2002.

Silva, R. A., Silva, N. M. and Menezes, P. R. V. 1974. "Ocorrência dos vírus da raiva na medula e no bulbo de equinos na doença natural e sua ausência nas diferentes regiões do sistema nervoso central e outros tecidos [*Occurrence of rabies viruses in the bone marrow and bulb of horses in natural disease and their absence in different regions of the central nervous system and other tissues*]." *Pesquisa Agropecuária Veterinária* 9, no. 1:29-31.

Simpson, C. F., Mayhew, I. G. 1980. "Evidence for *Sarcocystis* as the etiologic agent of equine protozoal myeloencephalites." *Journal Protozoal* 27, no. 1: 288-292.

Siqueira, R. F., Hansen, V. S., Martins, M. F. M., Leal, M. L. R. and Bondan, E. F. 2022. "Infecção pelo vírus da Febre do Nilo Ocidental em equinos no Estado de São Paulo [*West Nile Fever Virus Infection in Horses in São Paulo State, Brazil*]." *Acta Scientiae Veterinarie* 50, no. 1: 1-6. doi.org/10.22456/1679-9216.117796.

Smithburn, K. C., Hughes, T. P., Burke, A. W. and Paul, J. H. 1940. "A Neurotropic Virus Isolated from the Blood of a Native of Uganda." *The Amercian Journal of Tropical Medicine and Hygiene* 1, no. 4: 471-492.

Sousa, S. H., Teixeira Neto, R. A. L., Leonardo, A. C., Câmara, A. C. L. and Castro, M. B. 2018. "Neurological Changes in Horses Naturally Infected with *Halicephalobus gingivalis*." *Journal of Equine Veterinary Science* 60, no. 1 (January): 1-5. doi.org/10.1016/j.jevs.2017.10.006.

Sousa, S. K. H. 2013. "Doenças neurológicas em equinos do Distrito Federal e Goiás estudo retrospectivo (2003-2013) [*Neurological diseases in horses from the Federal District and Goiás retrospective study (2003-2013)*]." *Trabalho de conclusão de curso*. Universidade de Brasília – UnB. 65p.

Sousa, S. K. H., Sonne, L., Sant'Ana, F. J. F., Rels Júnior, J. L. 2015. "Encefalomielite equina do Leste no Distrito Federal e entorno [*Eastern Equine Encephalitis on Federal District of Brazil and Surrounding Areas*]." *Acta Scientiae Veterinariae* 43, no. 1268 (April):1-7.

Souza, P. G., Amaral, B. M. P. M. and Gitti, C. B. 2015. "Raiva animal na cidade do Rio de Janeiro: emergência da doença em morcegos e novos desafios para o controle [*Animal rabies in the city of Rio de Janeiro: emergence of the disease in bats and new challenges for control*]." *Revista do Instituto Adolfo Lutz* 73, no. 1: 119-124.

Souza-Lopes, O. and Sacchetta, L. A. 1978. "Isolation of Mucambo virus, a member of the venezuela equine encephalitis virus complex in the state of São Paulo." *Revista do Instituto de Medicina Tropical* 20, no. 2 (March): 82- 88.

Spohr, K. A. H., Borges, A. M. C. M., Ribeira, T. M. P., Jayme, V. S., Godoy, I., Nakazato, L., Dutra, V. and Aguiar, D. M. 2018. "Fatores de risco associados à prevalência de anticorpos anti-*Sarcocystis neurona*, *Neospora spp*. e *Toxoplasma gondii* em equinos de Roraima, Amazônia [*Risk factors associated to the prevalence of anti-Sarcocystis neurona, Neospora spp. and Toxoplasma gondii antibodies in horses from Roraima, Brazilian Amazon*]." *Pesquisa Veterinária Brasileira* 38, no. 7 (July): 1337-1343.

Stelmann, U. J. P. and Amorim, R. M. 2010. "Mieloencefalite protozoária equina [*Equine protozoal myeloencephalitis*]." *Veterinária e Zootecnia* 17, no. 2 (June): 163-176.

Stelman, U. J. P., Silva, R. C., Langoi, H., Borges, A. S. and Amorim, R. M. 2011. "Anticorpos contra *Toxoplasma gondii* em equinos com histórico de ataxia [*Antibodies Against* Toxoplasma Gondii *in Horses with History of Ataxia*]." *Revista Brasileira de Medicina Veterinária* 32, no. 4: 200-2002.

Stelmann, U. J. P., Ullmann, L. S., Langoni, H., Amorim, R. M. 2011. "Equine neosporosis: search for antibodies in cerebrospinal fluid and sera from animals with history of ataxia." *Revista Brasileira de Medicina Veterinária* 33, no. 2: 99-102.

Svoboda, W. K., Martins, L. C., Malanski, L. S., Shiozawa, M. M., Sphor, K. A. H., Hilst, C. L. S., Aguiar, L. M., Ludwing, G., Passos, F. C., Silva, L. R., Headley, S. A. and Navarro, I. T. 2014. "Serological evidence for Saint Louis encephalitis virus in free-ranging New World monkeys and horses within the upper Paraná River basin region, Southern Brazil." *Revista da Sociedade Brasileira de Medicina Tropical* 47, no. 3 (May): 280-286.

Sydenham, E. W., Marasas, W. F. O., Shephard, G. S., Thiel, P. G. and Hirooka, E. Y. 1992. "Fumonisin Concentrations in Brazilian Feeds Associated with Field Outbreaks of Confirmed and Suspected Animal Mycotoxicoses." *Journal of Agricultural and Food Chemistry* 40, no. 1: 994-997.

Taylor, K. and Paessler, S. 2013. "Pathogenesis of Venezuelan equine encephalitis." *Veterinary Microbiology* 167, no. 1-2 (November): 145-150.

Taylor, R. M., Work, T. H., Hurlbut, H. S., Rizk, F. 1956. "A study of the ecology of West Nile virus in Egypt." *American Journal of Tropical Medicine* 5, no. 4: 579-620.

Teixeira, L. A., Sandoval, M. R. C. and Takaoka, N. Y. 2004. "Instituto Pasteur de São Paulo: cem anos de combate à raiva [*Pasteur Institute of São Paulo: 100 years of fighting rabies*]." *História Ciência e Saúde* 11, no 3 (September-December): 751-766

Teixeira, R. B. C. T., Amorim, R. M., Borges, A. S., Gonçalves, R. C. and Chiachio, S. B. 2006. "Mieloencefalate Protozoária Equina – estudo de 10 casos [*Equine Protozoal Myeloencephalitis – Study of 15 cases*]." *Annual Conference of ABRAVEQ*, no. 1: 125-126.

Teixeira, T. F., Holz, C. L., Caixeta, S. P. M. B., Dezen, D., Cibulski, S. P., Silva, J. R., Rosa, J. C. A., Schimdt, E., Ferreira, J. C., Batista, H. B. C. R., Caldas, E., Franco, A. C. and Roehe, P. M. 2007. "Diagnóstico de raiva no Rio Grande do Sul, Brasil, de 1985 a 2007 [*Rabies diagnosis in the state of Rio Grande do Sul, Brazil, from 1985 to 2007*]." *Pesquisa Veterinária Brasileira* 28, no. 10(october): 515-520.

Ten Broeck, C., and Merrill, M. H. 1933. "A serological difference between and western equine encephalomyelitis virus." *Proceedings of the Society for Experimental Biology and Medicine* 31, no. 1 (November): 217-220.

Thiel, P. G., Shephard, G. S., Sydenham, E. W., Marasas, F. O., Nelson, P. E. and Terrance, M. W. 1991. "Levels of fumonisins B1 and B2 in feeds associated with confirmed cases of equine leukoencephalomalacia." *Jounal of Agriculture and Food Chemical* 39, no. 1 (January): 109-110. doi.org/10.1021/jf00001a021.

Torquato, R. B., K. Iamamoto, E. R. Fernandes, S. Achkar, S. R. Silva; I. S. S. Katz, and F. Guedes. 2020. "Detection of rabies virus antigen by the indirect rapid immunohistochemistry test in equines and comparisons with other diagnostic techniques." *Zoonoses and Public Health* 67, no. 6 (September): 651-657. 2020.

Torres, S. and Lima, E. Q. 1934. "Morcegos da família *Desmodontidae* e sen papel na trans-missáo de molestias aos animais [*Bats of the Desmodontidae family and their role in transmitting diseases to animals*] " *Revista do Departamento Nacional de Produção Animal* 1, no. 1: 25-40.

Trock, S. C., Meade, B. J., Glaser, A. L., Ostlund, E. N., Lanciotti, R. S., Cropp, B. C., Kulasekera, V., Kramer, L. D. and Komar 2001. "West Nile Virus Outbreak Among Horses in New York State, 1999 and 2000." *Emerging Infectious Diseases* 7, no. 4 (August): 745-748.

Tyska, D., Mallmann, A. O., Simões, C. T., Silva, C. R., Gressler, L. T. and Mallman, C. A. 2022. "Prediction of fumonisins B1 and B2 in corn distiller's dried grains with solubles through near-infrared reflectance spectroscopy." *Journal of The Science of Food and Agriculture*, no. 2 (February): 1-6. doi.org/10.1002/jsfa.11806.

U. S. Treasury Department, Public Health Service, Public Health Bull. 1935. *Report on the St. Louis outbreak of encephalitis.* no. 214, 944p.

Uzal, A. F., Navarro, M. A., Asin, J. and Henderson, E. E. 2022. "Clostridial diseases of horses: a review." *Vaccines* 10, no. 1 (February):1-21.

Valença, S. R. A., Andrade, M. R., Moré, G., Albuquerque, P. P. F., Pinheiro-Júnior, J. W. and Mota, R. A. 2019. "Low prevalence of infection by *Sarcocystis neurona* in horses from the State of Alagoas, Brazil." *Revista Brasileira de Parasitológica Veterinária* 28, no. 2 (April-June): 298-302.

Valim, A. C., Roncati, N. V., Costa, A. M. D., Ribeiro, T. F., Andrade, D. G. A. Amorim, R. M., and Borges, A. S. 2022. "Surto de Botulismo: primeira descrição da toxina D em Equinos no Brasil [*Botulism outbreak: first description of type D toxin in horses in Brazil*]." *Proceedings of the Annual Conference of ABRAVEQ* 2022, no. 1: 178-188.

Vargas, A. C. and Weiblen R. 1991. "Prevalência de anticorpos contra herpesvírus equino tipo -1 (HVE 1) em equinos de alguns municípios do Rio Grande do Sul [*Prevalence of antibodies against equine herpesvirus type -1 (HVE 1) in horses from some municipalities in Rio Grande do Sul*]." *A Hora Veterinária* 10, no. 59 (January): 5-8.

Vargas, E. A., Preis, R. A., Castro, L. and Silva, C. M. G. 2001. "Co-occurrence of aflatoxins B 1, B 2, G 1, G 2, zearalenone and fumonisin B 1 in Brazilian corn." *Food Additives and Contaminants* 18, no. 11 (November): 981–986.

Vasconcelos, P. F. C., Rosa, J. F. T., Rosa, A. P. A. T., Dégallier, N., Pinheiros, F. P. and Sá Filho, G. C. "Epidemiologia das Encefalites por Arbovirus na Amazônia Brasileira [*Epidemiology of arbovirus encephalitis in the Brazilian Amazon*]." *Revista do Instituto de Medicina Tropical* 33, no. 6 (December): 465-476.

Vasconcelos, R. O., Lemos, K. R., de Moraes J. R. E. and V. P. Borges. 2007. "*Halicephalobus gingivalis (H.deletrix)* in the brain of a horse." *Ciência Rural* 37, no. 4 (August): 1185-1187.

Vedovello, D., Drumound, B. P., Marques, R. E., Ullmann, L. S., Fávaro, E. A., Terzian, A. C. B., Figueiredo, L. T. M., Teixeira, M. M., Araújo-Júnior, J. P. and Nogueira, M.

L. 2015. "First genome sequence of St. Louis encephalitis virus (SLEV) isolated from a human in Brazil." *Archives of Virology* 160, no. 1 (March): 1189-1195.

Velasco-Villa, A., Mauldin, M. R., Shi, M., Escobar, L. E., Gallardo-Romero, N. F., Damon, I., Olson, V. A., Streicker, D. G. and Emerson. G. 2017. "The history of rabies in the Western Hemisphere." *Antiviral Research* 146, no. 1 (October): 221-232.

Vendruscolo, C. P., Frias, N. C., Carvalho, C. B., Sá, L. R. M., Beli, C. B. and Baccarin, R. Y. A. 2016. "Leuloencephalomalacia outbreak in horses due to consumption of contaminated hay." *Journal of Veterinary Internal Medicine* 30, no. 6 (November): 1879-1881. 10.1111/jvim.14588.

Vereecke, N., Carnet, F., Pronost, S., Vanchandevijl, K., Theuns, S. and Nawynck, H. 2021. "Genome Sequences of Equine Herpesvirus 1 Strains from a European Outbreak of Neurological Disorders Linked to a Horse Gathering in Valencia, Spain, in 2021." *Microbiology Resource Announcements* 10, no. 20 (December): 1-4.

Vidotto, O., Kano, F. S., Freire, R. L., Mitsuka, R., Ogawa, L. Boesi, G., Navarro, I. T. and Franciscon, F. S. G. 1997. "Ocorrência de anticorpos *anti-Toxoplasma gondi* em equinos procedentes de quarto estados (SP,PR.MS e MT) abatidos em Apucara, PR [*Occurrence of anti-*Toxoplasma gondii *antibodies in horses from four states (SP, PR, MS and MT) slaughtered in Apucarana, PR*]." *Semina Ciências Agrárias* 18, no. 1: 9-13.

Vieira, A., Kotait, I., Hardet, L., Kawai, J. G. C. and Takaoka. 2014. " Os desafios do controle da raiva e de outras encefalites [*The challenges of managing rabies and other encephalitis*]." *BEPA* 11 no. 121: 11-20.

Vieira, M. A. C. S., Romano, A. P. M., Borba, A. S., Silva, E. V. P., Chiang, J. O. and Azevedo, R. S. S. 2015. "West Nile Virus Encephalitis: The First Human Case Recorded in Brazil." *The American Journal of Tropical Medicine and Hygiene* 93, no. 2 (August): 377-379. 10.4269/ajtmh.15-0170.

Villalobos, E. M. C., Fruman, K. E., Lara, M. C. C. S. H., Cunha, E. M. S., Dedo, M. A., Busch, A. P., Barros-Filho, I. R., deconto, I., Dornbusch, P. T. and Biondo, A. W. 2012. "Detection of *Neospora* sp. antibodies in cart horses from urban areas of Curitiba, Southern Brazil." *Revista Brasileira de Parasitologia Veterinária* 21, no. 1 (January): 68-70.

Wada, M. Y., Rocha, S. M. and Maia-Elkahoury, A. N. S. 2011. "Situação da Raiva no Brasil, 2000 a 2009 [*Rabies situation in Brazil, 2000 to 2009*]." *Epidemiologia e Serviço de Saúde* 20, no. 4 (October): 509-518.

Weber, M. N., Mosena, A. C. S., Baumbach, L. F., Silva, M. S. Canova, R., Santos, D. L. R., Budaszwski, R. F., Oliveira, L. O., Soane, M. M., Saraiva, N. B., Belluco, F. T., Mazurek, B. A., Dihel, G. N., Gil, L. H. V. G., Borba, M. R., Coberlinni, L. G. and Canal, C. W. 2021. "Serologic evidence of West Nile virus and Saint Louis encephalitis virus in horses from Southern Brazil." *Brazilian Journal of Microbiology* 52, no. 2 (June): 1-11, 2021. doi.org/10.1007/s42770-021-00474-7.

Webster, L. T. and Fite G. L. 1933. "A virus encountered in the study of material from cases of encephalitis in the St. Louis and Kansas City epidemics of 1933." *Science* 78, no. 1:463-465.

Weiblen, R., Rabuske, M., Rebelato, M. C., Nobre, V. M. and Canabarro, T. F. 1994. "Abortion due to equine herpesvirus in southern Brazil." *Brazilian Journal of Medical and Biological Research* 27, no. 6 (June): 1317-1320.

Whitlock, R. and McAdams, S. 2006. "Equine Botulism." *Clinical Techinical Equine Pratice* 5, no. 1: 37-42.

Wilson, B. J. and Maronpot, R. R. 1971. Causative fungus agent of leucoencephalomalacia in equine animals. *Veterinary Records* 88, no. 1: 484-486.

Wilson, W. D. 1997. "Equine Herpesvirus 1 Myeloencephalopathy." *Veterinary Clinics of North America: Equine Pratice* 13, no. 1:53-72.

Xavier, J. G., Brunner, C. H. M., Sakamoto, M., Correa, B., Fernandes, W. R. and Dias, J. L. C. 1991. "Leucoencefalomalacia equina: relato de cinco casos [*Equine Leukoencephalomalacia: a report of five cases*]." *Brazilian Journal Veterinary Research Animal Science* 28, no. 2: 185-189.

Zanette, R. A. and Silva, G. M. 2009. "Aceturato de diminazeno no tratamento de eqüinos infectados naturalmente por *Trypanosoma evansi* no município de Cruz Alta - RS, Brasil [*Diminazene Aceturate in the Treatment of Horses Naturally Infected by Trypanosoma Evansi in the Municipality of Cruz Alta - RS, Brazil*]." *Medicina Veterinária e Zootecnia* 16, no. 1: 74-79.

Zanette, R. A., Silva, A. S., Costa, M. M., Monteiro, S. G., Santurio, J. M. and Lopes, S. T. A. 2008. "Ocorrência de Trypanosoma evansi em eqüinos no município de Cruz Alta, RS, Brasil [*Occurrence of* Trypanosoma evansi *in equines in Cruz Alta, RS, Brazil*]." *Ciência Rural* 38, no. 5 (August): 1468-1471.

Zimmerman, J. J., Karriker, L. A., Ramirez, A., Schwartz, K. J., Stevenson, G. W. and Zhang, J. 2019. "*Diseases of Swine || Herpesviruses.*" 548–575.

Zoppa, A. L. V., Crispim, R., Sinhorini, I. L., Benites, N. R., Silva, L. C. L. C. and Baccarin, R. Y. A. 2008. "Obstrução nasal por granuloma fúngico em eqüino: relato de caso [*Nasal obstruction caused by fungal granuloma in a horse: case report*]." *Arquivo Brasileiro de Medicina Veterinária e Zootecnia* 60, no. 2(April): 315-321.

Index

A

B

C

D

E

F

T

U

V

W

Editor's Contact Information

Selwyn Arlington Headley, DVM, MSc, PhD
Professor
Laboratory of Animal Pathology,
Department of Veterinary Preventive Medicine,
State University of Londrina, Paraná, Brazil
selwyn.headley@uel.br

List of Contributors

Amorim, Rogério Martins, DVM, MSc, PhD
Department of Veterinary Clinical Science (DCV),
School of Veterinary Medicine and Animal Science (FMVZ),
São Paulo State University (UNESP),
Botucatu, São Paulo, Brazil

Borges, Alexandre Secorun, DVM, MSc, PhD
Department of Veterinary Clinical Science,
School of Veterinary Medicine and Animal Science,
São Paulo State University (UNESP),
Botucatu, São Paulo, Brazil

Cerri, Fabrício Moreira, DVM
Department of Veterinary Clinical Science,
School of Veterinary Medicine and Animal Science
São Paulo State University (UNESP),
Botucatu, São Paulo, Brazil.

Danbirni, Samaila, DVM, MSc, PhD, FCVSN
Professor of Infectious Diseases,
Department of Veterinary Medicine,
Faculty of Veterinary Medicine,
Ahmadu Bello University,
Zaria, Nigeria

de Barros, Luiz Daniel, DVM, MSc, PhD
Professor of Parasitology and Parasitic Diseases,
Laboratory of Animal Protozoology,
Department of Veterinary Preventive Medicine,
State University of Londrina,
Londrina, PR, Brazil

de Souza Daniel, Amanda Gabrielle
School of Veterinary Medicine,
Federal University of Minas Gerais,
Belo Horizonte, Minas Gerais, Brazil

de Souza Rodrigues, Fernando, DVM, MSc, PhD
Professor of Parasitology and Parasitic Diseases,
Laboratory of Animal Protozoology,
Department of Veterinary Preventive Medicine,
State University of Londrina,
Londrina, PR, Brazil

Garcia, João Luis, DVM, MSc, PhD
Professor of Parasitology and Parasitic Diseases
Laboratory of Animal Protozoology,
Department of Veterinary Preventive Medicine,
State University of Londrina,
Londrina, PR, Brazil

Guedes, Roberto Maurício Carvalho, DVM, MS, PhD
Professor of Large Animal Clinics and Surgery,
School of Veterinary Medicine,
Federal University of Minas Gerais,
Belo Horizonte, Minas Gerais, Brazil

Lisbôa, Júlio Augusto Naylor, DVM, MSc, PhD
Professor of Large Animal Internal Medicine,
Department of Veterinary Clinics, CCA,
State University of Londrina,
Londrina, PR, Brazil

Lobayan, Sergio Ivan Jorge, DVM, MSc.
Professor of Parasitology and Parasitic Diseases,
School of Veterinary Medicine,
Faculty of Agricultural and Veterinary Sciences,
University of Salvador (USAL),
Corrientes, Argentina

Mshelia, Philip Wayuta, DVM, MS, PhD
Professor of Equine Medicine,
Department of Veterinary Medicine,
Equine Unit, Faculty of Veterinary Medicine,
Ahmadu Bello University,
Zaria, Nigeria

Queiroz, Gustavo Rodrigues, DVM, MSc, PhD
Professor of Large Animal Internal Medicine,
Pitagorás University, UNOPAR,
Arapongas, Paraná, Brazil

Sato, Jose Paulo Hiroji
School of Veterinary Medicine,
Federal University of Minas Gerais,
Belo Horizonte, Minas Gerais, Brazil

Schapiro, Javier Hernán, DVM, PhD
Professor of Parasitology and Parasitic Diseases,
School of Veterinary Medicine,
Faculty of Agricultural and Veterinary Sciences
University of Salvador (USAL), Buenos Aires, Argentina
Parasitology Area,
Institute of Pathobiology-IPVET, CICVyA,
National Institute of Agricultural Technology (INTA),
Buenos Aires, Argentina

Sears, Kelly, DVM, MS, PhD, DACVIM
Professor of Large Animal Medicine,
Carlson College of Veterinary Medicine,
Oregon State University,
Corvallis, Oregon, USA